Imaging of the Foot and Ankle

Imaging of the Foot and Ankle

Julia R. Crim, MD

Durham Radiology Associates, Durham, NC and
Clinical Assistant Professor of Radiology
Department of Radiology
Bowman Gray School of Medicine
Wake Forest University, Winston–Salem, NC

In collaboration with

Andrea Cracchiolo III, MD

Professor of Orthopedic Surgery
Department of Orthopedic Surgery
University of California at Los Angeles
Los Angeles, CA

Reginald L. Hall, MD

Assistant Professor in Orthopedic Surgery
Division of Orthopedic Surgery
Duke University, Durham, NC

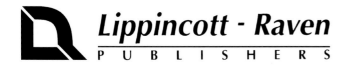 **Lippincott - Raven**
P U B L I S H E R S

Martin Dunitz

© Martin Dunitz Ltd 1996

First published in the United Kingdom in 1996 by Martin Dunitz Ltd,
The Livery House, 7–9 Pratt Street, London NW1 0AE

First published in the United States of America in 1996 by Lippincott–Raven
Publishers.

Library of Congress Cataloging-in-Publication Data applied for

ISBN 0-397-51463-8

Composition by Scribe Design, Gillingham, Kent, United Kingdom
Originated, printed and bound in Singapore by
Toppan Printing Company (S) Pte Ltd

TABLE OF CONTENTS

PREFACE

Disorders of the foot and ankle are very common, and in recent years significant strides have been made in understanding and treating them. However, the information available in the radiology literature has lagged behind orthopedic practice. As I became interested in radiology of the foot and ankle, it became evident that there was no text which addressed the many recent medical advances, especially in sports medicine, and no text which integrated all the current imaging modalities. This book is designed to fill that gap. Although it has been written primarily by a radiologist, I have drawn on the expertise of two orthopedists specializing in the foot and ankle, Drs Andrea Cracchiolo and Reginald Hall. Dr. Richard Gold also contributed his pre-eminent expertise and teaching file for the chapter on arthritis.

Some of the cases used as illustrations in this book were seen at a tertiary care university center. However, the majority were collected while I have been in private practice as a specialist in musculoskeletal radiology, at a primary care hospital with active orthopedic and rheumatologic services. My emphasis throughout the book is on cases which are pertinent to daily practice in radiology.

In order to comprehensively discuss disorders of the foot and ankle, and yet keep the book a reasonable size and price, I have sacrificed a discussion of congenital syndromes. I refer the interested reader to Taybi and Lachman, *Radiology of Syndromes, Metabolic Disorders, and Skeletal Dysplasias*, 3rd edn. (Year Book Medical Publishers: Chicago, 1990). My discussion of systemic disorders is intentionally brief, because patients with systemic disorders do not usually present with foot problems only, and I feel systemic disorders are better addressed in general musculoskeletal radiology texts such as Resnick's classic *Diagnosis of Bone and Joint Disorders* (2nd ed, WB Saunders Co: Philadelphia, 1988).

Many disorders in the foot have subtle radiographic findings, and many different entities have similar clinical presentations. For that reason, differential diagnosis is emphasized both in the text and in tables. Treatment of foot disorders is briefly discussed as well, because a knowledge of how injuries and disorders are treated aids the radiologist in constructing radiographic reports which provide the most useful information to the referring clinician.

There are a wide variety of imaging options available today, but cost-containment measures place an increasing pressure on utilization. It is as important for the radiologist to direct the imaging evaluation of a case as it is to read an individual study. After the plain film, what study should be performed next? For complex clinical problems, I have outlined the advantages and limitations of using different modalities. I have also included suggested MRI protocols for individuals who may lack experience with MRI of the extremities.

ACKNOWLEDGEMENTS

I would like to express my gratitude first to my husband, whose support made it possible for me to write this book while working a full time job, and despite the demands of two pregnancies and an active child. I also owe a debt of gratitude to those who taught me musculoskeletal radiology – Drs. Richard Gold and Larry Bassett at UCLA, and Dr. Donald Resnick at UCSD. The errors in this book are mine, but my inspiration came from their teaching.

My thanks go to Alan Burgess, my editor at Martin Dunitz, who was tireless in his efforts to bring the book to completion, with an attention to details as well as deadlines. Marion Tasker provided the fine illustrations, translating my very rough ideas into elegant line drawings. Dr. Andrew Collins at Duke University provided a number of cases of congenital foot abnormalities. Finally, I am indebted to the many orthopedists who asked me to answer their clinical questions, and provided the impetus for my research into imaging of the foot and ankle.

I. ANATOMY

The complex anatomy of the foot must be thoroughly understood in order to recognize radiographic abnormalities. In this chapter, a description of normal anatomy will be followed by a discussion of developmental anatomy and normal variants. The final section of this chapter is an atlas of normal cross-sectional anatomy.

ANKLE JOINT

The tibia and fibula articulate with the talus to form the ankle or talocrural joint (Fig. 1.1). The motions of the ankle are limited to dorsiflexion (extension) and plantar flexion (flexion). The ankle is sometimes referred to as a mortise joint, because the talus is analagous to a tenon held by the mortise of the tibia and fibula.

The plafond is the horizontal articular surface of the tibia, and the trochlea is the articular surface of the talar dome. The trochlea of the talus has three articular surfaces:
- superiorly it articulates with the plafond of the talus;
- medially it articulates with the medial malleolus of the tibia; and
- laterally it articulates with the lateral malleolus of the fibula.

The superior articular surface of the trochlea is slightly concave in the coronal plane, and there is a corresponding convexity of the plafond; therefore, even a slight lateral shift of the talus results in significant joint incongruity. The trochlea is wider anteriorly than posteriorly, which means that the trochlea is most tightly held by the mortise in dorsiflexion, and the ankle is more stable in dorsiflexion than in plantarflexion.

The medial malleolus can be divided into two tubercles, the larger anterior colliculus and the smaller posterior colliculus. The lateral malleolus lies within the peroneal groove (also known as the incisural notch) of the tibia. It extends further inferiorly than the medial malleolus. The posterior malleolus is the posterior margin of the tibia, and is not a well-defined anatomic structure.

Ligaments of the Ankle

The ankle is stabilized by three sets of ligaments: the medial and lateral collateral ligaments, and the tibiofibular syndesmosis.

Lateral collateral ligament
The lateral collateral ligament prevents inversion of the ankle and is the most frequently injured ligament. It is composed of three distinct ligaments, the anterior and posterior talofibular ligaments, and the calcaneofibular ligament. The calcaneofibular ligament may also serve to stabilize the subtalar joint.

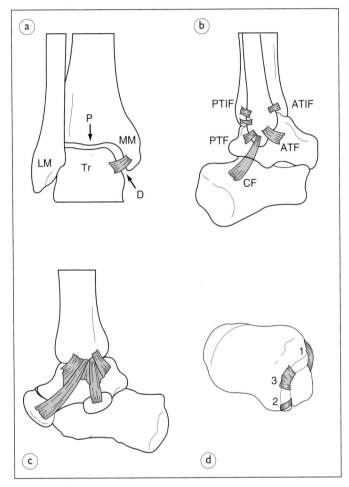

Fig. 1.1. Ankle joint. **a.** Anterior view. The plafond (P) of the tibia articulates with the trochlea (Tr) of the talar dome. The talar dome is held in place medially and laterally by the medial (MM) and lateral (LM) malleoli, and the medial and lateral collateral ligaments. Deep fibers of the deltoid ligament (D) are best seen on this view. **b.** Lateral view. There are three components to the lateral collateral ligament, the anterior talofibular (ATF), the posterior talofibular (PTF), and the calcaneofibular ligaments. The anterior (ATiF) and posterior (PTiF) tibiofibular ligaments, together with the interosseous ligament (not visible) maintain the fibula within the fibular notch of the tibia. **c.** Medial view. The deltoid ligament (D), arising from the medial malleolus, can be divided into deep fibers, which insert on the talus, and superficial fibers, which fan out to insert on the talus, navicular and sustentaculum tali. **d.** Axial view. The distal fibula lies within the peroneal groove (incisural notch) of the fibula, to which it is attached by the tibiofibular syndesmosis. There are three components of the syndesmosis, the ATiF, interosseous ligament (IL), and PTiF.

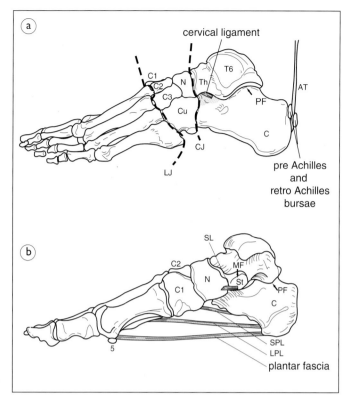

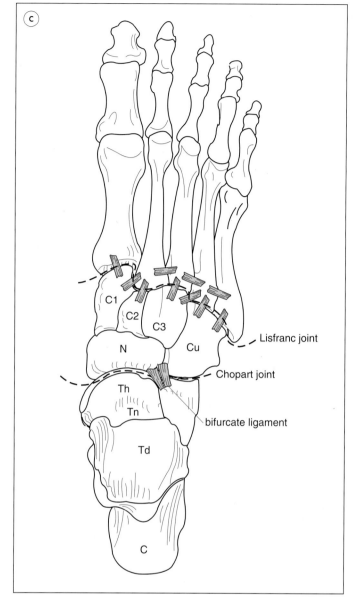

Fig. 1.2. Bones and ligaments of the foot **a.** Lateral view. **b.** Medial view. **c.** Anteroposterior view. See key (p. 17) for abbreviations.

Medial collateral ligament

The medial collateral or deltoid ligament prevents eversion at the ankle joint. It is divided into superficial and deep components. The fan-shaped superficial components extend anteriorly and posteriorly from the anterior colliculus of the medial malleolus to the talus, as well as to the navicular and the sustentaculum tali of the calcaneus. The deep fibers extend from the deep surface of the posterior colliculus to the subjacent talus, and they are the primary medial stabilizer of the ankle joint.

Tibiofibular syndesmosis

The tibiofibular syndesmosis maintains the position of the fibula within the peroneal groove of the tibia. It consists of the anterior and posterior inferior tibiofibular ligaments and the interosseous ligament. The posterior tibiofibular ligament can be divided into two portions: the posterior inferior tibiofibular ligament, which attaches to the lateral aspect of the tibia; and below it the inferior transverse ligament, which attaches to the posterior malleolus. The interosseous ligament is continuous with the interosseous membrane that extends along the lengths of the tibia and fibula. The three components of the tibiofibular syndesmosis allow slight flexibility of the mortise.

BONES AND JOINTS OF THE FOOT

Talus

The talus has three main portions, the body, the neck, and the head (Fig. 1.2). The posterior and lateral processes of the talus

arise from the body of the talus. The posterior process of the talus extends posterior to the subtalar joint. Its size is variable, and it may form a separate ossicle, the os trigonum. The posterior process has two tubercles between which the flexor hallucis longus tendon passes. The lateral process is usually larger than the medial.

No tendons insert on the talus, and 60% of the surface of the talus is covered with cartilage. The blood supply of the talus is chiefly via dorsal and plantar arteries that course posteriorly through the sinus tarsi and enter the talar neck. This renders the body of the talus vulnerable to avascular necrosis after displaced talar neck fractures. Vascular supply also enters via the deltoid ligament (to supply the medial quarter of the talar body) and via the posterior process.

Superiorly, the trochlea of the talus articulates with the plafond of the tibia. The lateral and medial aspects of the talar body articulate with the lateral and medial malleoli. Anteriorly, the head of the talus articulates with the navicular. Inferiorly, the talus articulates with the calcaneus in the subtalar (talocalcaneal) joint.

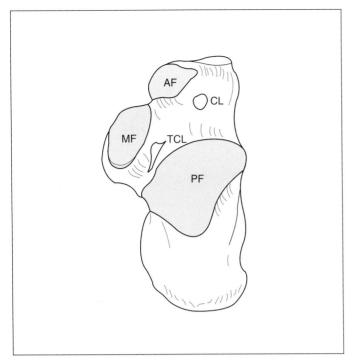

Fig. 1.3. Articular facets of the calcaneus, with attachment of interosseous talocalcaneal ligaments. Looking down on the disarticulated calcaneus from above, the three facets of the calcaneus can be seen. The posterior facet (PF) is the largest of the three; note that it has a greater anteroposterior dimension laterally than medially. The middle (MF) and anterior (AF) facets may be discerned as separate structures, or the AF may be contiguous with the MF. The ligament of the tarsal canal (TCL) attaches to the calcaneus between the sustentaculum tali and the posterior facet. The cervical ligament (CL) attaches anterolateral to it. (Adapted from McMinn et al.[1])

Subtalar Joint

The subtalar joint is divided into three facets and two joints (Fig. 1.3; see Fig. 1.2). The middle and anterior facets form a common cavity with the talonavicular joint, and together are designated the talocalcaneonavicular joint. The posterior facet is a joint cavity that is separate from the middle and anterior facets, though it sometimes communicates with the ankle joint. The posterior facet is the largest facet. It transmits about half the force of weight bearing during ambulation, with half transmitted at the metatarsophalangeal joints. It is diagonally oriented from posterosuperior to anteroinferior. The articular surface of the talus is concave, and the corresponding calcaneal surface is convex. The lateral talocalcaneal ligament is a small ligament at the lateral aspect of the posterior facet, which acts to restrict separation of the articular surfaces. The middle facet is located medially between the sustentaculum tali of the calcaneus and the medial talus. The most posterior portion of the sustentaculum tali is nonarticular. The anterior facet is small, and is sometimes continuous with the middle facet.

Sinus Tarsi

Anterior to the posterior facet, the lateral portions of the talus and calcaneus are divided by the sinus tarsi (tarsal sinus). The

posteromedial portion of the sinus tarsi, just behind the sustentaculum tali, is called the tarsal canal. The sinus tarsi contains fat, the artery of the tarsal canal (which supplies the talus), and ligaments.

There are two talocalcaneal ligaments within the tarsal sinus. The ligament of the tarsal canal is located posteromedially, between the posterior and middle subtalar facets. The cervical ligament extends from the lateral aspect of the calcaneus to the talar neck. Both serve as stabilizers of the subtalar joint.[1,2] The extensor retinaculum also inserts in the tarsal sinus, but it is probably not an important stabilizer of the subtalar joint. Its fibers course from the superolateral aspect of the tarsal sinus inferiorly and medially.

Calcaneus

The calcaneus is the largest of the tarsal bones. The anterior process of the calcaneus is joined to the navicular and cuboid via the bifurcate ligament. A sulcus is present on the superior surface of the calcaneus, within the tarsal sinus. Laterally, the peroneal tubercle separates the tendons of the peroneus brevis and longus. The posterior portion of the calcaneus is sometimes called the tuberosity or posterior process. The weight of the heel is borne on rounded medial and lateral tuberal processes that are located on the posterior process of the calcaneus. The calcaneus articulates with the talus superiorly and the cuboid anteriorly.

Midtarsal Joint

The hindfoot is composed of the talus and calcaneus. It is divided from the midfoot, which is composed of the remaining tarsal bones, by a compound joint that is variously called the midtarsal joint, the transverse tarsal joint, or the joint of Chopart.

The midfoot consists of the calcaneocuboid joint and the talonavicular portion of the talocalcaneonavicular joint. Inversion and eversion as well as dorsiflexion and plantarflexion take place at the midtarsal joint. The talonavicular joint is stabilized by the spring ligament and posterior tibial tendon medially, by the bifurcate ligament laterally, and by the dorsal talonavicular ligament. The calcaneocuboid joint is stabilized by the short plantar (plantar calcaneocuboid) ligament.

Navicular

The navicular bone forms the keystone of the longitudinal and transverse arches of the foot. Its position is stabilized by the spring ligament and by the tibialis posterior tendon, which insert on its medial tuberosity.

Cuneiforms

There are three cuneiform bones, which, as their name implies, are wedge-shaped in configuration. They are referred to as the first, second, and third cuneiforms or the medial, middle, and lateral cuneiforms. They all articulate posteriorly with the navicular. Anteriorly the medial cuneiform articulates with the first metatarsal, the middle cuneiform with the second metatarsal, and the lateral cuneiform with the third metatarsal. The lateral cuneiform articulates laterally with the cuboid. They are stabilized by their shape, which prevents inferior subluxation, as well as by ligaments between them and the cuneiforms and adjacent bones and between each other. The cuneonavicular joint usually forms one common cavity and is rarely injured in isolation.

Cuboid

The cuboid articulates posteriorly with the calcaneus and laterally with the fourth and fifth metatarsals. Medially it articulates with the navicular and the lateral cuneiform. At its lateral aspect is a groove under which passes the peroneus longus tendon.

Tarsometatarsal Joint

The tarsometatarsal joint (also known as the Lisfranc joint) is a compound joint. There are three synovium-lined joint cavities: a medial cavity for the first toe, an intermediate cavity for the second and third toes, and a lateral cavity for the fourth and fifth. Intermetatarsal joints between the second to fifth toes are continuous with the tarsometatarsal joints. There is no intermetatarsal joint between the first and second metatarsals. The Lisfranc joint acts in flexion and extension. It is stabilized by the recessed position of the base of the second metatarsal, and by the tarsometatarsal ligaments. There is no ligament between the first and second metatarsal bases, and so this is a point of weakness. The obliquely oriented Lisfranc ligament, between the first cuneiform and the second metatarsal, stabilizes this region.

Metatarsals

The first three metatarsals articulate proximally with the corresponding cuneiforms, while the two lateral metatarsals articulate with the cuboid. Distally, the metatarsals articulate with the corresponding proximal phalanges. Each metatarsal can be divided into a base, a shaft, a neck, and a head.

Joints of the Digits

The metatarsophalangeal (MTP) joint and interphalangeal (proximal interphalangeal or PIP and distal interphalangeal or DIP) joints are simple hinge joints. The anterior attachment of the plantar fascia is at the MTP joints. The plantar surface of the MTP and IP joints has a thickened plate called the plantar ligament, to which the flexor tendon sheaths attach. The sesamoids of the toes lie within the plantar ligament. Medial and lateral collateral ligaments are present. Dorsally, the extensor tendons largely replace the fibrous joint capsule.

Sesamoids are present at the first MTP joint. The medial sesamoid is frequently bipartite or multipartite, the lateral sesamoid is usually unipartite. The sesamoids articulate with concave facets, separated by an intersesamoidal ridge, on the

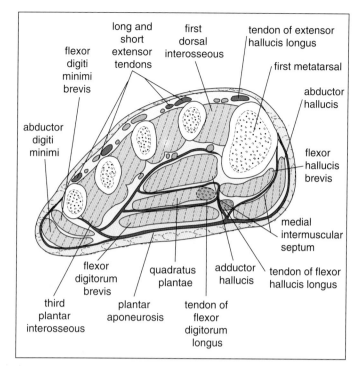

Fig. 1.4. Compartments of the foot. Coronal cross-section of the forefoot shows its division into medial, middle, and lateral compartments. In the hindfoot and midfoot, the compartments are less well defined.

metatarsal head. The articulation of the sesamoids with the metatarsal is a true synovial joint. There is an associated bursa at the plantar aspect of the joint. Sesamoids at the other MTP and IP joints are inconstant; the most commonly seen is a sesamoid at the fifth MTP.

Phalanges
There are two phalanges of the first toe, and three phalanges of the second to fifth toes. The middle and distal phalanges of the fifth toe are often congenitally fused. The second digit of the foot maintains a relatively stable position, with abduction and adduction of the forefoot occuring relative to its axis.

MAJOR PLANTAR LIGAMENTS

Plantar Calcaneonavicular or Spring Ligament

The plantar calcaneonavicular ligament, also called the spring ligament, is vital in maintaining the medial longitudinal arch of the foot. It extends from the undersurface of the sustentaculum tali to the inferior and medial aspect of the navicular. At its navicular insertion, the fibers of the spring ligament blend with the anterior fibers of the deltoid ligament. The deltoid ligament and the posterior tibial tendon help support the spring ligament.[3]

Plantar Aponeurosis

The plantar aponeurosis arises as a fairly narrow band from the tuberosity of the calcaneus. As it extends distally, it fans out into

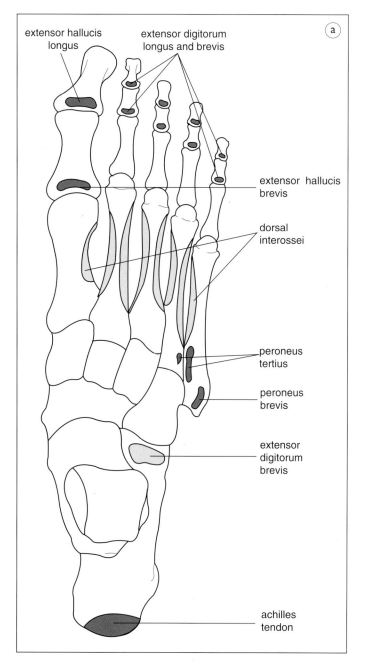

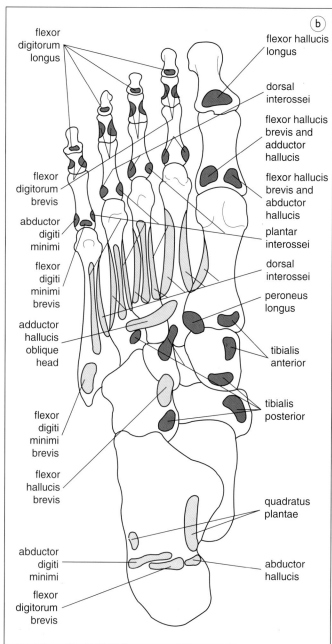

Fig. 1.5. Muscle attachments in the foot. **a.** Dorsal surface. Muscle origins are shown in red, and insertions are in black. **b.** Plantar surface. (Adapted from Hollinshead.[5])

separate components to each of the digits. These components partially blend with the flexor tendon sheaths, and the remaining portions continue to attach to the deep transverse metatarsal ligament, the bases of the proximal phalanges, and the skin. At the level of the metatarsal heads, the superficial transverse metatarsal ligament crosses the foot superficial to the plantar fascia.

Long and Short Plantar Ligaments

The long and short plantar ligaments arise from the plantar aspect of the calcaneus. The long plantar ligament inserts on the cuboid, and the bases of the second to fourth metatarsals. The short plantar ligament inserts on the cuboid. They aid in maintaing the longitudinal arch of the foot.

Intermuscular Septae

Septae arise from the plantar fascia and divide the foot into lateral, intermediate and medial compartments (Fig. 1.4). Infection will generally be limited to one compartment by the intermuscular septae.

BURSAE OF THE FOOT

Bursae are synovium-lined sacs that facilitate normal motion of tendons and cushion areas of stress. Important bursae are present anterior and rarely posterior to the Achilles tendon, beneath the calcaneal tuberosity, inferomedial to the first MTP joint, and inferolateral to the fifth MTP joint.[4]

EXTRINSIC MUSCLES OF THE FOOT

There are three groups of extrinisic foot muscles: anterior, lateral, and posterior. Accessory muscles are uncommon, and are discussed in Chapter 7 as causes of pain and dysfunction. Attachments of the extrinsic and intrinsic muscles on the foot are shown schematically in Fig. 1.5.

Anterior Compartment

The anterior muscles arise from the anterior aspect of the tibia, interosseous membrane, and fibula, and are extensors of the foot. They are innervated by the deep peroneal nerve, which runs with the anterior tibial artery. At the level of the ankle, the neurovascular bundle lies between the extensor hallucis longus and the extensor digitorum longus. The anterior tibial artery becomes the dorsalis pedis artery in the foot.

The most medial of the anterior muscles is the tibialis anterior, which inserts on the plantar aspect of the first cuneiform and metatarsal. In addition to dorsiflexing the foot, it also acts to invert and abduct. The extensor hallucis longus inserts on the distal phalanx of the first toe. It primarily dorsiflexes the first toe, and it is only a weak dorsiflexor of the foot. The extensor digitorum longus divides into four tendons, which insert on the four lateral toes. Each tendon forms one middle and two lateral bands as it reaches the proximal phalanx of the toe. The middle band inserts on the middle phalanx, and the lateral bands come together and insert on the lateral phalanx. The peroneus tertius is an inconstant muscle that inserts on the bases of the fourth and fifth metatarsals. The extensor digitorum longus and peroneus tertius act together to dorsiflex, evert, and abduct the foot.

The extensor muscles are all tendinous by the point where they cross the ankle joint. The tendons are held in place as they change from a vertical to a horizontal course by the superior and inferior extensor retinacula.

Lateral Compartment

There are two lateral muscles, both innervated by the superficial peroneal nerve. Vascular supply is by the peroneal artery. Both muscles act to evert the foot, and both are weak flexors. The peroneus longus arises from the proximal and mid-fibula. It covers the peroneus brevis, which arises from the distal fibula. The tendons course together behind the posterior malleolus, where they share a common tendon sheath. They are held against the lateral aspect of the ankle by the superior and inferior peroneal retinacula. The calcaneofibular ligament lies deep to the peroneal tendons.

The peroneus brevis inserts on the base of the fifth metatarsal. The peroneus longus extends below the cuboid to course across the plantar aspect of the foot and insert on the first cuneiform and the base of the first metatarsal. It may contain a sesamoid bone, the os peroneale, which is seen at the lateral aspect of the cuboid.

Posterior Compartment

The posterior muscles are divided into superficial and deep compartments by the deep transverse fascia. The lower part of this fascia thickens at the ankle to form the flexor retinaculum. The muscles are supplied by the tibial nerve. The popliteal artery divides just below the knee into the anterior and posterior tibial arteries, and the posterior tibial artery sends off the peroneal artery. At the ankle, the posterior tibial artery runs with the tibial nerve behind the medial malleolus, between the flexor digitorum longus and the flexor hallucis longus. In the foot, the neurovascular bundle divides into medial and lateral plantar branches.

Superficial group

There are three superficial muscles, the gastrocnemius, the soleus, and the plantaris. The gastrocnemius arises from medial and lateral heads on the femoral epicondyles, while the soleus arises from the posterior aspects of the proximal tibia and fibula. The two muscles join to form the Achilles or calcaneal tendon, which inserts on the posterior process of the calcaneus and acts to flex the ankle.

The plantaris muscle arises from the posterolateral aspect of the femur, and forms a long tendinous band, which sometimes blends with the Achilles tendon and sometimes inserts medial or anteromedial to it on the calcaneus.

Deep group

There are three flexors of the foot in the deep compartment. They all course behind the medial malleolus, where their orientation changes from vertical to horizontal. Their position is maintained by the flexor retinaculum, and each tendon is protected by a separate tendon sheath in this region. The tendon sheath of the flexor hallucis longus often communicates with the ankle joint, and therefore fluid within the tendon sheath does not necessarily indicate that there is an abnormality of the flexor hallucis longus tendon. The tibial nerve and posterior tibial artery lie between the flexor digitorum longus and the flexor hallucis longus, within the flexor retinaculum. The tunnel formed by the flexor retinaculum superficially and the tibia and calcaneus deep to the tendons is called the tarsal tunnel. Space-occupying lesions within the tarsal tunnel can cause pain and dysfunction of the posterior tibial nerve or its branches (tarsal tunnel syndrome; see Chapter 8.)

The tibialis posterior arises from the posterior aspect of the tibia, the interosseous membrane and the medial aspect of the fibula. Its tendon inserts on the navicular, with smaller slips to the cuneiforms and second, third, and fourth metatarsal bases. At its navicular insertion, the tibialis posterior lies superficial to the anterior fibers of the deltoid ligament. The flexor digitorum longus arises from the posterior aspect of the tibia and divides into four slips which insert on the distal phalanges of the second to fifth toes. The flexor hallucis longus arises from the posterior surface of the tibia. At the ankle it courses medially, and then extends beneath the sustentaculum tali, which acts as a pulley. It inserts on the distal phalanx of the first toe.

RETINACULA

The flexor retinaculum extends from the medial malleolus to the calcaneus, and encloses the extrinsic flexor tendons, which are contained within tendon sheaths at this point, and the posterior tibial neurovascular bundle. The extensor retinaculum overlies the extrinsic extensor tendons, as well as the anterior tibial artery and vein and the deep peroneal nerve. There are two medial bands, which attach to the medial malleolus and to the medial plantar fascia. The bands join over the dorsum of the foot, and they insert on the lateral and superior surface of the calcaneus in the tarsal sinus.

There are two retinacula overlying the peroneal tendons, which lie within a common tendon sheath. The superior peroneal retinaculum extends from the lateral malleolus to the calcaneus. The inferior peroneal retinaculum is attached at both ends to the lateral aspect of the calcaneus. It blends superiorly with the extensor retinacula.

INTRINSIC MUSCLES OF THE FOOT

The names of most of the intrinsic muscles of the foot describe the action of the muscle. In the following discussion, a muscle's action is described only for the cases where it is not clear from its name.

Dorsal

There is only one anterior intrinsic muscle, the extensor digitorum brevis. It arises from the dorsolateral calcaneus and divides into four tendons extending to the first to fourth toes.

Plantar

Plantar intrinsic muscles can be divided into four layers, numbered from the most superficial to the deepest layer. All are innervated by the medial or lateral branch of the plantar nerve.

First plantar layer

Three muscles form the superficial layer. The most medial is the abductor hallucis, which arises from the medial aspect of the calcaneal tuberosity, and attaches to the medial aspect of the base of the first proximal phalanx. Its tendon, and that of the flexor hallucis brevis, attach to the medial sesamoid of the first toe.

The flexor digitorum brevis arises mainly from the medial aspect of the calcaneal tuberosity and divides into four tendons, which course immediately superficial to the flexor digitorum longus tendons and insert on the four lateral toes. The tendon to the fifth toe may be congenitally absent.

The abductor digiti minimi arises from the lateral aspect of the calcaneal tuberosity and inserts on the base of the fifth proximal phalanx. An accessory muscle, the abductor ossis metatarsi quinti, may be present, attaching to the tuberosity of the fifth metatarsal.

Second plantar layer

This layer contains the tendons of the flexor digitorum and flexor hallucis longus, as well as intrinsic muscles. The quadratus plantae arises from two heads, one on the medial side of the calcaneal tuberosity and one on the lateral side. It inserts into the lateral margin of the flexor digitorum longus. The muscle is occasionally absent. The four lumbricals arise from the tendons of the flexor digitorum longus. They insert with the extensor tendons on the

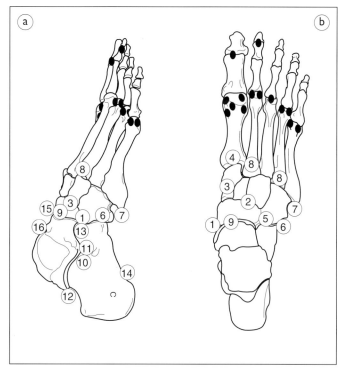

Fig. 1.6. Location of accessory centers of ossification and sesamoids in the foot. **a.** Anterior view. **b.** Lateral view. (Adapted from Koehler et al.[6])

1. Os tibiale externum
2. Processus uncinatus
3. Os intercuneiforme
4. Pars peronae metatarsalia I
5. Cuboides secundarium
6. Os peroneum
7. Os vesalianum
8. Os intermetatarseum
9. Os supratalare
10. Talus accessories
11. Os sustentaculum
12. Os trigonum
13. Calcaneus secundarium
14. Os subcalcis
15. Os supranaviculare
16. Os talotibiale

dorsal surface of the proximal phalanges. They extend the proximal interphalangeal joints and flex the metatarsophalangeal joints, and their absence results in claw toe deformity.

Third plantar layer

The flexor hallucis brevis has a tendinous origin from the cuboid and lateral cuneiform. It has a medial and lateral head, inserting on the base of the first proximal phalanx. The medial head, together with the abductor hallucis, contains the medial sesamoid of the great toe. The lateral head blends with the two heads of the abductor hallucis, and contains the lateral sesamoid of the first toe. The adductor hallucis has an oblique and a transverse head. The oblique head arises from the bases of the second, third, and fourth metatarsals and the long plantar ligament. The transverse head arises from the deep transverse metatarsal ligaments.

The flexor digiti minimi brevis arises from the tuberosity of the fifth metatarsal and inserts on the base of the fifth proximal phalanx.

Fourth plantar layer

There are seven interosseous muscles in the fourth layer, three plantar and four dorsal. The three plantar interossei arise respectively from the medial aspects of the third, fouth, and fifth

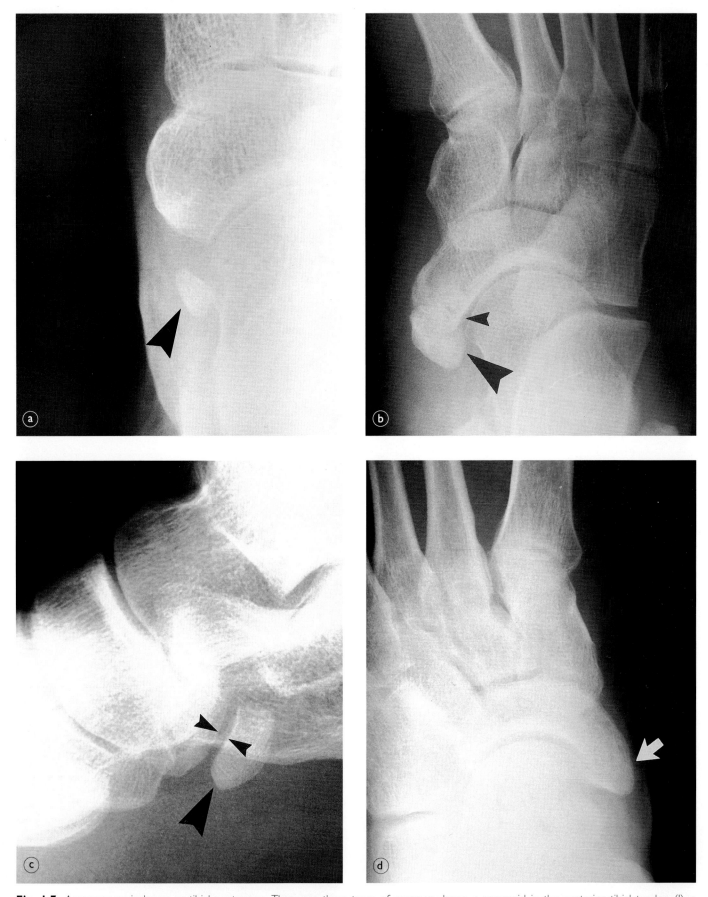

Fig. 1.7. Accessory navicular or os tibiale externum. There are three types of accessory bone, a sesamoid in the posterior tibial tendon (I), a bone articulating with the navicular by a synchondrosis (II), and an assimilated center (III). **a.** Type I accessory navicular (arrowhead). The small sesamoid is separated from the tuberosity of the navicular. **b, c.** Type II accessory navicular. AP and lateral radiograph show the type II accessory navicular (large arrowheads) and the synchondrosis (small arrowheads). **d.** Type III accessory navicular, AP radiograph. The tuberosity of the navicular is larger than is usually seen, owing to assimilation of the accessory ossification center.

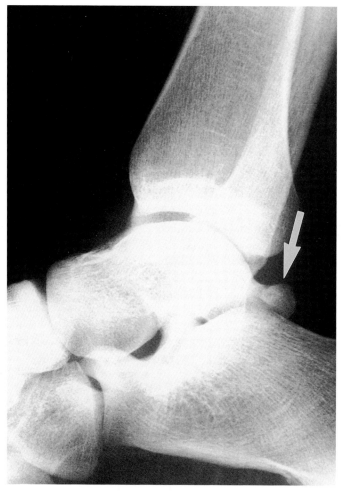

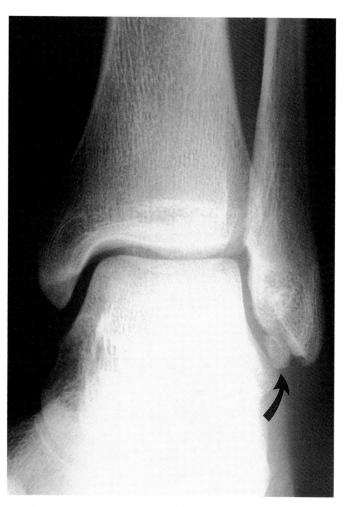

Fig. 1.8. Lateral radiograph of hindfoot showing os trigonum (arrow), a separate ossification center of the posterior process of the talus.

Fig. 1.9. Mortise radiograph. Os subfibulare (arrow).

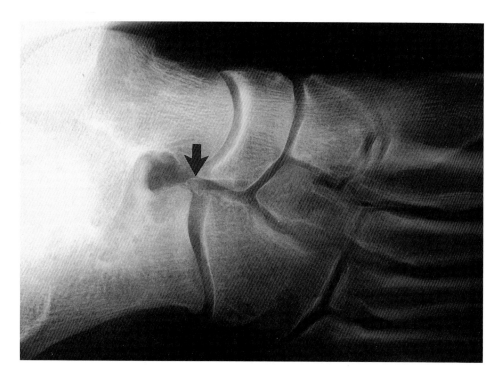

Fig. 1.10. Oblique radiograph. The calcaneus secondarium (arrow) is located at the anterior process of the calcaneus.

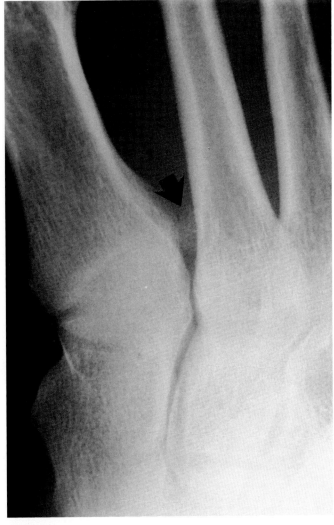

Fig. 1.11. AP radiograph. Os intermetatarsum (arrow) is located between the first and second metatarsal bases.

metatarsals, and they insert on the medial bases of the third, fourth, and fifth proximal phalnages. They adduct the forefoot. The four dorsal interossei have dual heads arising from two adjacent metatarsals. The first and second dorsal interossei insert on the medial and lateral aspects of the base of the second proximal phalanx. The third and fourth dorsal interossei insert on the lateral aspect of the third and fourth proximal phalanges, respectively. The dorsal interossei abduct the forefoot. Adduction and abduction occur relative to the second ray, which is the least mobile.

ALIGNMENT AND MOTION OF THE FOOT

The architecture of the foot can be thought of in terms of longitudinal and transverse arches. The medial foot forms the higher portion of the arches, with the head of the talus as a keystone in the arch.

When a person is standing, motions of the foot are complex. If the medial aspect of the foot moves inferiorly, this is pronation, a combination of eversion of the hindfoot and abduction of the forefoot. The opposite motion, inversion and adduction, is called supination.

NORMAL BONY VARIANTS

Accessory Ossicles

There are numerous accessory centers of ossification and variable sesamoids in the foot (Fig. 1.6). It can be difficult to differentiate an old nonunited fracture from an accessory ossicle. In general, the contour of a nonunited fragment will closely mirror the donor site in the adjacent bone. The two pieces can be thought of as fitting like pieces of a jigsaw puzzle. The accessory ossicle, on the other hand, is usually round or oval and will not conform so closely to the contour of the adjacent bone.

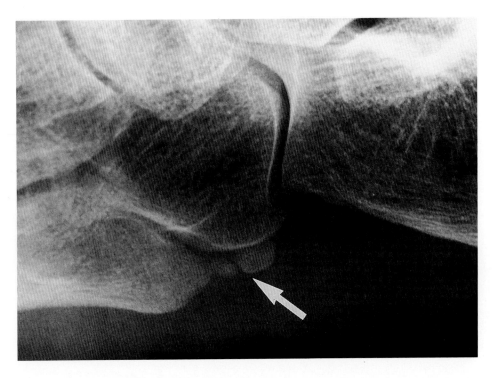

Fig. 1.12. Lateral radiograph. Bipartite os peroneum (arrow) in the tendon of the peroneus longus.

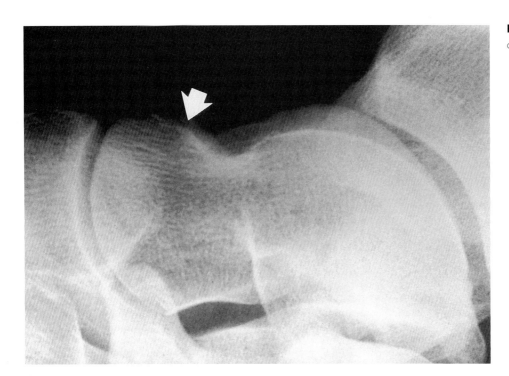

Fig. 1.13. Lateral radiograph. Dorsal ridge of the talar neck (arrow).

Frequently, a reliable distinction between an accessory center of ossification and a post-traumatic ossicle cannot be made. The well-corticated margins of either an accessory ossicle or a nonunited fragment distinguish them both from a fragment caused by acute fracture. Several of the more common ossicles are illustrated in Figs 1.7–1.12.

Accessory ossicles can be associated with pain. This is especially true of the bone that is known in the radiology literature as the os tibiale externum, and in the orthopedic literature as the accessory navicular.[7–9] The os tibiale externum arises at the medial aspect of the navicular bone, and it can have three different configurations (see Fig. 1.7). Type I is a sesamoid in the tibialis posterior tendon. Type II is united with the navicular by a synchondrosis, which may fracture (see Chapter 4). Type III is assimilated with the underlying navicular, resulting in a prominent medial tuberosity.

A medial malleolar accessory ossification center is present bilaterally in 13% of children, and unilaterally in an additional 7%, but it usually unites with the main portion of the epiphysis in adolescence. It can be painful.[10]

Pain is also associated with the os peroneum.[11]

The posterior process of the talus arises as a separate center of ossification between the ages of eight and 11 years, and it usually fuses with the body of the talus within a year of its appearance.[12] When it persists, it is known as the os trigonum (see Fig. 1.8). In dancers or other athletes with an os trigonum or a prominent posterior process of the talus, repeated plantar flexion can lead to os trigonum syndrome, pain and impingement of the flexor hallucis longus[13] (see Chapter 7).

Other Bony Variants

A dorsal ridge, which can be prominent, is normally seen on the neck of the talus[13] (Fig. 1.13). It must be differentiated from

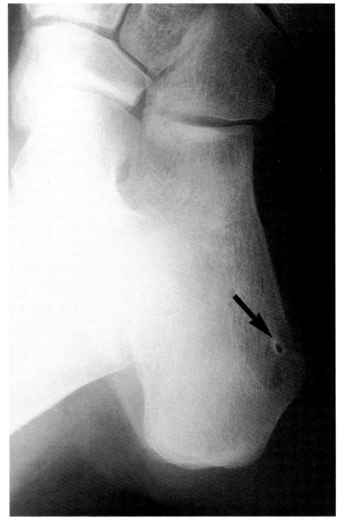

Fig. 1.14. Oblique radiograph. Nutrient foramen (arrow) of the calcaneus.

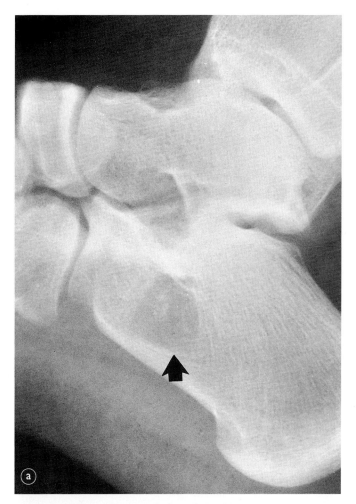

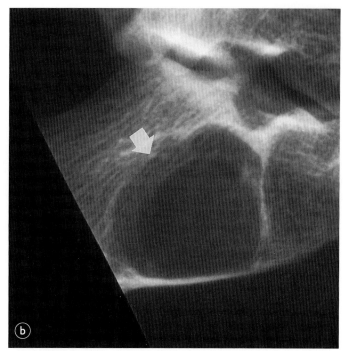

Fig. 1.15. a. Lateral radiograph of calcaneal pseudocyst (arrow). This normal rarefaction of trabeculae seen below the sustentaculum tali can mimic a lytic lesion. Careful inspection of the radiograph will disclose that the 'margins' of the pseudocyst are normal trabeculae rather than a rim of reactive bone. b. Lateral radiograph of simple cyst (arrow) of calcaneus for comparison. In contrast to the appearance of the pseudocyst, a rim of reactive bone will form around a true bone cyst. Lipomas are sometimes seen in this location, and will also have a sclerotic rim.

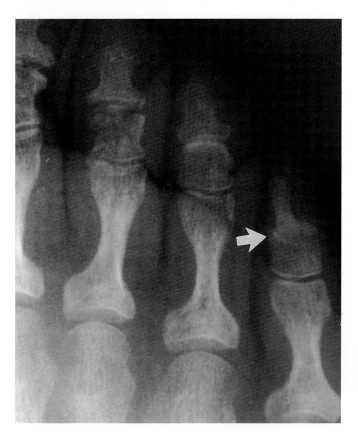

Fig. 1.16. Failure of segmentation of the middle and distal phalanges of the fifth toe. AP radiograph.

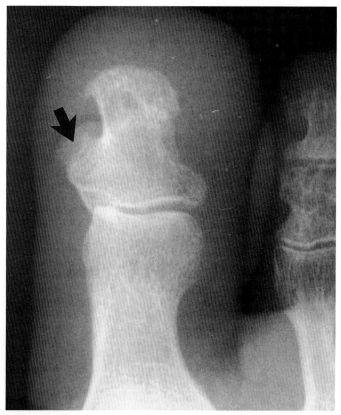

Fig. 1.17. Exostosis of the medial aspect of the first distal phalanx. AP radiograph.

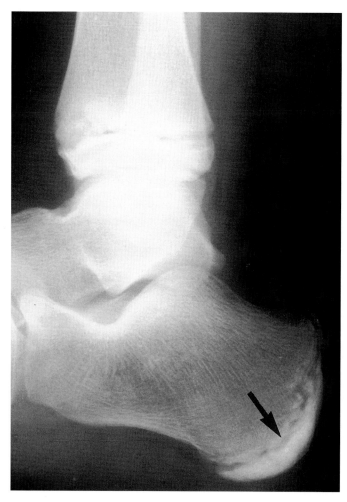

Fig. 1.18. Sclerotic appearance of the normal calcaneal apophysis (arrow) on lateral radiograph.

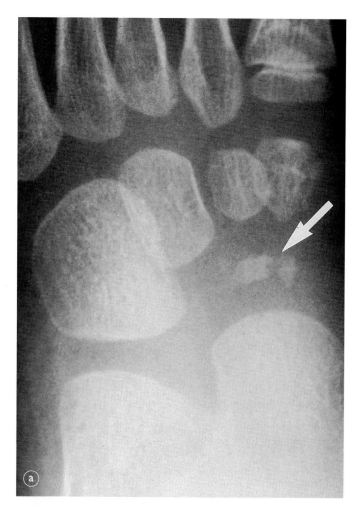

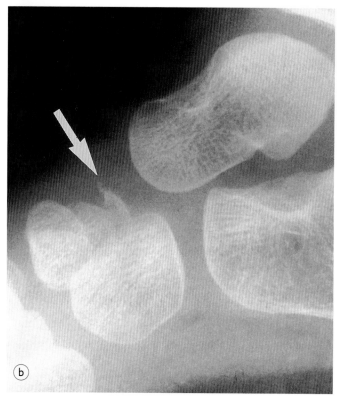

Fig. 1.19. Fragmented, sclerotic appearance of the navicular. **a.** AP radiograph. **b.** Lateral radiograph. This patient was asymptomatic, indicating that the finding is a normal variant, but an identical appearance can be seen in osteonecrosis (see Chapter 5).

the more proximally located dorsal spur, which can cause dorsal ankle impingement (see Chapter 6), and the more distally located talonavicular osteophytes and talar beaks (see Chapter 5). In the calcaneus, the plantar vascular foramen may mimic a small bony defect (Fig. 1.14). There is a normal rarefaction of trabeculae in the midportion of the calcaneus, called the calcaneal pseudocyst[15] (Fig. 1.15), which can mimic a lytic lesion.

A common variant in the forefoot is failure of segmentation of the mid and distal phalanges of the fifth toe (Fig. 1.16). Prominence of the ungual tufts is more variable than in the hands. A medial projection of the base of the distal phalanx of the first toe (Fig. 1.17) may represent a stress response rather than a normal variant,[16] but it is so common it may be considered a normal variant.

DEVELOPMENTAL ANATOMY

Table 1.1 shows the age of appearance of ossification centers in the foot in Scandinavian children. Ossification is normally seen at birth in the calcaneus and talus. The calcaneal ossification center appears between 22 and 25 weeks' gestation, and the talus between 25 and 31 weeks' gestation. The cuboid center may appear before birth (37 weeks' gestation) or shortly thereafter.[17]

Table 1.1 (From Silverman[17])

Ossification centre	Boys					Girls				
	First appearance	25%	50%	75%	100%	First appearance	25%	50%	75%	100%
Calcaneus	0	0	0	0	0	0	0	0	0	0
Talus	0	0	0	0	0	0	0	0	0	0
Cuboideum	0	0.8	2.0	3.7	7.0	0	0.6	1.7	2.5	5.0
Third cuneiform	0	4.1	5.0	7.4	20.0	0	2.7	4.2	5.3	9.0
First cuneiform	7	19.0	25.5	38.3	51.5	8	11.4	20.6	24.3	32.0
Navicular	7	23.6	31.4	36.3	51.5	9	20.1	22.5	25.4	35.0
Distal epiphysis of tibia	12	31.6	38.1	51.5	—	13–15	22.6	25.9	35.1	51.5
Distal epiphysis of fibula	1	3.9	5.7	6.7	10.0	3	4.7	5.6	6.6	7.0
First metatarsal epiphysis	6	9.7	10.8	22.5	35.0	1	7.3	8.8	10.7	20.0
Second metatarsal epiphysis	22–24	28.3	31.9	33.8	35.0	8	17.8	20.0	22.2	26.0
Third metatarsal epiphysis	28–30	34.8	39.0	45.2	51.5	13–15	23.1	25.9	28.6	32.0
Fourth metatarsal epiphysis	28–30	37.5	39.5	49.0	57.5	19–21	25.5	29.1	32.0	35.0
Fifth metatarsal epiphysis	28–30	42.9	47.5	51.5	—	19–21	28.4	32.0	35.9	51.0
First proximal phalangeal epiphysis	28–30	43.7	48.2	55.7	—	19–21	32.1	35.0	43.0	57.5
Second proximal phalangeal epiphysis	9	24.3	28.8	32.7	45.5	8	17.2	19.6	20.0	29.0
Third proximal phalangeal epiphysis	13–15	17.2	21.9	25.8	29.0	8	11.0	14.9	18.8	23.0
Fourth proximal phalangeal epiphysis	13–15	14.7	20.8	23.4	29.0	8	10.9	12.3	16.8	23.0
Fifth proximal phalangeal epiphysis	13–15	16.0	21.8	22.4	29.0	8	11.0	13.3	19.3	23.0
First middle phalangeal epiphysis	16–18	23.5	28.8	32.7	45.5	8	18.0	21.0	23.0	26.0
Second middle phalangeal epiphysis	13–15	21.7	24.3	28.6	35.0	10	11.0	16.9	20.0	26.0
Third middle phalangeal epiphysis	10	15.2	25.3	29.0	35.0	10	11.2	17.5	23.4	—
Fourth middle phalangeal epiphysis	9	17.7	26.2	35.0	—	10	12.4	22.4	26.3	—
Fifth middle phalangeal epiphysis	9	29.0	35.1	47.4	—	12	20.0	25.9	35.7	—
First distal phalangeal epiphysis	8	12.9	14.0	19.6	26.0	8	9.1	10.2	13.2	26.0
Second distal phalangeal epiphysis	13–15	34.2	39.5	47.3	—	10	22.4	29.1	33.0	57.5
Third distal phalangeal epiphysis	16–18	35.2	41.5	47.1	—	13–15	20.0	29.3	34.4	51.5
Fourth distal phalangeal epiphysis	16–18	37.1	41.7	46.8	—	13–15	22.6	29.5	35.4	51.5
Fifth distal phalangeal epiphysis	9	36.7	39.5	49.5	—	12	23.1	30.1	36.0	51.5

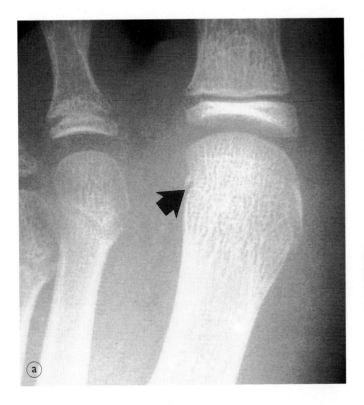

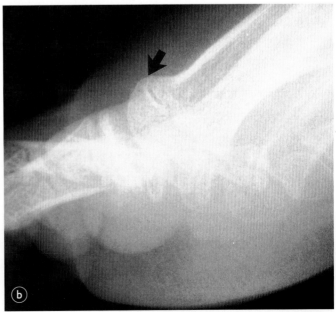

Fig. 1.20. Pseudoepiphysis (arrow) of the distal first metatarsal. **a.** AP radiograph. **b.** Lateral radiograph. The epiphysis of the first metatarsal is proximally located.

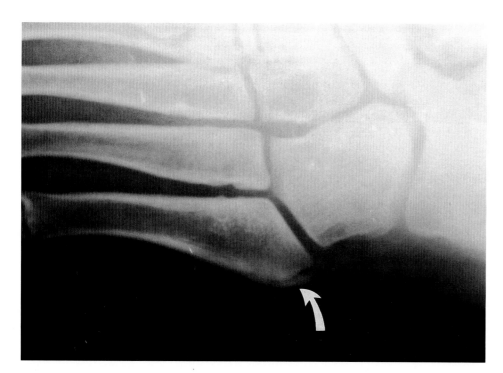

Normally developing bones in children may mimic abnormal conditions radiographically. The calcaneal apophysis may appear sclerotic and fragmented (Fig. 1.18). This appearance was formerly called Sever's disease and was thought to be due to osteonecrosis, but it is now considered a normal variant. The navicular may appear sclerotic and fragmented in children (Fig. 1.19). It is considered a normal variant as long as the child is asymptomatic, but it can also be a manifestation of osteonecrosis (see Chapter 6). A pseudoepiphysis can form at the nonepiphyseal end of a metarsal or phalanx[18] (Fig. 1.20). The apophysis of the fifth metatarsal is vertically oriented (Fig. 1.21), which differentiates it from fractures of the tuberosity, which are transversely oriented.

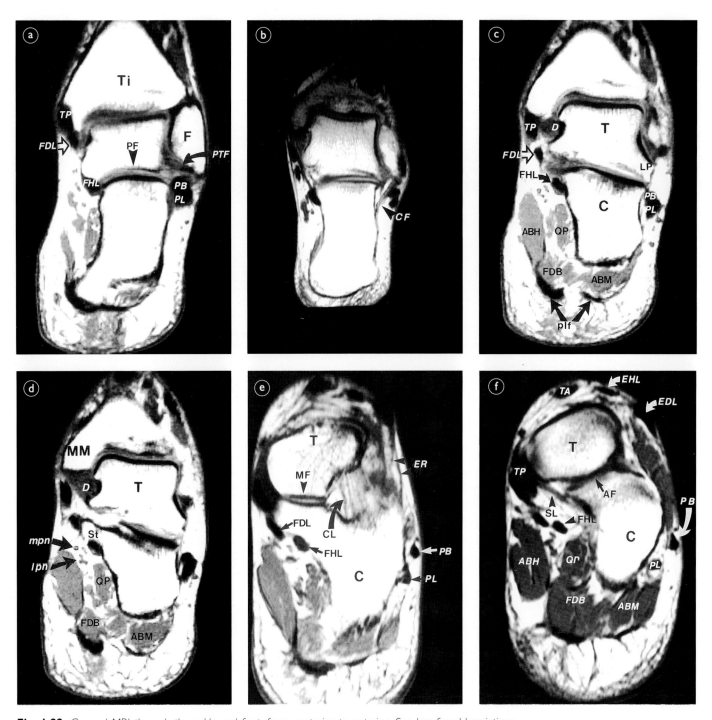

Fig. 1.22. Coronal MRI through the ankle and foot, from posterior to anterior. See key for abbreviations.
a. Section through midportion of the posterior subtalar facet (PF). **b.** Similar section to (a), but angled posteriorly to show the calcaneofibular ligament (CF), which courses posterolaterally from its lateral malleolar attachment to insert on the calcaneus. Peroneal tendons are immediately superficial to the CF. **c.** Ankle and subtalar joint. Deep fibers of the deltoid ligament (D) are seen inserting on the body of the talus. The lateral process (LP) of the talus extends below the lateral malleolus. **d.** Posterior portion of the sustentaculum tali (ST). Note that this portion of the ST does not articulate with the talus. **e.** Middle subtalar facet. Cervical ligament (CL) courses obliquely through the sinus tarsi. **f.** Anterior subtalar facet. A portion of the spring ligament (SL), extending from the sustentaculum tali to the navicular, is seen.

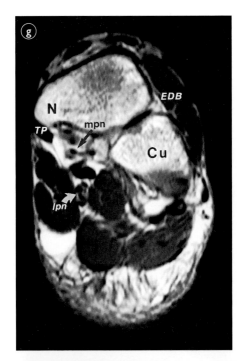

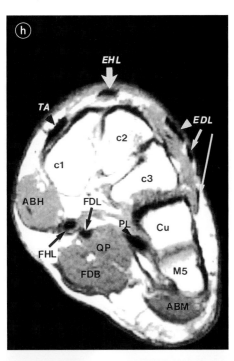

Fig. 1.22. *Continued*
g. Cuboid and navicular. The tibialis posterior (TP) inserts on the tuberosity of the talus. **h.** Cuneiforms. The peroneus longus (PL) tendon is coursing medially towards its insertion on the first metatarsal. The extensor digitorum longus tendons (EDL) cover the extensor digitorum brevis. **i.** Metatarsal shafts. The flexor digitorum brevis (FDB) tendons are superficial to the flexor digitorum longus (FDL) tendons. **j.** First metatarsophalangeal joint. The sesamoids are symmetrically positioned beneath the first metatarsal head.

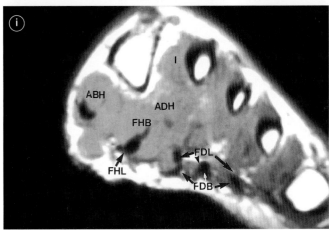

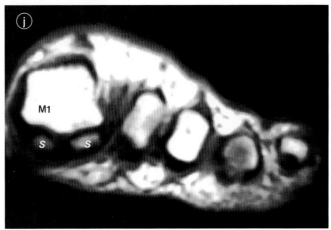

KEY TO ABBREVIATIONS

ABH	abductor hallucis	Cu	cuboid	M 1-5	metatarsals 1-5	St	sustentaculum tali
ABM	abductor digiti minimi	D	deltoid ligament	MF	middle subtalar facet	T	talus
ADH	adductor hallucis	dp	dorsalis pedis artery and vein	MM	medial malleolus	TA	tibialis anterior
AF	anterior subtalar facet	EDB	extensor digitorum brevis	mpn	medial plantar neurovascular bundle	Tb	talar body
AG	angle of Gissane	EDL	extensor digitorum longus			TCL	ligament of the tarsal canal
anb	anterior tibial neurovascular bundle	EHL	extensor hallucis longus	N	navicular	Td	talar dome
		ER	extensor retinaculum	P	phalanx	Th	talar head
AT	Achilles tendon	F	fibula	P	plafond	Ti	tibia
ATF	anterior talofibular ligament	FDB	flexor digitorum brevis	PB	peroneus brevis	Tn	talar neck
ATiF	anterior tibiofibular ligament	FDL	flexor digitorum longus	PF	posterior subtalar facet	tnb	posterior tibial neurovascular bundle
BL	bifurcate ligament	FHL	flexor hallucis longus	PL	peroneus longus		
C	calcaneus	I	interosseous muscle	plf	plantar fascia	TP	tibialis posterior
c1	medial cuneiform	IPR	inferior peroneal retinaculum	PTF	posterior talofibular ligament	Tr	trochlea of talus
c2	middle cuneiform	LM	lateral malleolus	PTiF	posterior tibiofibular ligament	TS	tarsal sinus
c3	lateral cuneiform	Lp	lateral process of talus	S	sesamoid		
CF	calcaneofibular ligament	LPL	long plantar ligament	SL	spring ligament		
CJ	Chopart joint	lpn	lateral plantar neurovascular bundle	SPL	short plantar ligament		
CL	cervical ligament			SPR	superior peroneal retinaculum		

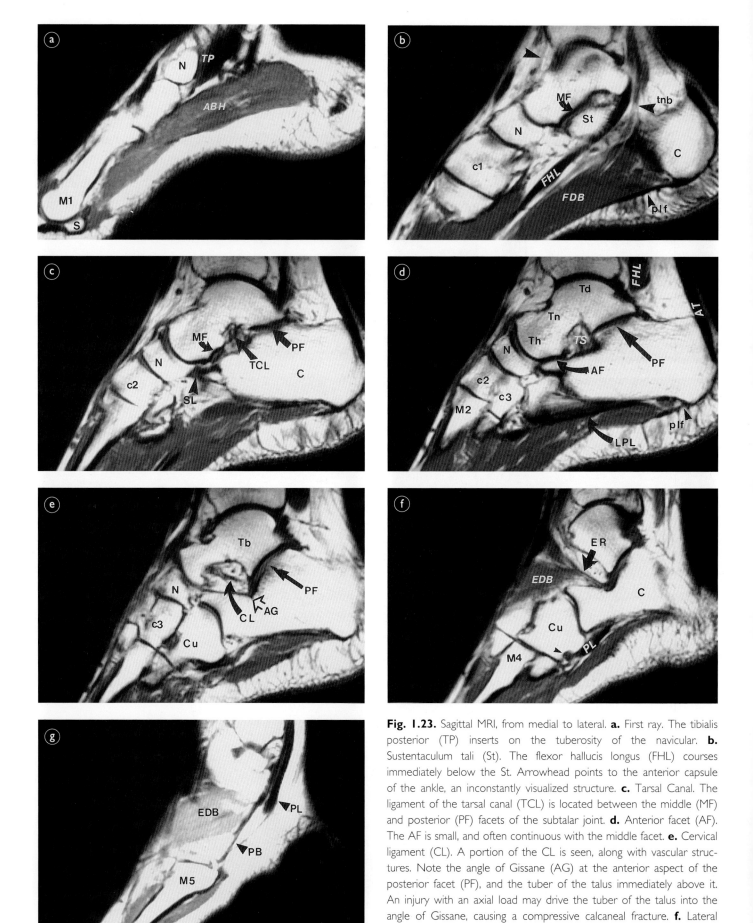

Fig. 1.23. Sagittal MRI, from medial to lateral. **a.** First ray. The tibialis posterior (TP) inserts on the tuberosity of the navicular. **b.** Sustentaculum tali (St). The flexor hallucis longus (FHL) courses immediately below the St. Arrowhead points to the anterior capsule of the ankle, an inconstantly visualized structure. **c.** Tarsal Canal. The ligament of the tarsal canal (TCL) is located between the middle (MF) and posterior (PF) facets of the subtalar joint. **d.** Anterior facet (AF). The AF is small, and often continuous with the middle facet. **e.** Cervical ligament (CL). A portion of the CL is seen, along with vascular structures. Note the angle of Gissane (AG) at the anterior aspect of the posterior facet (PF), and the tuber of the talus immediately above it. An injury with an axial load may drive the tuber of the talus into the angle of Gissane, causing a compressive calcaneal fracture. **f.** Lateral aspect of tarsal sinus, showing extensor retinaculum. The peroneus longus (PL) extends below the groove (arrowhead) at the lateral aspect of the cuboid. **g.** Peroneus brevis (PB). PB inserts on the tuberosity of the fifth metatarsal (M5).

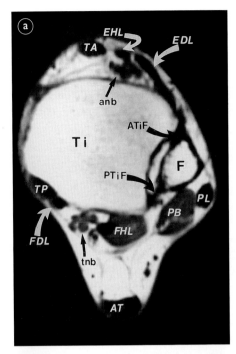

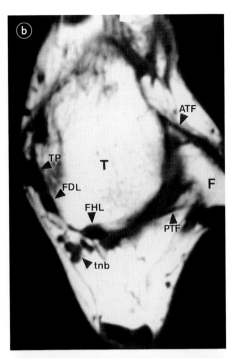

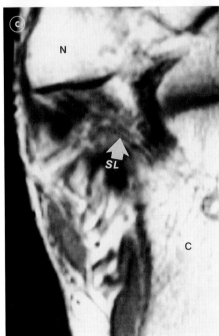

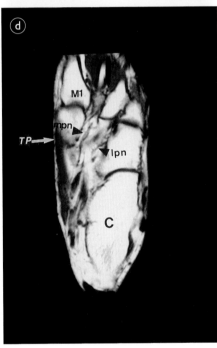

Fig. 1.24. Axial MRI, from superior to inferior. **a.** Tibiofibular syndesmosis, showing anterior (ATiF) and posterior (PTiF) tibiofibular ligaments. The relative position of the extrinsic flexors of the foot, from medial to lateral, can be remembered by the mnemonic Tom, Dick, and Harry. [Tom – tibialis posterior (TP), Dick – flexor digitorum longus (FDL), Harry – flexor hallucis longus (FHL).] FHL is still muscular at the level of the ankle joint, while the TP and FDL are tendinous. **b.** Talofibular ligaments. The anterior talofibular ligament (ATF) has an oblique orientation, anteriorly, medially and inferiorly from the fibula to the talus. Axial sections obtained along the long axis of the talus will usually show it in its entirety on one or two images. Posterior talofibular ligament (PTF) is transversely oriented. **c.** Spring ligament (SL). Several distinct fibrous bands of the SL can be seen extending from the calcaneus (C) to the navicular (N). **d.** Medial (mpn) and lateral (lpn) plantar nerves. The plantar nerve usually divides into medial and lateral branches in the region of the tarsal tunnel.

REFERENCES

1. McMinn RMH, Hutchings RT, Logan BM. *Color Atlas of Foot and Ankle Anatomy* (Appleton–Century–Crofts: East Norwalk, Connecticut, 1982).

2. Kjaersgaard-Anderson P, Wethelund JO, Helmig P, et al. The stabilizing effect of the ligamentous structures in the sinus and canalis tarsi on movement in the hindfoot. *Am J Sports Med* 1988; **16:**512–6.

3. Rule J, Yao L, Seeger LL. Spring ligament of the ankle: normal MR anatomy. *Am J Roentgen* 1993; **161:**1241–4.

4. Hartmann. The tendon sheaths and synovial bursae of the foot. *Foot Ankle* 1981; **1:**247-69.

5. Hollinshead WH. *Textbook of Anatomy*, 3rd edn. (Harper and Row: Philadelphia, 1974).

6. Koehler A, Zimmer EA. *Borderlands of the Normal and Early Pathologic in Skeletal Roentgenology*, 11th edn. (Grune and Stratton: New York, 1968).

7. Sella EJ, Lawson JP, Ogden JA. The accessory navicular synchondrosis. *Clin Orthop* 1986; **209:**280–5.

8. Sella EJ, Lawson JP. Biomechanics of the accessory navicular synchondrosis. *Foot Ankle* 1987; **8:**156–63.

9. Grogan DP, Gasser SI, Ogden JA. The painful accessory navicular: a clinical and histopathological study. *Foot Ankle* 1989; **10:**164–9.

10. Powell HDW. Extra centre of ossification for the medial malleolus in children: incidence and significance. *J Bone Joint Surg* 1961; **43B:**107–13.

11. Sobel M, Pavlov H, Geppert MJ, Thompson FM, DiCarlo EF, Davis WH. Painful os peroneum syndrome: a spectrum of conditions responsible for plantar lateral foot pain. *Foot Ankle* 1994; **15**:112–24.

12. McDougall A. The os trigonum. *J Bone Joint Surg* 1955; **37B:**257–65.

13. Marotta JJ, Micheli LJ. Os trigonum impingement in dancers. *Am J Sports Med* 1992; **20:**533–6.

14. Resnick D. Talar ridges, osteophytes and beaks: a radiologic commentary. *Radiology* 1984; **151:**329–32.

15. Sirry A. The pseudo-cystic triangle in the normal os calcis. *Acta Radiol* 1951; **36:**516–20.

16. Lee M, Hodler J, Haghighi P, Resnick D. Bone excrescence at the medial base of the distal phalanx of the first toe: normal variant, reactive change, or neoplasia? *Skeletal Radiol* 1992; **21:**161–5.

17. Silverman FN. *Caffey's Pediatric X-Ray Diagnosis: an Integrated Imaging Approach*, 8th edn. (Year Book Medical Publishers: Chicago, 1985).

18. Ogden JA, Ganey TM, Light TR, Belsole RJ, Greene TL. Ossification and pseudoepiphysis formation in the 'nonepiphyseal' end of bones of the hands and feet. *Skeletal Radiol* 1994; **23:**3–13.

2. IMAGING TECHNIQUES

PLAIN RADIOGRAPHS

Ankle

Three views of the ankle are routinely obtained, the anteroposterior (AP), the mortise, and the lateral.

AP view
Because the ankle is externally rotated 20° relative to the knee and the axis of the first toe, an AP radiograph, obtained with the knee and first toe facing forward, does not optimally demonstrate the medial and lateral gutters of the ankle (Fig. 2.1A). The medial malleolus of the tibia is well seen, with the larger anterior and smaller posterior colliculus overlapping. There is approximately a 1 cm overlap between the fibula and the tibia at the level of the plafond. The lateral malleolus of the fibula extends further inferiorly than the medial; the angle formed between the articular surface of the plafond and a line extending from the lateral to the medial malleolus (talocrural angle, chapter 3), should measure 83° ± 4°.

Mortise view
To obtain a radiograph that optimally shows both the medial and lateral gutters of the joint, the foot must be internally rotated 15–20°.[1] This is known as the mortise view (Fig. 2.1B). In the mortise view, the medial and lateral malleoli are equidistant from the film cassette. The ankle is dorsiflexed so that the widest portion of the talar dome is seen. On the mortise view, the joint space should be equal medially, superiorly, and laterally. The distance between the incisural notch of the tibia and the medial margin of the fibula should measure less than 5 mm. The tibia and fibula should overlap approximately 1 mm at the level of the plafond. If the ankle is overly rotated, there may be no overlap seen between the fibula and tibia (Fig. 2.1C). This technical problem can be differentiated from true widening of the syndesmosis, because if the problem is technical both gutters are not well seen.

Overrotation of the mortise view is a common error made by radiology technologists, and it is promoted by at least one textbook of radiographic positioning, which recommends a 45° internal rotation of the foot for this view.

Lateral view
On the lateral radiograph (Fig. 2.1D), the medial and lateral malleoli overlap. The hindfoot is well seen on the lateral study of the ankle. The base of the fifth metatarsal should be included in either this view or the mortise view so that fractures of the fifth metatarsal, which can mimic ankle fractures, can be seen on a routine ankle series.

Foot

Three views are routinely obtained: the anteroposterior (AP), the lateral, and the oblique (Fig. 2.2). The AP view is obtained with the plantar surface of the foot against the cassette. For the oblique view, the medial aspect of the foot is placed against the film cassette, with the lateral aspect of the foot elevated at an angle of about 30°. The lateral view is obtained with the lateral aspect of the foot against the cassette. If alignment of the foot is of concern, the AP and lateral views should be obtained with the patient standing (see Chapter 10).

On the AP view of the foot, the medial cortex of the base of the second metatarsal should always line up exactly with the medial cortex of the second cuneiform.[2] On the oblique radiograph, the lateral margin of the third metatarsal will line up with the lateral margin of the third cuneiform, and the medial margin of the fourth metatarsal with the medial margin of the cuboid. The base of the fifth metatarsal will project beyond the cuboid.

Subtalar Joint

The posterior and middle facets of the subtalar joint are usually well seen on the lateral view of the foot or ankle (Fig. 2.3A). The sustentaculum tali forms an elongated rectangle, and the middle facet lies above it. The posterior facet partially overlaps the middle facet on this projection. The subtalar joint can be further evaluated with the axial or Harris view. This view is obtained with the ankle dorsiflexed, the film cassette behind the heel, and a beam directed 45° cephalad through the heel (Fig. 2.3B). A 45° oblique view of the subtalar joint can also be obtained (Fig. 2.3C).

Sesamoids of First Toe

The articulation between the first metatarsal head and its sesamoids can be seen with the sesamoid view (Fig. 2.4). This view can be obtained either with the patient prone, and the toes dorsiflexed against the cassette, or with the patient supine, and the toes held in plantarflexion by a piece of cloth held by the patient and looped under the toes.

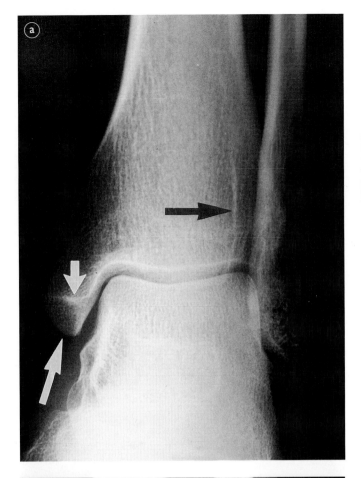

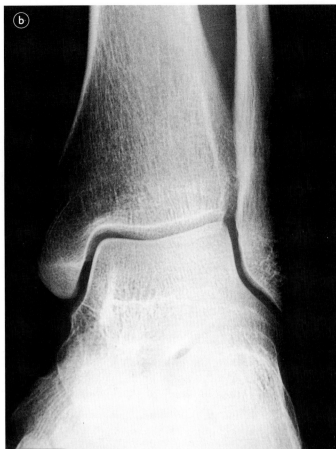

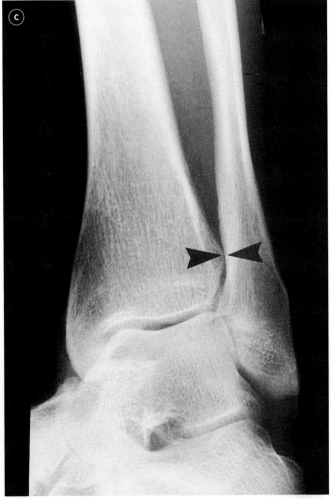

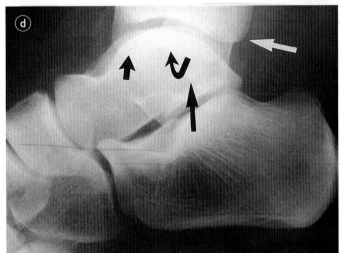

Fig. 2.1. Normal radiographic appearance of the ankle. **a.** AP radiograph. The peroneal groove of the tibia is demarcated medially by a line of cortical bone (black arrow). The distance from this line to the medial margin of the fibula should be ≤ 5 mm. Overlap between tibia and fibula should measure 1 cm at the widest portion of the tibia (at the level of the black arrow). Short white arrow points to posterior colliculus of the medial malleolus, and long white arrow to anterior colliculus. **b.** Mortise radiograph. The joint space appears equal medially, superiorly and laterally. There is 1 mm overlap between the tibia and fibula. c. Overly rotated 'mortise' radiograph. The normal overlap between the tibia and fibula immediately above the ankle joint is lost (arrowheads) because of overrotation. **d.** Lateral radiograph. The medial and lateral malleoli overlap. Short straight arrow – anterior colliculus, curved arrow – posterior colliculus, and long straight arrow – lateral malleolus. Posterior malleolus is an ill-defined region at the posterior lip of the tibia (white arrow).

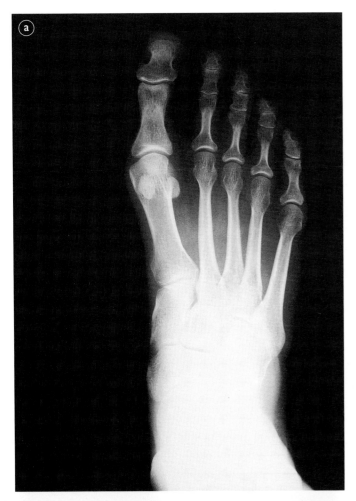
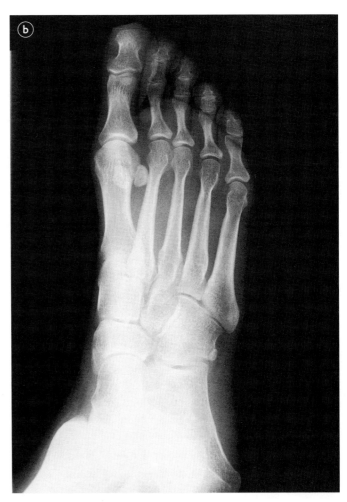
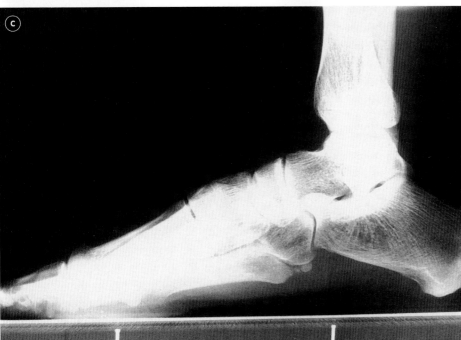

Fig. 2.2. Normal radiographic appearance of the foot. **a.** AP radiograph. The intercuneiform joints and the tarsometatarsal joints may be poorly seen; this is due to the obliquity of the joints, and should not be mistaken for fusion of the joint. It is difficult to obtain an optimal radiograph of both the hindfoot and the forefoot, due to differences in tissue thickness. For this radiograph, as well as (b), a wedge filter, thicker toward the toes, was used. **b.** Oblique radiograph. **c.** Lateral radiograph.

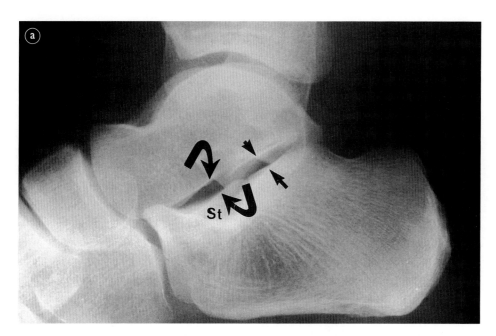

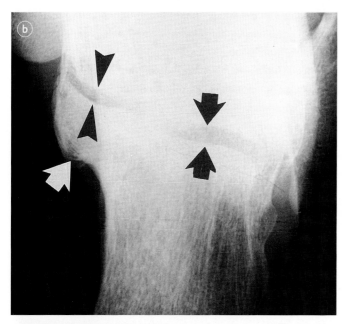

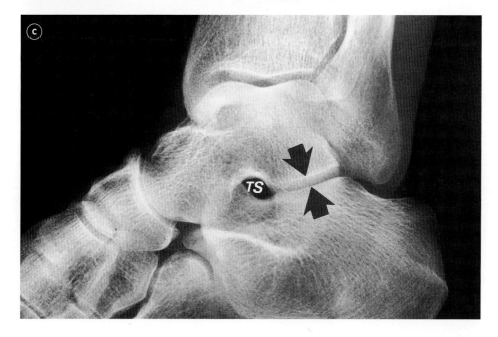

Fig. 2.3. Subtalar joint. **a.** Lateral radiograph. The posterior subtalar facet (straight arrows) and middle subtalar facet (curved arrows) are seen on a lateral radiograph if the X-ray beam is centered on the foot. The sustentaculum tali (St) of the calcaneus is a rectangular medial projection of the calcaneus which supports the middle subtalar facet. **b.** Harris view. Both the posterior facet (straight arrows) and middle facet (arrowheads) can be seen. White arrow points to sustentaculum tali. **c.** 45° oblique radiograph. This provides an additional view of the posterior facet (arrows), and shows the tarsal sinus (TS).

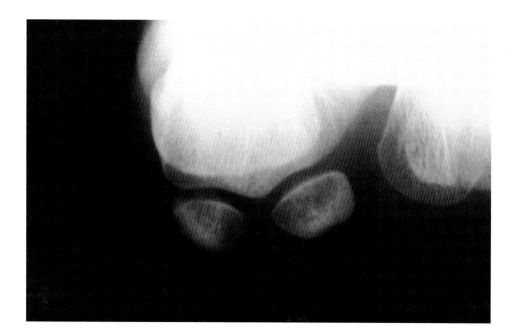

Fig. 2.4. Sesamoid view. The medial and lateral sesamoids of the first toe are symmetrically positioned at the medial and lateral facets of the first metatarsal head.

NUCLEAR MEDICINE STUDIES

^{99m}Technetium Bone Scans

Scans are performed with 10–20 mCi of ^{99m}technetium-labelled diphosphonate (generally methylene diphosphonate) administered intravenously. The diphosphonate initially distributes throughout the body in an amount proportional to blood flow. As the tracer is cleared by the kidneys, the soft tissue accumulation of tracer declines, and the diphosphonate is taken up in bone in an amount dependent on the degree of osteoblastic activity.[3]

A ^{99m}technetium bone scan is routinely obtained 2–4 hours after injection of the radionuclide. At this time, any process that results in increased osteoblastic activity will demonstrate increased accumulation of technetium ('hot spots') relative to normal bone (Table 2.1). Decreased activity leads to photopenic areas, known as 'cold spots', on bone scan (Table 2.2).

The three-phase bone scan was developed to increase the specificity of bone scanning for osteomyelitis. The first phase of the scan is a radionuclide angiogram, with images obtained every 3–6 seconds over the area of clinical concern to assess relative blood flow compared to the contralateral extremity. The second phase is a blood pool image obtained immediately after the angiogram. This shows soft-tissue activity due to hyperemia. The third phase is obtained after 3–4 hours and primarily reflects bone uptake of radionuclide due to osteoblastic activity. Although the specificity of three-phase bone scan for osteomyelitis is superior to that of single-phase bone scans, there are many other causes of positive three-phase scans (Table 2.3). As discussed in Chapter 6, the specificity of bone scan for osteomyelitis is increased by adding a fourth phase, at 24 hours after injection.

^{111}Indium-Labelled White Blood Cell Scans

Indium scans are performed using 0.5–1.0 mCi of ^{111}indium oxine-labelled leukocytes. Imaging is performed 18–24 hours after injection. The labelled white cells are sequestered in the spleen, liver, bone marrow, and any site where there are increased numbers of white blood cells. Indium scans are primarily used to diagnose infection. Noninfectious inflammatory processes may also show localized accumulation of the ^{111}indium-labelled leukocytes. Spatial definition is poor, and in the small bones of the foot it may be difficult to determine if activity is in the bone or the soft tissue. A detailed discussion of its uses and limitations in osteomyelitis of the foot is found in Chapter 6.

Table 2.1. Causes of 'Hot Spots' on single phase ^{99m}technetium bone scan.
Osteomyelitis
Cellulitis
Neuropathic joint
Fracture (including healed fractures)
Recent surgery (even if limited to soft tissues)
Primary or metastatic bone tumors
Arthritis (both degenerative and inflammatory)
Reflex sympathetic dystrophy
Avascular necrosis and bone infarction (reparative phase)
Radiation therapy
Myositis ossificans and other heterotopic ossification

Table 2.2. Causes of 'cold spots' on ^{99m}technetium bone scan.
Fractures less than 24 hours old
Early infection (especially in children)
Multiple myeloma
Purely lytic metastatic tumors (especially lung, renal, neuroblastoma)
Early avascular necrosis or infarction
Attenuation by overlying metal, plaster cast, etc.

Table 2.3. Causes of positive three-phase ⁹⁹ᵐtechnetium bone scan.

Osteomyelitis

Cellulitis

Neuropathic joint

Acute fracture

Fracture nonunion

Recent bone surgery

Vascular tumor (some sarcomas and metatastases, osteoid osteoma, hemangioma)

Reflex sympathetic dystrophy

Inflammatory arthritis (e.g. gout, rheumatoid arthritis)

Myositis ossificans (active)

ARTHROGRAPHY

Arthrography utilizes positive contrast (iodinated contrast agents), negative contrast (air), or both to demonstrate joint abnormalities that are not normally evident on plain radiographs. Today, arthrography of the ankle joint is primarily used (in conjunction with polydirectional tomography or CT) to look for osteochondritis dissecans and intra-articular loose bodies. Cartilage and intra-articular loose bodies are seen because they are outlined by contrast.

In the past, arthrography was used to evaluate ligamentous tears caused by ankle sprains. Ligamentous tears can be inferred when contrast extends beyond the normal confines of the joint. This technique is rarely used today because most ankle sprains are treated conservatively, so precise localization of the site of tear is not needed to guide treatment. The need for more precise diagnosis is limited to the chronically painful sprain, but in this setting arthrography has a high incidence of false-negative results. False-negative arthrograms occur in chronic sprain because fibrous tissue forms at the site of ligamentous injury, preventing extravasation of contrast from the site of ligamentous rupture. MRI is preferable in the chronically painful sprain, both to evaluate the ligaments and to rule out other abnormalities.

Technique of Ankle Arthrography

The ankle can be entered with a 23 or 25 gauge needle, using an anterior approach. The ankle is placed in the lateral position. The dorsalis pedis artery is palpated, and the site of entry is made medial to the artery. The needle is angled slightly cephalad from an entry point just below the joint. This approach allows the needle tip to slip under the anterior lip of the tibia. In general, for a single contrast arthrogram, 8–10 cm³ of iodinated contrast will be used, and for a double contrast arthrogram, 1 cm³ of iodinated contrast, 0.2 cm³ of epinephrine 1:1000 (if the patient is to undergo CT scan), and 8–10 cm³ of air will be used. Arthrography can be performed with air only if the patient is allergic to iodine. CT arthrograms should not be performed with full strength single contrast technique, because loose bodies will be obscured. They can be performed as double

contrast examinations, air only, or with dilute single contrast (e.g., Isovue® 240 diluted 1:3 with normal saline).

After injection, the ankle should be passively exercised for a few seconds. AP, lateral, and internal and external oblique radiographs are routinely obtained (Fig. 2.5). For the evaluation of osteochondritis dissecans or a loose body, tomograms or CT in addition to plain radiographs are strongly recommended (see Chapter 4).

Dedicated hypocycloidal tomography machines are often not available today, despite their proven efficacy in bone radiology. However, the polydirectional tomographic capabilities of many machines designed for intravenous pyelograms will provide adequate bone images. Linear tomography should be avoided if possible because of streak artifacts.

Normal Findings on Ankle Arthrography

Anterior and posterior recesses of the joint will normally fill on arthrography, and should have a smooth contour. Note that the joint capsule attaches to the tibia aprroximately 1 cm above the articular surface. Distally, it extends to the junction of the talar neck and head. Medially and laterally, contrast extends below but not beyond the malleoli. Contrast may extend between the tibia and fibula for up to 2.5 cm.[4] In about 20% of normal ankles, there is communication between the ankle joint and the flexor hallucis longus and flexor digitorum longus tendon sheaths.[5] In about 10% of normal ankles, there is communication between the ankle and posterior subtalar joints.

COMPUTERIZED AXIAL TOMOGRAPHY

Computerized axial tomography (CT) scanning employs thinly collimated X-ray beams arranged circumferentially around the body. Computer analysis of the attenuation of the X-ray beams measures the degree to which small areas of tissue, called pixels, attenuate the X-ray beam. The attenuation of a given pixel correlates to the density of the tissue in the pixel, and this attenuation is measured in Hounsfield units (HU). HU range from -1000 (air) to +1000 (cortical bone). Water is approximately 0 HU. The absolute HU measurement varies between CT scanners, but in general muscle will be 20–40 HU, blood 40–50 HU, and fat -50 to -100 HU.

Although CT can differentiate between 2000 different levels of beam attenuation, the human eye can only distinguish about 20 shades of grey. Therefore, CT data is manipulated to provide images with a gray scale appropriate to the tissues being examined. The width of the grey scale setting is know as the CT window. The middle grey level is known as the center. For example, a window of 400 with a center of 50 will show all tissues with an attenuation above 250 HU as white, and all tissues below -150 as black.

In the musculoskeletal system, two types of windows are usually employed:

- soft-tissue windows; and
- bone windows.

A soft-tissue window is centered around the density of muscle, with a fairly narrow window width (e.g. center 40 HU

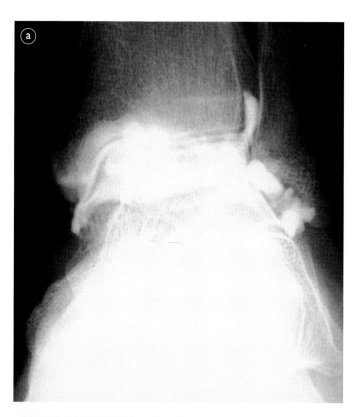

Fig. 2.5. Normal arthrography. **a.** AP radiograph. The articular cartilage is outlined by contrast. Note that the contrast does extend a short distance superiorly between the tibia and fibula. It does not extend beyond the tips of the malleoli. **b.** Lateral radiograph. Anterior and posterior recesses are seen, and have a smooth appearance. **c.** Lateral complex motion tomogram, 3 mm thick. No filling defects are present in the contrast.

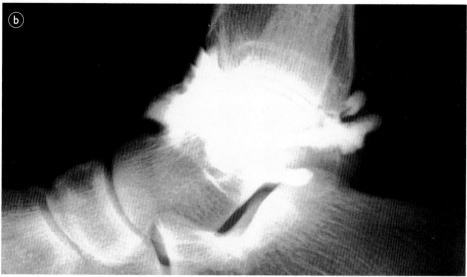

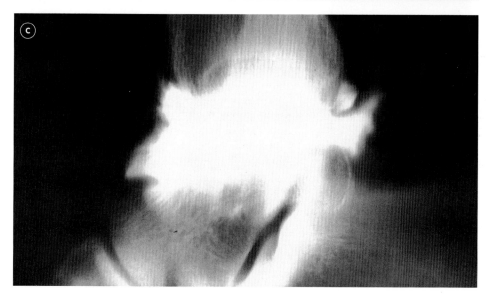

and window width 350–450 HU), in order to optimize visualization of differences in attenuation between muscle, fluid, soft-tissue masses, blood, etc.

A bone window is chosen to enhance visualization of bone trabeculae, fracture lines, periosteal new bone, and cortical abnormalities. It will have a wide window (e.g. 2000 HU), centered at about 500 HU. CT scans obtained after arthrography are often best seen on an intermediate window with a width of about 1000 HU.

Musculoskeletal CTs should be viewed at both bone and soft-tissue windows. If a fracture case is viewed only at bone windows, important soft-tissue injuries may be overlooked. Soft-tissue windows are also needed to see bone-marrow infiltration. Conversely, fracture lines or cortical breakthrough due to tumor or osteomyelitis may not be evident on soft-tissue window, but are easily identified on bone windows.

CT scans of the foot and ankle can be performed in either the axial or the coronal plane, and for most clinical purposes both projections should be obtained. To obtain axial images, the patients lies supine in the scanner, with the lower extremities extended and the feet in a comfortable position. Motion should be minimized by using tape and cushions to help hold the feet. For coronal images, the knees are flexed, and the feet are placed flat against the CT gantry. Again, cushioning and tape are helpful in maintaining the patient's position. Feet can be scanned through plaster or fiberglass casts or splints, but the presence of the cast or splint may prevent positioning for direct coronal scans. In that case, reformatted images should be performed in the coronal plane. The CT gantry should be angled to obtain the optimal scan plane.

On most current CT scanners, CT data can easily be reformatted into any desired plane. When spiral CT is available, excellent detail can be obtained by scanning the patient with 3 mm thick spiral cuts, having the computer reanalyze the images as 1 mm cuts, and then reformatting the thinner images in the desired plane. If spiral CT is not available, excellent reformatted images can be obtained from 2 mm thick contiguous axial images or 3 mm thick images with a 1 mm slice overlap.

Three-dimensional CT is an option that can be helpful for users unfamiliar with cross-sectional imaging. However, fracture lines tend to be less obvious on three-dimensional images than on conventional images.

MAGNETIC RESONANCE IMAGING

There are many sources explaining the physics of magnetic resonance imaging (MRI), but a detailed understanding is not necessary to interpret MR scans. The following discussion is limited to several key concepts with which the MRI user must be familiar.[6]

MRI uses a series of magnetic pulses that excite mobile protons (hydrogen atoms) in a chosen cross-sectional volume (slice). As the protons return to their base state, they emit magnetic signals whose characteristics depend on the interaction of the proton with adjacent molecules. The signal elicited by a magnetic pulse depends on the concentration of mobile protons, the nature of the adjacent tissue, and the type of pulse administered.

Table 2.4. Signal intensity of common tissues on T1-weighted and T2-weighted MRI sequences

Tissue type	T1-weighted images	T2-weighted images
cortical bone	low	low
fat (incl. fatty marrow)	high	intermediate-high
red marrow	low	intermediate
muscle	low	intermediate
tendon, ligament, fascia	low	low
low-protein fluid	low	high
high-protein fluid	high	high

The signals emitted by the protons are interpreted by computer in terms of variables which are designated T1 relaxation and T2 relaxation. An imaging sequence is called T1-weighted or T2-weighted according to the relative contribution of T1 and T2 relaxation to the image. A tissue will have a short T1 and appear bright on T1-weighted images if hydrogen nuclei are closely associated with macromolecules such as protein or fat, or if a paramagnetic substance such as gadolinium or methemoglobin is present. A tissue will have a long T2 and appear bright on T2-weighted images if a large amount of free water is present (Table 2.4).

Tumors, infection, cysts, and edema all appear bright on T2-weighted images because of the increased amount of free water present. The signal elicited from flowing blood will vary according to the velocity of the blood and multiple other factors. The appearance of hemorrhage will vary over time;[7] the stages of evolution of a hematoma are less predictable in the musculoskeletal system than in the brain.

In a MRI sequence, the frequency of the applied magnetic pulse is varied along one axis (frequency-encoding axis) and the phase of excitation along the second axis (phase-encoding axis). This causes slight variations in the signals emitted by protons at different locations, so that the origin of a signal can be localized to create a two-dimensional image.

Types of Sequences

There are several common types of MRI sequences: spin echo (SE), inversion recovery (IR), and gradient echo (GRE). A shorthand is employed to describe the sequence used, and it will be seen throughout this book on captions of MRI images. By convention, an MRI sequence can be described by the type of sequence (e.g. SE), followed by a description of how it is weighted (either T1-weighted, T2-weighted, or balanced), and the magnetic pulse sequence used (TR/TE for SE images, TR/TE/TI for inversion recovery images, and TR/TE/flip angle (FA) for gradient echo sequences).

Spin echo (SE) images are the most commonly obtained. Signal characteristics of a given tissue depend on pulse repetition time (TR) and echo time (TE) in spin echo sequences. Sequences can be either T1-weighted or T2-weighted. T1-weighting depends primarily on a short TR, and T2-weighting depends primarily on a long TE. A T1-weighted spin echo image will generally have a TR of 600 milliseconds or less to maximize T1 effects, and will minimize T2-weighting with a short (25 milliseconds or less) TE. A T2-weighted image will have a TE of 60 milliseconds or above, preferably at least 80 milliseconds, and will minimize T1-weighting with a long (2000 milliseconds or greater) TR.

Today, T2-weighted sequences generally employ two echoes, for instance TE 20 and TE 80, obtained during the same TR. The first echo will have minimized T1-weighting, owing to the long TR, and minimized T2-weighting, owing to the long TE. The images obtained from this first echo are often referred to as spin density, proton density, or intermediate images. Signal intensities on this sequence will be intermediate between T1 and T2. Fat Suppression techniques are now available on spin echo images. They can be useful in increasing conspicuity of lesions in fatty marrow, and improving visualizaton of articular cartilage.[8] Fast spin echo (FSE) techniques with a TR of 3000–4000 and TE>100 are another technique, and are used to decrease the amount of time needed to acquire a T2-weighted image. FSE has a serious potential pitfall in the musculoskeletal system, however. Fat has a brighter appearance on FSE T2-weighted images than on SE, and so abnormalties occuring within fatty marrow or other fat-containing areas may be obscured.

Inversion recovery sequences use an inversion magnetization pulse with an inversion time TI, in addition to TE and TR. The sequence is described by the TR/TE/TI, in that order. Because of the added pulse, this sequence takes a long acquisition time, and the number or slices per scan is limited. Short tau inversion recovery (STIR) images are commonly used in the musculoskeletal system. They suppress signal caused by fat, and increase the visibility of abnormalities within fatty marrow.

Gradient echo (GRE) images are obtained with a variety of techniques,[9] and may be either slices of tissue similar to SE images ('two-dimensional' GRE), or acquisitions of an entire volume of data ('three-dimensional' GRE), which can be reformatted in any plane. There are multiple acronyms in use to describe different gradient echo sequences. The greater the flip angle used, the greater the T1-weighting of a sequence.

Contrast agents , usually employing the element gadolinium, may be used to increase conspicuity of a lesion.[10] The enhancement of a lesion, with the exception of lesions of the central nervous system, is dependent primarily on blood flow. Therefore, inflammatory processes such as osteomyelitis, vascular benign tumors such as osteoblastoma, and malignant neoplasms will all show enhancement following gadolinium administration.

Factors Affecting Quality of MRI Images

The quality of an MRI image will depend on the signal to noise ratio (SNR), which is the amount of magnetic signal received from the tissue relative to the amount of 'noise' present.

Signal-to noise ratio is greatly enhanced by the use of surface coils, which should be used for all examinations of the foot and ankle. Most systems have an extremity coil that will fit the foot, but a head coil may also be used.

Patient motion is a major cause of image noise, and care should be given to positioning the foot comfortably and maintaining its position with tape and padding in order to minimize motion. Any movement by the patient during the acquisition of a sequence will degrade all of the images in that sequence. If necessary, sedation should be used to decrease motion by the nervous or claustrophobic patient or by the patient who is unable to lie still because of pain. At our institution, we routinely administer 2–5 mg of Versed to an adult patient, adding 50-100 mg of Fentanyl if the patient is experiencing pain.

SNR can be increased by performing two or more sequential acquisitions of data (referred to as acquisitions (acq) or excitations (NEX)), which are averaged by the computer. This will increase examination time, but a compensatory time reduction may be achieved by employing a rectangular field of view for a body part that is wider in one axis than in another; this is especially useful in coronal images of the foot.

Resolution can be increased by decreasing the field of view (FOV), and by increasing the matrix of a sequence.

Artefacts

Artefacts are a common problem in MRI, and it is important to recognize them. Pulsation artefact is spurious signal propagated from arterial pulsations (see Fig. 11.17). Chemical shift artefact occurs between two tissues of different compositions (see Fig. 11.9). Metal artefact occurs because of distortion of the local magnetic field by metal in the body. Even tiny shreds of metal (for instance, those left behind after a fixation screw is removed) cause this artefact. A low signal area larger than the metal itself is seen, often containing bands of high signal intensity (see Fig. 5.57).

Wraparound artefact can occur when the FOV is smaller than the body part being imaged. It is decreased by surface coils, which decrease signal reception by tissues not in the coil. Special techniques are available on many scanners to eliminate wraparound.

MRI Hazards

MRI is contraindicated in patients with cardiac pacemakers and defibrillators, some heart valves, cochlear implants, magnetic ocular implants, and intracerebral vascular clips, among others.[12] All patients undergoing MRI should be screened.

A metallic foreign body in the eye is a contraindication to MRI, but patients may not be aware if one is present. At our institution, all patients who have performed metal work are screened with AP, Waters, and lateral views of the orbits. If there is a history of previous intraorbital metal, a CT of the orbits is obtained prior to MRI.

REFERENCES

1. Goergen TG, Danzig LA, Resnick D. Roentgenographic evaluation of the tibiotalar joint. *J Bone Joint Surg* 1977; **59A:**874–7.

2. Stein RE. Radiological aspects of the tarsometatarsal joints. *Foot Ankle* 1983; **3:**286–9.

3. Mettler FA, Guiberteau MJ. Skeletal system. In: *Essentials of Nuclear Medicine Imaging*. (WB Saunders: Philadelphia, 1991), Chapter 11.

4. Arner O, Ekengren K, Hulting B et al. Arthrography of the talocrural joint: anatomic, roentgenographic and clinical aspects. *Acta Chir Scand* 1957; **113:**253–9.

5. Goergen TG, Resnick D. Arthrography of the ankle and hindfoot. In: Dalinka MK (ed). *Arthrography*. (Springer: New York, 1980), pp 137–53. .

6. Pykett IL, Newhouse JH, Buonanno FS, et al. Principles of nuclear magnetic resonance imaging. *Radiology* 1982; **143:**157–65.

7. Bradley WH. MR appearance of hemorrhage in the brain. *Radiology* 1993; **189:**15-26.

8. Mirowita SA. Fast scanning and fat-suppression MR imaging of musculoskeletal disorders. *Am J Roentgenol* 1993; **161:**1147–57.

9. Elster AD. Gradient-echo MR imaging: techniques and acronyms. *Radiology* 1993; **186:**1–8.

10. Saini S, Modic MT, Hahn PF. Advances in contrast-enhanced MR imaging. *Am J Roentgenol* 1991; **156:**235-54.

11. Shellock FG, Curtis JS. MR imaging and biomedical implants, materials and devices: an updated review. *Radiology* 1991; **180:**541-50.

3. ANKLE TRAUMA

ANATOMY

The ankle joint is a hinge joint that normally allows flexion (commonly called plantar flexion) and extension (dorsiflexion) only. There are three sets of ligaments, the medial and lateral collateral ligaments and the syndesmotic tibiofibular ligaments, which maintain the integrity of the joint and help prevent inversion and eversion as well as anterior and posterior translation. The anatomy of the ankle is discussed in detail in Chapter 1.

Neer[1] has popularized the concept that the tibia, fibula, talus, and ankle ligaments form a vertical ring. As in any ring, a single break is stable, and two breaks are required to destabilize it (Fig. 3.1). Consideration of the integrity of this ring is important in evaluating ankle fractures.

TYPES OF INJURY

Injuries to the ankle can be divided into malleolar fractures, sprains, and pilon fractures. Malleolar fractures and sprains occur because of supination or pronation injury, whereas pilon fractures are the result of axial load injury. Fracture-dislocations can be considered as part of the continuum of malleolar fractures.

MALLEOLAR FRACTURES

Malleolar fractures can be most simply described by the number of malleoli involved (unimalleolar, bimalleolar or trimalleolar). The fractures can be more completely understood by either of the two classifications of malleolar fractures in common use, the Lauge-Hansen classification and the Danis–Weber classification (the AO classification). Both systems have limitations, and the radiologist's description of an ankle fracture should not be limited to designating its category in either classification. Numerous eponyms, with which the radiogist should be familiar, are also used for ankle fractures (Table 3.1).

Terminology

The terms inversion and eversion describe motion in a single plane. Since ankle injuries occur when the foot is planted on the ground, the motion of the foot is complex and is better described by the terms supination and pronation, and these are used in the Lauge-Hansen system. Supination refers to inversion

of the hindfoot with adduction of the forefoot – the medial arch of the foot is elevated. Pronation refers to eversion of the hindfoot with abduction of the forefoot – the medial arch of the foot is depressed.

It should be noted that displacement of bones is always described in terms of the motion of the distal part relative to the proximal part. Therefore, rotational injuries occurring with the foot planted on the ground and internal rotation of the leg are referred to as lateral or external rotation injuries.

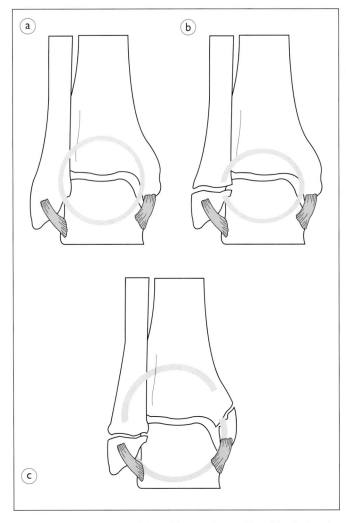

Fig. 3.1 Neer's concept of the ankle as a ring. **a.** The tibia, fibula, talus and ligaments form a stable ring in the coronal plane. **b.** A single break in the ring does not cause instability. **c.** Two breaks in the ring result in an unstable configuration. (Adapted from Neer.[1])

Table 3.1 Eponymic ankle fractures.	
Bosworth	fibular fracture with posterior dislocation
Duputreyn	fracture of fibula 4–10 cm above syndesmosis, syndesmotic rupture
Maisonneuve	fracture of proximal fibula, syndesmotic rupture
Marmor-Lynn	triplane fracture tibia
Pott	fracture of fibula 2–6 cm above syndesmosis, syndesmosis intact (this fracture is rare)
Tillaux	fracture of tibial attachment of anterior tibiofibular ligament
Volkmann	fracture of tibial attachment of posterior tibiofibular ligament
Wagstaffe–Le Fort	fracture of fibular attachment of anterior tibiofibular ligament

The Lauge-Hansen classification of fractures

Lauge-Hansen performed cadaveric studies of ankle fractures and proposed a classification into four basic types of injuries.[2,3] This system, modified by Arimoto and Forrester,[4] is widely used today, at least in an abbreviated form.

The Lauge-Hansen system designates basic types of ankle injury with a two-part descriptor. The first term refers to the position of the foot at the time of injury (supination or pronation). The second term describes the force acting on the talus (abduction, adduction, or external rotation). Within each category, injuries occur in a predictable sequence, and the stages of injury are designated numerically (Table 3.2). A fifth category of injury, pronation–dorsiflexion (PD), was added later[5] to describe axial load injuries, but is not in common use. Therefore, the stages of pronation–dorsiflexion injury are listed in Table 3.2 but are not discussed further. Axial load injuries are known as pilon fractures, and are discussed separately below.

Table 3.2. Lauge-Hansen Classification. (Adapted from Arimoto and Forrester.[4])

Supination–adduction (10–20% of ankle fractures)
SA-1 – transverse traction fracture of lateral malleolus below level of plafond, or LCL rupture
SA-2 – plus near-vertical fracture of the medial malleolus

Supination–external rotation (40–75% of ankle fractures)
SER-1 – rupture anterior tibiofibular ligament*
SER-2 – plus spiral fracture of lateral malleolus near level of plafond
SER-3 – plus rupture of posterior tibiofibular ligament or avulsion of its attachment to the posterior tibia
SER-4 – plus rupture of deltoid ligament or transverse or oblique fracture of the medial malleolus

Pronation–abduction (5–20% of ankle fractures)
PA-1 – transverse fracture of medial malleolus or rupture of deltoid ligament
PA-2 – plus rupture of both anterior and posterior tibiofibular ligaments and posterior tibial fracture
PA-3 – plus oblique fracture of fibula, generally just above the plafond

Pronation–external rotation (7–20% of ankle fractures)
PER-1 – rupture of deltoid ligament or avulsion of medial malleolus
PER-2 – plus rupture of anterior tibiofibular ligament and interosseous ligament
PER-3 – plus high spiral fracture of the fibula
PER-4 – plus fracture of the posterior tibia at the attachment of the posterior tibiofibular ligaments, or rupture of the ligaments

Pronation–dorsiflexion
PD-1 – medial malleolar fracture
PD-2 – plus fracture anterior tibial margin
PD-3 – plus fracture of the fibula above the plafond
PD-4 – plus transverse fracture of the posterior tibia, connecting to the vertical fracture of the anterior tibia from stage 2

*rarely, avulsion of its tibial attachment (Tillaux fracture) or its fibular attachment (Wagstaff–Le Fort fracture).

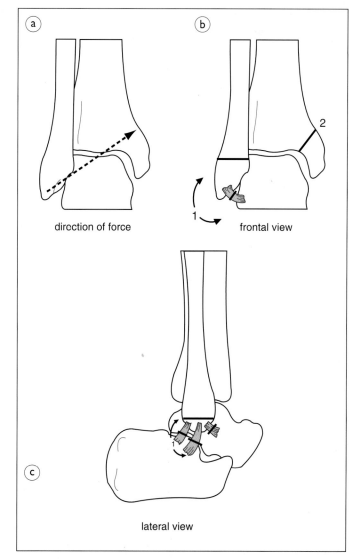

Fig. 3.2. Mechanism of supination-adduction injury. **a.** A linear force starts laterally and extends superomedially. **b.** Frontal and **c.** lateral diagrammatic representations. The first injury (1) is an avulsion of the lateral malleolus or LCL rupture. This is followed by a near vertical fracture of the medial malleolus (2).

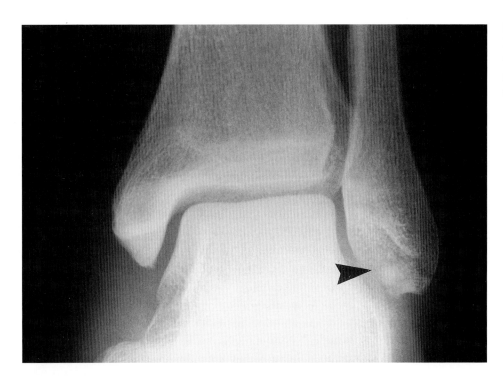

Fig. 3.3. Supination–adduction injury. Mortise radiograph of SA-1. There is a transverse fracture of the tip of the lateral malleolus (open arrow). The medial malleolus is intact.

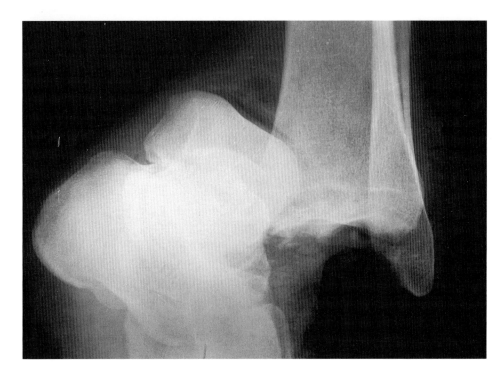

Fig. 3.4. Supination–adduction injury. AP radiograph of SA-2 fracture dislocation. There is rupture of the lateral collateral ligaments, and fracture of the medial malleolus.

Figures 3.2, 3.5, 3.9 and 3.12 schematically demonstrate how each injury can be visualized as a sequence of events occuring in a logical order, progressing from the point of initial injury along the direction of the force acting on the foot.

In supination–adduction (SA) injury (Figs 3.2–3.4), supination of the foot first puts tension at the lateral aspect of the ankle, causing a transverse, avulsion type fracture of the lateral malleolus or a rupture of the lateral collateral ligament. The talus is adducted and impacts on the medial malleolus, causing a shear fracture that is near-vertical in orientation. There may also be impaction of the medial aspect of the tibial plafond.

Supination–external rotation (SER) injuries (Figs 3.5–3.8) are the most common type of injury. The rotational force on the supinated foot begins anterolaterally with the rupture of the anterior tibiofibular ligaments, continues posteriorly to cause a spiral fracture of the lateral malleolus and then a rupture of the posterior tibiofibular ligament or a fracture of its tibial attachment, and continues medially to fracture the medial malleolus or rupture the deltoid ligament.

Supination-external rotation stage 4 (SER-4), if there is rupture of the deltoid ligament instead of a medial malleolar fracture, will appear radiographically similar to SER-2. However, SER-2 is

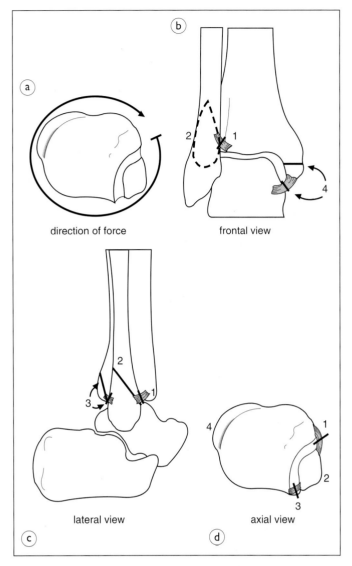

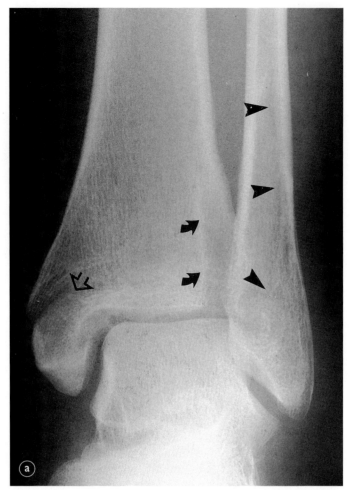

Fig. 3.5. Mechanism of supination–external rotation injury. **a.** A rotational force begins at the anterolateral aspect of the ankle, and progresses posteriorly, then medially. **b–d.** Frontal, lateral and axial diagrams. The first injury (1) is rupture of the anterior tibiofibular ligament, followed by spiral fracture of the lateral malleolus (2), rupture of the posterior tibiofibular ligament or a fracture of its tibial attachment (3), and fracture of the medial malleolus or deltoid ligament rupture (4).

Fig. 3.6. Stage 4 supination-external rotation injury. **a.** AP radiograph. As is characteristic of this injury, the spiral fracture of the distal fibula (arrowheads) is difficult to see on the AP view. The distance from the incisural notch of the tibia (curved arrows) to the medial margin of the fibula is slightly increased (6 mm), indicating tibiofibular diastasis. There is an oblique fracture of the medial malleolus (open arrow), which is minimally displaced.

stable while SER-4 is unstable, because SER-4 represents two breaks in the vertical ring. Widening of the medial gutter of the mortise indicates deltoid ligament tear (Fig. 3.7).

In pronation-abduction (PA) injury (Figs 3.9–3.11), pronation stresses the medial aspect of the joint and causes an avulsion of the medial malleolus or deltoid ligament tear. The dome of the talus impacts on the fibula, causing first rupture of the tibiofibular ligaments and then a short, oblique fracture of the fibula. There may be lateral impaction of the tibial plafond. The fibular fracture is frequently comminuted at its lateral aspect.

Pronation–external rotation (PER) injury (Figs 3.12 and 3.13) involves a rotational stress that starts medially with rupture of the deltoid ligament or transverse fracture of the medial malleolus, and progresses anterolaterally to cause rupture of the anterior tibiofibular ligament. As the stress progresses posteriorly, there is a high fracture of the fibula, with rupture of the interosseous ligament superiorly to the point of fracture. Finally, there is fracture of the attachment of the posterior tibiofibular ligament or rupture of the ligament. Extreme external rotation can lead to posterior dislocation of the fibula (Bosworth fracture).

Duputreyn's fracture is a fibular fracture 4–10 cm above the plafond. It is usually caused by a PA or PER injury, less commonly by SER injury.[6] Maisonneuve fracture (Fig. 3.13) is a type of PER fracture in which the fibular fracture is located in the proximal to midshaft of the fibula. When there are radiographic signs of PER injury (isolated fracture of the medial or posterior malleolus, or widening of the medial mortise) without

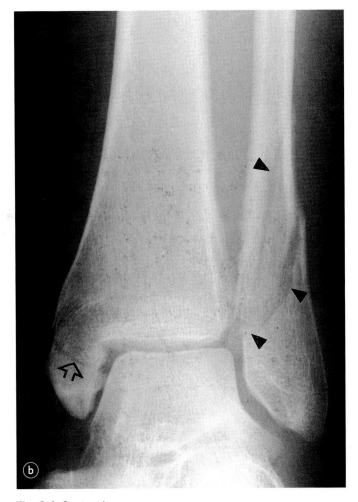

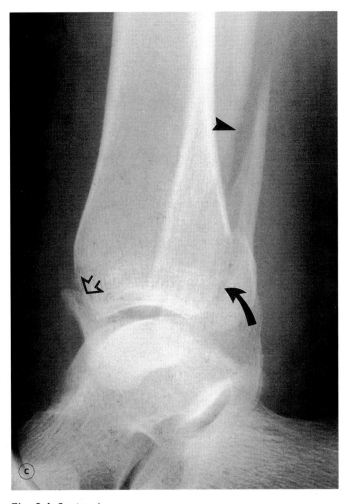

Fig. 3.6 *Continued*

b. Mortise radiograph shows both the medial (open arrow) and lateral (arrowheads) malleolar fractures well. The oblique fracture of the fibula in this injury originates medially at the level of the plafond, and extends superolaterally and posteriorly.

Fig. 3.6 *Continued*

c. On the lateral radiograph, the small posterior malleolar fragment (curved arrow) is appreciated, as well as the medial (open arrow) and lateral (arrowhead) malleolar fractures.

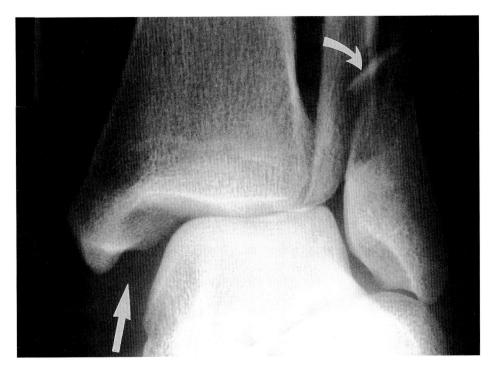

Fig. 3.7. Stage 4 supination–external rotation injury without medial malleolar fracture, mortise view. The medial gutter of the joint is widened (straight arrow) owing to deltoid ligament rupture. The joint widening differentiates this injury from an SER-2 fracture. The fibula is shortened owing to overriding of the fibular fracture (curved arrow).

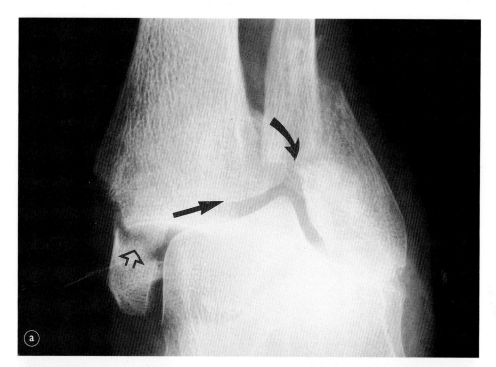

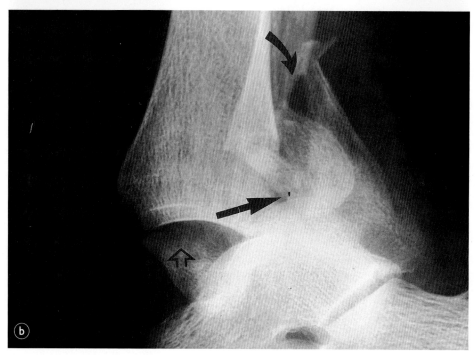

Fig. 3.8. Stage 4 supination-external rotation fracture-dislocation. **a.** Mortise radiograph. **b.** Lateral radiograph. There is an oblique fracture of the medial malleolus (open arrow), a fracture of the lateral malleolus (curved arrow) with overriding and valgus angulation, and a large posterior malleolar fragment (straight arrow).

evidence of fibular fracture on ankle radiographs, then radiographs of the entire tibia and fibula should be obtained to exclude a Maisonneuve fracture.

The most important radiographic factor in distinguishing the different types of fracture within the Lauge-Hansen system is the fracture of the lateral malleolus, when this is present (Fig. 3.14):

- in SA injuries, a transverse avulsion fracture is seen below the level of the tibial plafond;
- in SER injuries, the spiral fracture is best seen on the lateral radiograph and occurs at or above the level of the plafond;
- in PA injuries, the short oblique fracture runs upwards from medial to lateral, is best seen on the anteroposterior radiograph, and is above the level of the plafond;

- in PER injuries, the fibular fracture is high, often about 6 cm above the plafond or even higher, and downwards from anterior to posterior.

Danis–Weber classification

A classification system designed to optimize internal fixation of ankle fractures was proposed by Danis,[7] modified by Weber,[8] and popularized by the AO–ASIF (Arbeitsgemeinschaft für Osteosynthesefragen – Association for the Study of Internal Fixation) Group. It is variously known as the Weber, Danis–Weber, AO, or AO–ASIF classification.

This system divides fractures into three groups based on the integrity of the tibiofibular syndesmosis (Fig. 3.15). Disruption of

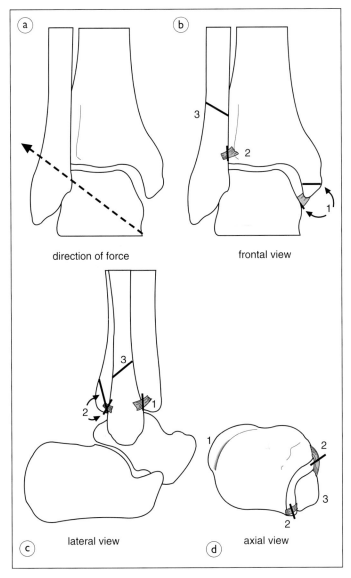

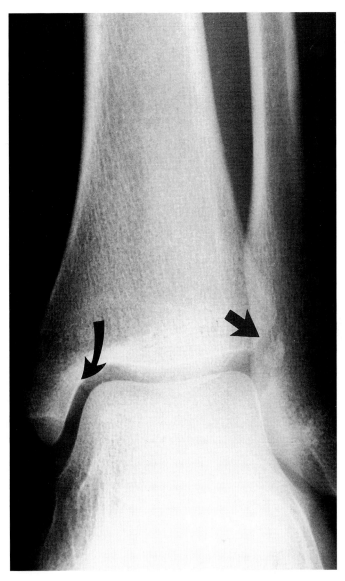

Fig. 3.9. Mechanism of pronation-abduction injury. **a.** A linear force starts medially and progresses superolaterally. **b–d.** Frontal, lateral and axial diagrams. The first injury is an avulsion of the medial malleolus or deltoid ligament tear (1). The dome of the talus impacts on the fibula, causing rupture of the tibiofibular ligaments (2) and then an impaction fracture of the fibula (3).

Fig. 3.10. Stage 2 pronation–abduction injury. AP radiograph shows a small avulsion of the tibial attachment of the posterior tibiofibular ligament (arrow), called a Volkmann's fragment. Nondisplaced medial malleolar fracture is faintly visible (curved arrow). The lack of a fibular fracture distinguishes this from SER-4.

the syndesmosis leads to ankle stability and is therefore an important prognostic factor in ankle fractures.

A fibular fracture below the plafond, or alternatively a rupture of the lateral collateral ligament, is designated type A. The tibiofibular syndesmosis is intact. These fractures are treated conservatively unless other concommitant fractures result in instability.[9] A Weber type B fracture is at the level of the plafond, so there is partial rupture of the syndesmosis. These may be treated with closed reduction if anatomic reduction can be obtained, but they may need open reduction and internal fixation (ORIF). A Weber type C fracture is above the level of the plafond, so there is complete rupture of the syndesmosis, and these are almost always treated with internal fixation.

Table 3.3. Correlation between Weber and Lauge-Hansen Classifications

Lauge-Hansen type	Weber type
supination-adduction	A
supination-external rotation 2–4*	B or C
pronation-abduction 3*	C
pronation-external rotation 3–4 *	C

* SER-1, PA-1, PA-2, PER-1 and PER-2 have no correlate in the Weber classification

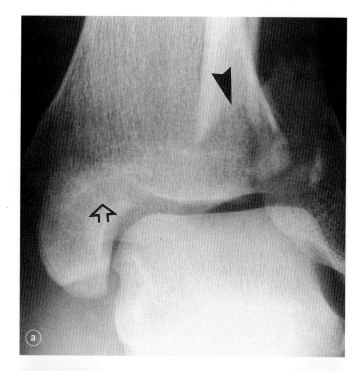

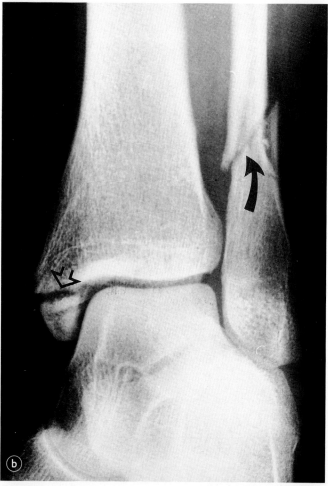

Fig. 3.11. Stage 3 pronation–abduction injury. **a.** AP radiograph. There is a transverse fracture of the medial malleolus (open arrow) and a short, oblique fracture of the fibula (arrowhead). **b.** Mortise radiograph in another patient. The fibular fracture in this patient is about 6 cm above the mortise, and PER fractures will also be seen at this level. The orientation of the fibular fracture (see Fig. 3.14) usually allows differentiation between these two, similar-appearing fractures.

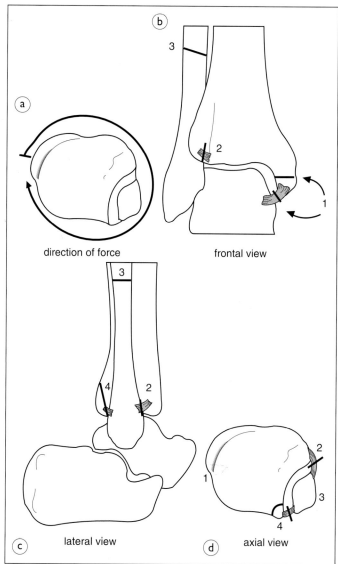

Fig. 3.12. Mechanism of pronation-external injury. **a.** A rotational force starts medially, extending anterolaterally and then posteriorly. **b–d.** Frontal, lateral and axial diagrams. The first injury is rupture of the deltoid ligament or transverse fracture of the medial malleolus (1), followed by rupture of the anterior tibiofibular ligament (2), high fracture of the fibula (3) and fracture of the attachment of the posterior tibiofibular ligament or rupture of the ligament (4).

Different mechanisms of injury as described by the Lauge-Hansen system tend to result in fibular fractures at predictable levels relative to the tibial plafond. This means that there is a correlation, although an imperfect one, between the Lauge-Hansen and the Weber classifications (Table 3.3). One major difference in classification is that Weber considered fractures at the level of the tibial plafond to be due to pronation. These are usually SER fractures as classified by the Lauge-Hansen system, whereas PA fibular fractures are slightly higher.

Other factors in malleolar fractures

Neither the Weber nor the Lauge-Hansen system is ideal for describing malleolar fractures. The Lauge-Hansen system is

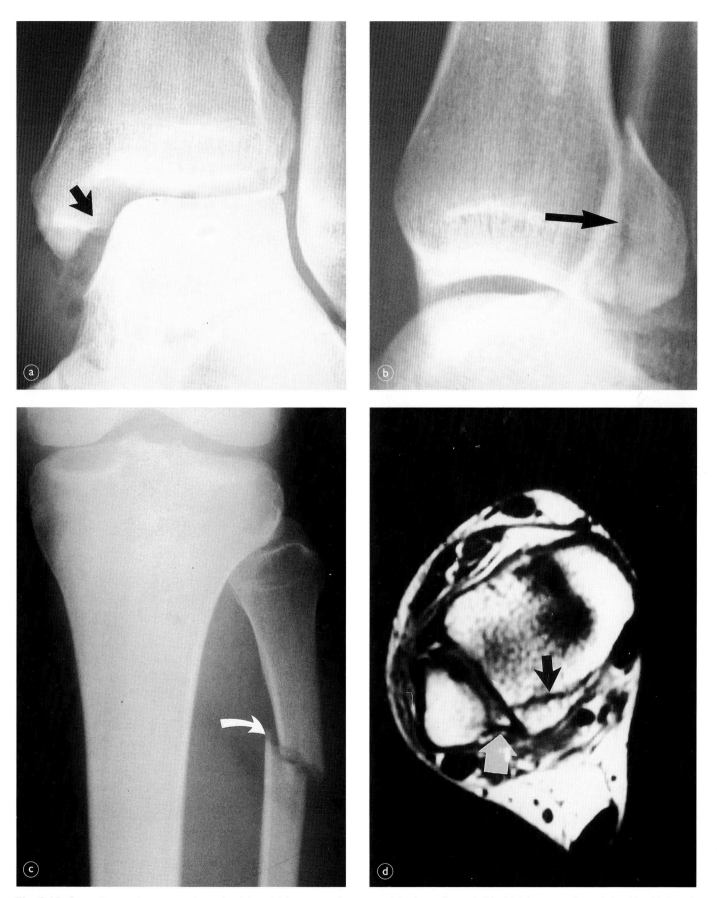

Fig. 3.13. Stage 4 pronation–external rotation injury, Maisonneuve fracture. **a.** Mortise radiograph. Medial joint space (arrow) is wide. Air in soft tissue is from deep abrasions. There is loss of the normal overlap between the fibula and tibia, indicating rupture of the syndesmosis. **b.** Lateral radiograph. Fracture of the posterior malleolus is seen (arrow). **c.** AP radiograph of the proximal leg shows oblique fibular fracture (curved arrow). **d.** Axial SE 600/28 MRI at the level of the plafond. The relationship of the fracture (arrow) to the posterior tibiofibular ligament (white arrow) is well seen.

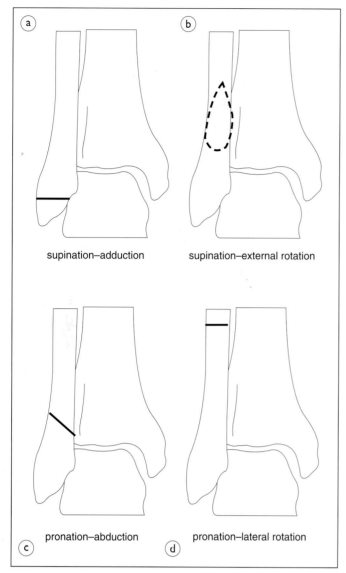

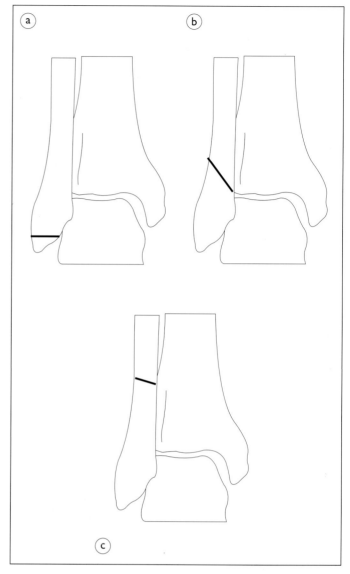

Fig. 3.14. Schematic representation of appearance of fibular fractures in different types of injury. **a.** Supination–adduction. The fibular fracture is transverse, and below the level of the plafond. **b.** Supination-external rotation. The fibular fracture is spiral, usually originating at the level of the plafond although it may be higher. It is often difficult to see on the AP radiograph. **c.** Pronation–abduction. The fibular fracture is oblique from inferomedial to superolateral, and slightly above the ankle joint. **d.** Pronation–external rotation. The oblique fibular fracture is high in position relative to the ankle joint and extends from posteroinferiorly to anterosuperiorly. (Modified from Arimoto and Forrester.[4])

Fig. 3.15. Danis–Weber classification of ankle fracture. **a.** Type A – fibular fracture below the tibial plafond, or rupture of the lateral collateral ligaments. **b.** Type B – fibular fracture at the level of the plafond. **c.** Type C – fibular fracture above the level of the plafond.

somewhat cumbersome and of limited prognostic value.[10] It does provide more clinical information and can direct the physician to the sites of ligamentous injuries associated with different fractures.[11]

The Weber classification is easy to use, but only partially describes the ankle injury. Other factors besides the fracture of the lateral malleolus are important in determining treatment and predicting prognosis.[8–15] It is important to realize that the stability of the ankle mortise is not solely dependent on the tibiofibular syndesmosis, but also on the integrity of the vertical ring

formed by the ankle (see Fig. 3.1), as well as on anteroposterior stability.

A factor in determining prognosis is the size of a posterior malleolar fragment. Large posterior malleolar fragments (more than 25% of the articular surface), even if there is adequate internal fixation, have a higher risk of premature ankle osteoarthritis than small fragments.[12–15]

Fractures that involve the medial malleolus[12] and even small fractures of the posterior malleolus[15] have been found to have a worse prognosis than isolated lateral malleolar fractures.

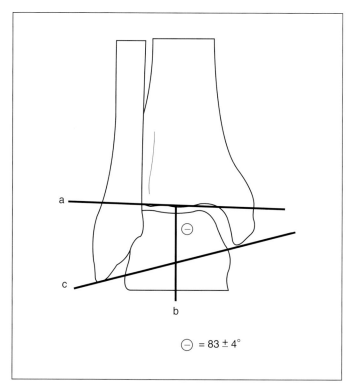

Fig. 3.16. Measurement of talocrural angle, to detect fibular shortening. A line (a) is drawn along the tibial plafond, and a second line (b) is drawn perpendicular to it. A third line (c) joins the lateral and medial malleoli. The superomedial angle between line b and line c should measure 83°±4°.

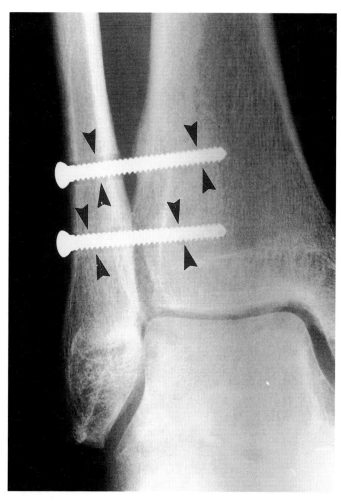

Fig. 3.17. Unstable pronation–external rotation injury one month following open reduction and internal fixation. Two syndesmosis screws maintain normal mortise width during healing. AP radiograph. Owing to normal superoinferior motion of the fibula relative to the tibia, circumferential lucencies (arrowheads) have developed surrounding the screws. The lucencies should not be mistaken for a sign of infection.

It is important in reporting radiographs of ankle fractures not to stop with a classification, but to describe all fracture fragments and their alignment, any associated widening of the mortise, any subluxation or dislocation, and also the percentage of the articular surface that is involved with posterior malleolar fractures.

Treatment

Nondisplaced fractures are usually treated with immobilization. Displaced fractures are usually treated by AO–ASIF principles, with rigid fixation designed to restore anatomic alignment and the integrity of the syndesmosis.

Imaging of Malleolar Fractures

Plain radiography is the mainstay of imaging, since it is fast, readily available, and accurate. The three standard views of the ankle are obtained as discussed in Chapter 2, and may be supplemented by the poor or off-lateral view[16] for better visualization of the posterior malleolus.

Owing to the frequency of ankle injury, overuse of radiographs is a significant problem in cost. Stiell et al[17] developed several criteria for the use of ankle radiographs which they found to be 100% sensitive and 40% specific in detecting malleolar fractures. The criteria used were:

- pain near the malleoli if the patient is over 55 years; or
- localized bone tenderness of the posterior edge or tip of either malleolus; or
- the patient is unable to bear weight both immediately after the injury and in the emergency department.

Shortening of the fibula is an important finding in lateral malleolar fractures, as it may lead to premature osteoarthritis if not corrected. The talocrural angle (Fig. 3.16), which should measure 83°±4°, is often used as an indication of fibular shortening. Magid et al[18] found that there was a wide variability in talocrural angle, and recommended that the uninjured ankle be used as a control. The incisural notch of the fibula is a useful landmark and should be located at the level of the plafond. However, it is not always well visualized. Rotational displacement of the fibula can be detected by CT.[18]

Widening of the joint space indicates joint instability. Three areas should be evaluated for joint space widening: the medial and lateral gutters, the tibiofibular syndesmosis, and the superior

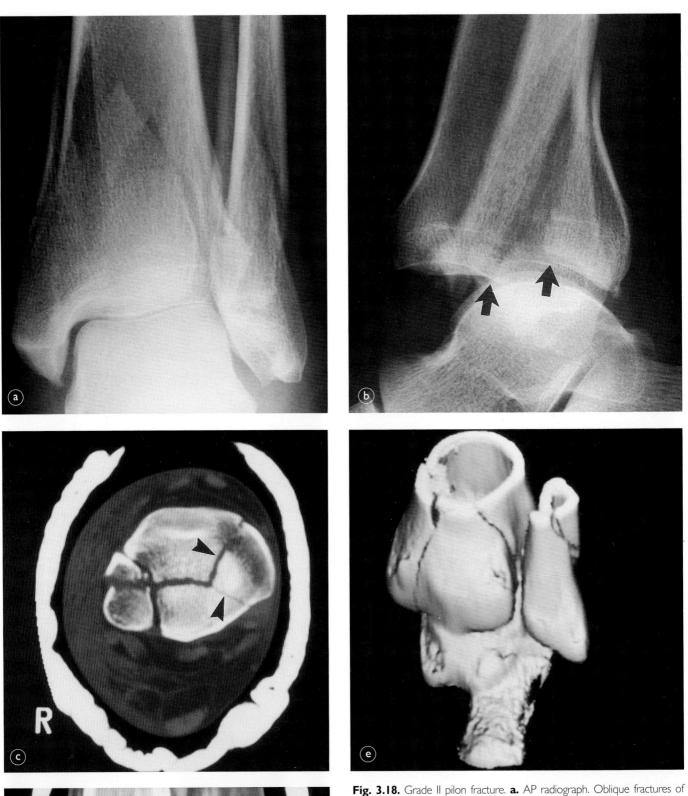

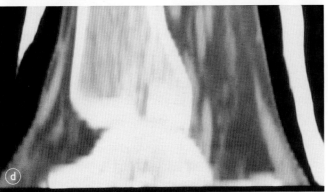

Fig. 3.18. Grade II pilon fracture. **a.** AP radiograph. Oblique fractures of the tibia and fibula are seen, but disruption of the tibial articular surface is not evident on this view. **b.** Lateral radiograph. There is wide diastasis of the tibial fracture fragments at the articular surface (arrows show fracture margins), and depression of the posterior fragment. **c.** Axial CT immediately above mortise shows that the main fracture line is coronally oriented. The comminuted medial fragment (arrowheads) was not evident on plain radiographs. CT images were obtained following closed reduction; 3 mm spiral scans were obtained, from which 1 mm slices were generated by computer, and used for reformatted images. **d.** Reformatted sagittal CT shows the coronally oriented fracture line. **e.** Three-dimensional CT viewed from posteriorly most clearly shows the orientation of the fracture lines.

articular surface. A measurement of 4 mm is usually used as the upper limit of normal for the medial joint space on the mortise view,[19] but the space can be slightly wider in large patients. Rather than relying on absolute measurements, it is better to compare the width of the medial and lateral gutters on a good mortise radiograph. Widening of the medial gutter indicates tear of the deltoid ligament. The tibiofibular syndesmosis should be considered widened if there is less than 1 cm of overlap between the tibia and fibula on the anteroposterior view, or less than 1 mm of overlap on the mortise view.[20] The distance between the medial aspect of the fibular notch of the tibia and the medial cortex of the fibula can also be measured, and should be less than 5 mm. Widening of the syndesmosis indicates disruption of the tibiofibular ligaments. The surface of the talar dome should be parallel to the tibial plafond; a talar tilt suggests lateral collateral ligament injury, as discussed below in the section on ankle sprains.

Following reduction, radiographs are used both to monitor healing and to check that reduction is maintained. Any hardware is examined radiographically for evidence of mechanical failure or infection. It should be noted that, because of the normal superior–inferior motion of the fibula relative to the tibia, lucencies usually develop surrounding syndesmosis screws (Fig. 3.17), and such lucencies should not be interpreted as a sign of infection. In order to prevent metal fatigue fracture from tibiofibular motion, the syndesmosis screws are almost always removed after sufficient healing has taken place.

Polydirectional tomography or CT is useful to evaluate the extent of articular disruption, and can alter surgical planning.[18] MRI may be used (see Fig. 3.13d) both to show fractures and to identify ligamentous ruptures, but usually adds little to information that can be deduced from plain radiographs by use of the Lauge-Hansen system. MRI does not demonstrate small intra-articular fractures as well as CT does, but it can be used to evaluate suspected injury to the posterior tibial or peroneal tendons, which can be associated with malleolar fractures (Chapter 7).

DISLOCATIONS OF THE ANKLE

Dislocations of the ankle can be seen in either the mediolateral or the anteroposterior plane (see Figs 3.4, 3.9). They are almost always associated with malleolar fractures. Neurovascular compromise is common.

AXIAL LOAD INJURIES TO THE TIBIA (PILON FRACTURES)

Axial load injuries may occur in motor vehicle accidents or when a standing person falls from a height. They are generally termed pilon fractures.[21-25] Prognostically, it is important to determine the degree of articular displacement and the amount of comminution present. The simple classification system described by Ruedi and Allgower[25] is widely used. In this system:

- a grade I fracture has no significant articular displacement;
- a grade II fracture has displacement of articular surface without significant comminution; and
- a grade III fracture has severe comminution and impaction.

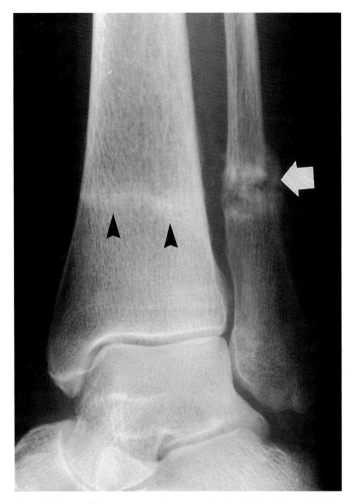

Fig. 3.19. Insufficiency stress fractures of the distal tibia and fibula. Mortise radiograph. A sclerotic band (arrowheads) crossing the tibia represents callus formation at the fracture site. The fibular fracture shows periosteal callus (arrow) as well.

Pilon fractures are caused by substantial forces and are often associated with other fractures – calcaneal, pelvic, spine, or tibial plateau.[21]

Imaging of Pilon Fractures

Plain radiography (Fig. 3.18ab) often underestimates the severity of pilon fractures. CT (Fig. 3.18cde) is valuable in evaluating the degree of displacement and comminution of the articular surface, and it is an asset in surgical planning.[21]

STRESS FRACTURES

Stress fractures can be divided into insufficiency and fatigue fractures.

Insufficiency Fractures

These are due to normal stresses on abnormal bone. They occur commonly in osteoporotic or osteomalacic persons. They have

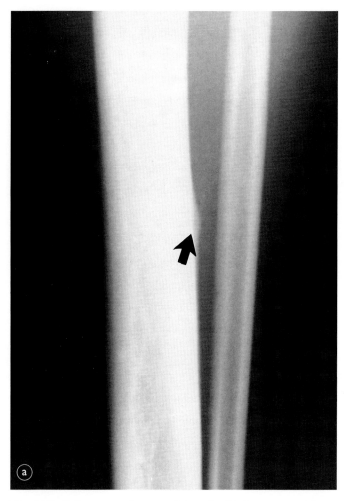 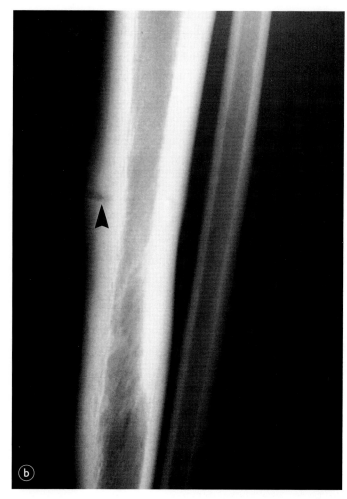

Fig. 3.20. Fatigue stress fracture of the mid tibia in a young athlete. **a.** AP radiograph. The tibia is markedly dense relative to the fibula, due to reactive new bone formation. A more focal area of periosteal new bone (arrow) is seen at the fracture site. **b.** lateral radiograph. The linear configuration of the lucency in the anterior cortex (arrowhead) distinguishes a fracture from an osteoid osteoma which has a round, lucent nidus.

been reported in the distal tibia and calcaneus as a complication of disuse osteoporosis caused by immobilization for traumatic ankle fractures.[26]

Fatigue Fractures

These are due to repeated stress on normal bone. They tend to occur in runners and other athletes. Patients complain of pain exacerbated by exercise and relieved by rest. Local tenderness is usually present at the fracture site.

Imaging of Stress Fractures

Radiographs are normal early in the course of the fracture. Later, a lucent fracture line or a sclerotic line due to callus formation may be seen (Fig. 3.19). Periosteal new bone is usually prominent. The fracture line may not traverse the entire bone (Fig. 3.20). Because of the chronicity of symptoms and the surrounding bony reaction, a stress fracture is sometimes mistaken for an osteoid osteoma. The radiographic differentiation between the two lies in the fact that stress fractures have a linear lucency

representing the fracture line, whereas osteoid osteomas have a round, lucent nidus. If this distinction is not evident on plain radiographs, polydirectional tomography is ideal for further evaluation.

Three-phase [99m]technetium bone scan demonstrates the sensitive but nonspecific findings of increased flow and blood pool activity, and intense focal activity at the fracture site. Stress fractures are a frequent finding on bone scans performed for occult pain of the foot or ankle.

MRI demonstrates a low-signal fracture line, surrounded by marrow edema.[27,28] CT scan can often demonstrate stress fractures, but in the ankle it is difficult to show the fracture line because both the CT image and the fracture line are in the horizontal plane.

ANKLE SPRAIN

Injuries to the lateral collateral ligament are very common and represent the typical ankle sprain, occuring because of supination injury often combined with internal rotation of the foot. There are three components of the lateral collateral ligament – the anterior and posterior talofibular ligaments, and the calcaneofibular ligament. The anterior talofibular ligament is the first ligament to rupture, followed by the calcaneofibular ligament. The posterior talofibular ligament is rarely injured.[29]

The deltoid ligament is strong, and isolated deltoid sprain is rare compared to tensile fractures of the medial malleolus. Injury to the deltoid ligament can occur as part of a malleolar fracture or syndesmosis sprain.

Treatment

Primary repair of the ruptured ligaments is rarely performed, because it has not been shown to have superior results to nonoperative management.[30] Instead, patients are treated with early progressive weight bearing. Patients may be immobilized with a cast or cast brace, or may be merely protected against repeat inversion with an air cast or equalizer.

Differential Diagnosis

There are numerous other injuries that can be misdiagnosed as 'ankle sprain' (Fig. 3.21 and Table 3.4). These should be considered both at the time of acute injury and in cases where chronic pain or instability follow an inversion injury of the ankle. In the acute setting, films should be scrutinized for unsuspected fractures of the foot (Fig. 3.21). When patients develop chronic pain following an ankle sprain, CT[31] or MRI should be considered to rule out other occult lesions (see Tables 3.4 and 7.7). Chip fractures around the ankle must be differentiated from accessory ossicles (see Chapter 1).

Imaging of Ankle Sprain

Anteroposterior and mortise radiographs in ankle sprain demonstrate lateral soft-tissue swelling. A joint effusion may be present (Fig. 3.22), but in more severe sprains, radiographically evident ankle effusions are uncommon, because the fluid leaks out of the ruptured ankle capsule. Plain radiographs should also be used to screen for other injuries that mimic ankle fracture. Mortise views in plantar and dorsiflexion are useful for increasing visibility of small osteochondral fractures of the talar dome. A small flake of bone at the lateral aspect of the fibula is a sign of peroneal tendon subluxation or dislocation with avulsion of the attachment of the peroneal retinaculum.

Stress radiographs can be performed (Fig. 3.23) to evaluate stability.[32] Sensitivity will be increased if local anesthesia – either an ankle block or a peroneal nerve block – is used. Inversion stress is performed with the foot in plantar flexion. The degree of talar tilt normally present on inversion stress radiographs averages 7° and is rarely more than 10°.[32] In a few cases, an asymptomatic ankle may have a tilt of up to 27°.[33,34] The degree of talar tilt in a normal ankle is usually within 10° of the contralateral side.[33] Anterior stress (the anterior drawer sign) will demonstrate abnormal anterior translation of the talus with ligamentous injury. It should be noted that these tests may be falsely normal in acute injury, especially if they are not performed with anesthesia. Stress testing cannot differentiate between rupture of the talofibular ligament alone and rupture of both the talofibular and the calcaneofibular ligaments.[33]

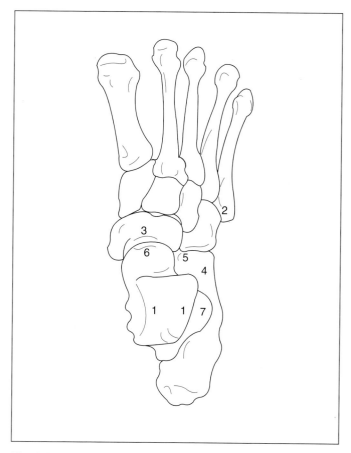

Fig. 3.21. Sites of foot fractures that can mimic ankle sprain. These fractures are discussed in Chapter 4. 1. Osteochondral fracture of the medial or lateral talar dome. 2. Fracture of the base of the fifth metatarsal (avulsion of peroneus brevis insertion). 3. Dorsal chip fracture of the navicular. 4. Avulsion of the origin of the extensor digitorum brevis from the lateral aspect of the calcaneus. 5. Fracture of the anterior process of the calcaneus. 6. Avulsion of the anterior joint capsule from its insertion on the neck of the talus. 7. Fracture of the lateral process of the talus.

Table 3.4. Differential diagnosis of ankle sprain	
Fracture	osteochondral fracture of talar dome
	medial impingement lesions tibial plafond
	fracture base fifth metatarsal
	chip fracture dorsal navicular
	avulsion extensor digitorum brevis origin
	fracture anterior process of calcaneus
	fracture lateral process talus
Ligamentous injury	syndesmosis sprain
	talo-calcaneal ligament rupture (tarsal sinus syndrome)
Tendon injury	peroneal tendon rupture
	dislocation of posterior tibial tendon

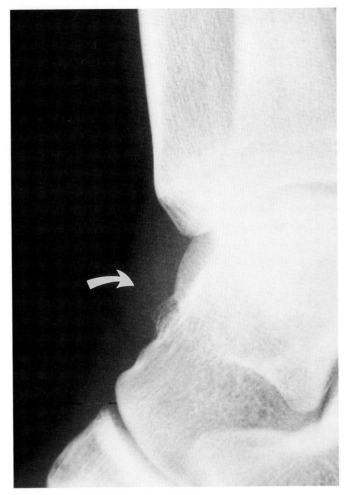

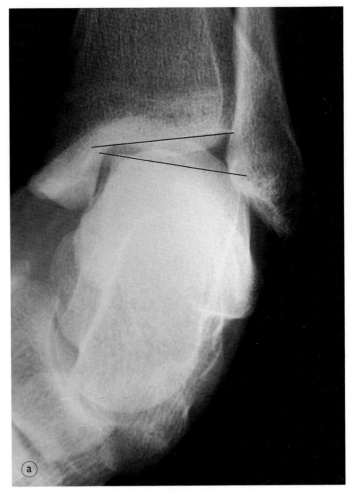

Fig. 3.22. Joint effusion in ankle sprain. Lateral radiograph. Joint effusions are often difficult to detect. They are seen anteriorly, as a soft-tissue density between the bony structures of the ankle and the extrinsic extensor tendons. Posteriorly, effusions are masked by the belly of the flexor hallucis longus muscle, which creates a soft-tissue fullness on radiographs.

Fig. 3.23. a. AP radiograph of a patient with chronic instability shows 15° of talar tilt when inversion stress is applied.

Arthrography can be used to evaluate ankle sprains (see Fig. 4.4). Extension of contrast beneath the tip of the lateral malleolus indicates rupture of the lateral collateral ligament. Arthrography can be falsely normal unless performed at the time of the acute injury.[35,36] Tenography can also be performed.[37] However, these studies are rarely indicated today, since most sprains are managed functionally.[29] MRI can also demonstrate ligamentous injury (Fig. 3.24a).[38,39] MR arthrography using intra-articular gadolinium has been shown to have greater sensitivity than noncontrast-enhanced MRI[39] in detecting ligamentous tears, but it is not yet FDA approved. CT arthrography can detect ligamentous tears that are occult on conventional arthrography (Fig. 3.24b).

SYNDESMOSIS SPRAIN

The syndesmosis sprain without associated malleolar fracture is an uncommon injury, occurring when the ankle is pronated and externally rotated.[40–42] Along with the syndesmotic injury, the deltoid ligament and anterior tibiofibular ligament are injured.

There is tenderness over the deltoid ligament and the anterior tibiofibular ligament. Recognition of the injury is important, since it can lead to chronic ankle instability if not treated with open reduction and internal fixation.[40]

Imaging of Syndesmosis Sprain

On radiographs, widening of the mortise is usually seen, but some cases are occult. In radiographically occult cases, radionuclide bone scan has been used to confirm the diagnosis.[42] Plastic deformity of the fibula or high fibular fracture may be present. Periosteal new bone at the distal syndesmosis (Fig. 3.25) is suggestive of prior syndesmosis injury.

OSTEOCHONDRAL INJURY OF THE TIBIAL PLAFOND

Osteochondral fractures of the talar dome (see Chapter 4) can occur as a result of inversion injuries. A similar osteochondral

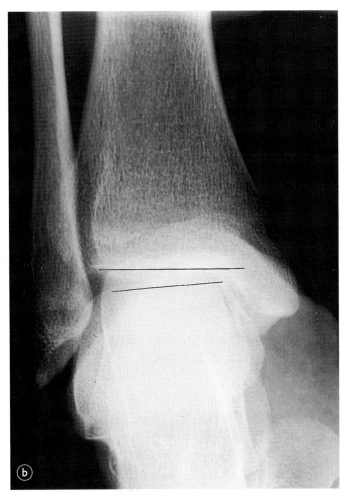
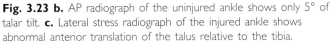

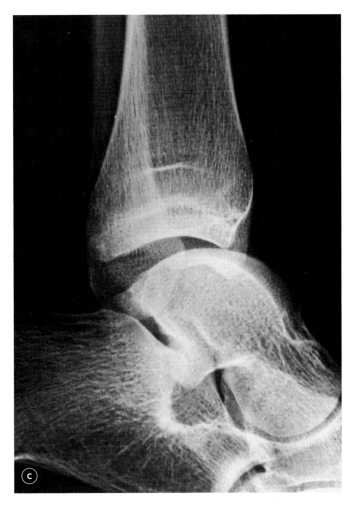

Fig. 3.23 b. AP radiograph of the uninjured ankle shows only 5° of talar tilt. **c.** Lateral stress radiograph of the injured ankle shows abnormal anterior translation of the talus relative to the tibia.

injury of the medial tibial plafond has been described,[43] and this may be a cause of chronic ankle pain. This lesion has not been described in the MRI literature, but it should have a similar appearance to osteochondral fractures of the talar dome.

SALTER–HARRIS FRACTURES

The physeal plate is an area of relative weakness in the immature skeleton, and fractures involving the physis (Salter–Harris fractures)[44] (Fig. 3.26) are common. Type II injuries are the most common, making up 73–75% of Salter-Harris fractures. Type I make up 6–8.5%, type III 6.5–8%, type IV 10–12%, and type V less than 1%.[45] Usually the fractures are the result of a single episode of trauma, but stress fractures can occur, especially at the distal fibula.[45]

Type II fractures of the ankle may result in limb shortening, although they rarely cause growth disturbance elsewhere.[45] Fractures of types IV and V have a high risk of limb shortening. The injured portion of the epiphysis may fuse prematurely,

creating a bony bridge called a physeal bar, which prevents further growth at that site.

The distal tibial epiphysis begins to fuse in its central portion when a child is approximately 12.5 years old. Fusion progresses medially, then laterally, and is completed about age 14. This sequence favors the formation of a particular type of Salter–Harris IV fracture, the triplane fracture (Figs 3.28, 3.29) in adolescents.[45–48] This accounts for 6% of fractures of the distal tibial epiphysis.[45] It is caused by an external rotation injury. A variant, the medial triplane fracture, is thought to occur because of adduction and axial loading.

The triplane fracture consists of a sagittally oriented fracture of the epiphysis, a transverse fracture through the unfused portion of the epiphysis, and an oblique coronal fracture of the posterior metaphysis. The fracture may have two or three fragments, and accordingly can be classified into two-part or three-part fractures (Fig. 3.27). When the medial portion of the physis is fused, the fracture is characteristic of the two-part variety,[46] extending through the lateral portion of the growth plate and sparing the medial portion. The medial triplane

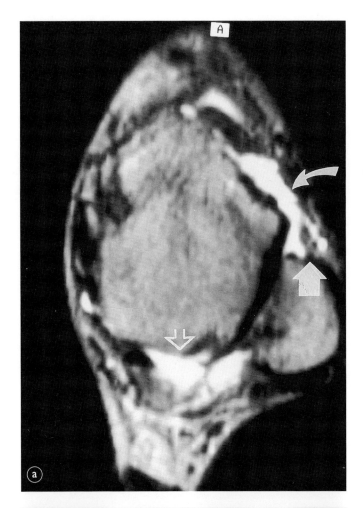

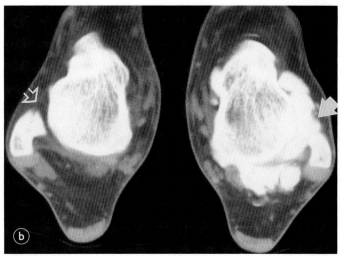

Fig. 3.24. Tear of the anterior talofibular ligament. **a.** Axial MRI SE 2200/80 in a patient with chronic ankle pain. A stump of the anterior talofibular ligament (arrow) is seen adjacent to the fibula. Fluid (curved arrow) extends through the gap in the ligament anteriorly. The joint effusion can also be seen posteriorly (open arrow). **b.** Axial CT arthrogram in a second patient. Plain arthrogram was normal, and CT was performed to evaluate for occult cartilage abnormality in a patient with chronic ankle pain following sprain. A stump of the anterior talofibular ligament (closed arrow) is visible, and contrast extends anteriorly through the gap in the ligament. Formation of scar tissue, preventing extension of contrast beneath the fibular tip, caused the false-negative plain arthrogram. Open arrow shows normal anterior talofibular ligament on the uninjured side.

Fig. 3.25. Old syndesmosis sprain in patient complaining of ankle pain and instability. Mortise view. Mature periosteal new bone (arrow) is seen along the syndesmosis. The mortise is widened, with loss of the normal overlap between the tibia and fibula.

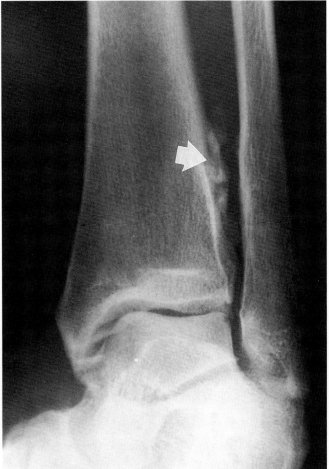

fracture and the classic three-part triplane fractures occur in slightly younger patients who have a completely open physeal plate.

The juvenile Tillaux fracture is a fracture of the lateral portion of the epiphysis without metaphyseal fracture.

Imaging of Salter–Harris Fractures

Plain radiographs

When there is no evidence of intra-articular extension, imaging evaluation is generally limited to plain radiographs. Salter–Harris I fractures can be detected when there is displacement of the epiphysis or widening of the growth plate. Radiographs of the unaffected ankle are useful in the detection of subtle widening of the physeal plate. Stress radiographs can be performed to elicit widening of the growth plate, but they may aggravate the injury.[45] Type V fractures tend to go undetected, as they have no radiographic findings until the onset of growth disturbance.

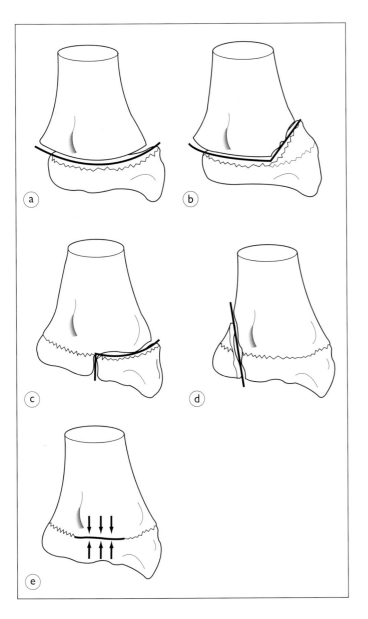

Fig. 3.26. Salter–Harris classification of physeal plate injury. **a.** Type I. Transverse fracture extends along the physis. **b.** Type II. A triangular metaphyseal fragment (Thurston-Holland fragment) accompanies the transverse physeal fracture. Although in most sites complications of this fracture are uncommon, premature fusion can be seen in the ankle. **c.** Type III. A vertical fracture extends through the epiphysis. Displacement of more than 2 mm is associated with growth disturbance and joint incongruity. **d.** Type IV. A vertical fracture extends through both the epiphysis and metaphysis. e. Type V. Crush injury to the growth plate. Premature fusion is characteristic.

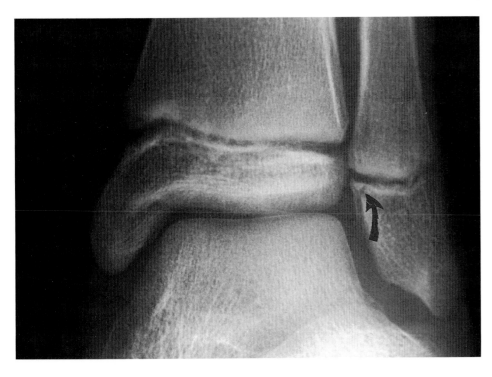

Fig. 3.27. Non-displaced Salter–Harris type III fracture of the fibula. Mortise radiograph. There is a fracture through a small portion of the epiphysis (arrow). Even if the growth plate fracture is not evident radiographically a chip fracture of the epiphysis adjacent to the physis indicates a fracture of the growth plate.

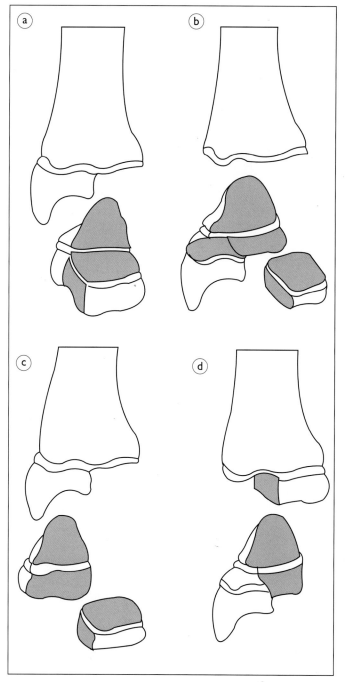

Fig. 3.28. Diagrammatic representation of triplane fractures of the tibia. **a.** two-part triplane fracture. **b.** classic three-part triplane fracture. **c.** variant three-part pattern. **d.** medial triplane fracture. (From Marymount et al,[42] used with permission.)

The presence of a metaphyseal fracture line that extends to the physis usually implies that a physeal fracture is present, even if the epiphysis is not displaced. An exception is the metaphyseal 'corner' fragment seen in child abuse.[45] In child abuse, fractures are generally multiple, they are often first imaged in the subacute stage, and periosteal new bone formation along the diaphysis of the bone is commonly seen.

CT and polydirectional tomography

CT, with direct coronal images or two- or three-dimensional reformatting (Fig. 3.29) has become the standard in evaluating articular disruption in triplane fractures. Polydirectional tomography or CT can be used to detect the location of a post-traumatic physeal bar, facilitating surgical correction of the bar.

MRI

MRI has been used to evaluate fractures through the growth plate. Jaramillo et al[49] found that MRI changed the Salter–Harris classification in six of 26 fractures. MRI can detect type V fractures[50] because of the presence of subperiosteal hematoma. A physeal bar will be seen as a zone of fat-containing marrow traversing the physis.

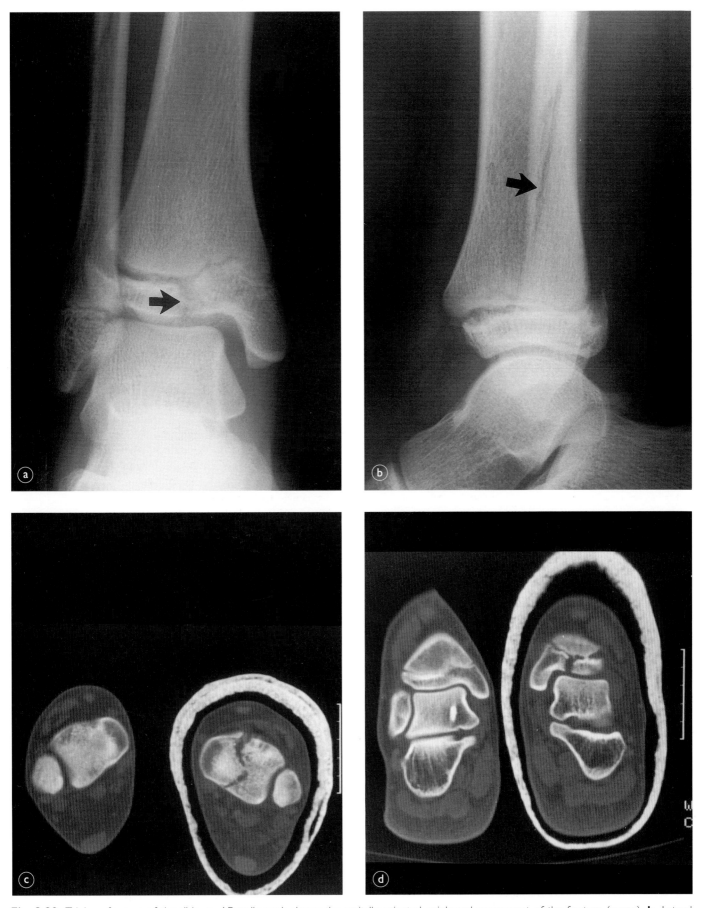

Fig. 3.29. Triplane fracture of the tibia. **a.** AP radiograph shows the sagitally oriented epiphyseal component of the fracture (arrow). **b.** Lateral radiograph shows the slightly posterior displacement of the physis, and the oblique coronal fracture of the metaphysis (arrow). **c.** Axial CT through the epiphysis demonstrates the epiphyseal component of the fracture. **d.** Direct coronal CT shows the degree of separation of the fragments at the articular surface.

REFERENCES

1. Neer CS. Injuries of the ankle joint—evaluation. *Conn State Med J* 1953; **17**:580-7.

2. Lauge-Hansen N. Fractures of the ankle: analytic historic survey as the basis of new experimental, roentgenologic and clinical investigations. *Arch Surg* 1948; **56**:259-317.

3. Lauge-Hansen N. Fractures of the ankle. II. Combined experimental-surgical and experimental roentgenologic investigations. *Arch Surg* 1950; **60**:947-85.

4. Arimoto HK, Forrester DM. Classification of ankle fractures: an algorithm. *Am J Roentgenol* 1980; **135**:1057-63.

5. Lauge-Hansen N. Fractures of the ankle. V. Pronation–dorsiflexion fracture. *Arch Surg* 1953; **67**:813.

6. Pankovich AM. Fractures of the fibula proximal to the distal tibiofibular syndesmosis. *J Bone Joint Surg [Am]* 1978; **60A**:221-35.

7. Danis, R. Les fractures malleolaires. In: Danis R (ed). *Théorie et pratique de l'ostéosynthèse*, (Masson: Paris, 1949), 133-65.

8. Weber, BG. *Die Verletzungen des obern Sprunggelenkes*, 2nd edn. (Hans Huber: Bern, Stuttgart, Vienna, 1972).

9. Lindsjo U. Operative treatment of ankle fracture-dislocations: a follow-up study of 306/321 consecutive cases. *Clin Orthop* 1985; **199**:28-38.

10. Lindsjo U. Classification of ankle fractures: Lauge-Hansen or AO system. *Clin Orthop* 1985; **199**:12-16.

11. Daly PJ, Fitzgerald RH, Melton LJ, et al. Epidemiology of ankle fractures in Rochester, Minnesota. *Acta Orthop Scand* 1987; **58**:539-44.

12. Broos PLO, Bisschop APG. Operative treatment of ankle fractures in adults: correlation between types of fracture and final results. *Injury* 1991; **22**:403-6.

13. Bauer M, Bergstrom B, Hemborg A, et al. Malleolar fractures: nonoperative versus operative treatment. *Clin Orthop* 1985; **199**:17-27.

14. Boggs LR. Isolated posterior malleolar fractures. *Am J Emerg Med* 1986; **4**:334-6.

15. Jaskulka RA, Ittner G, Schedl R. Fractures of the posterior tibial margin: Their role in the prognosis of malleolar fractures. *J Trauma* 1989; **29**:1565-70.

16. Mandell J. Isolated fractures of the posterior tibial lip at the ankle as demonstrated by an additional projection, the 'poor' lateral view. *Radiology* 1971; **101**:319-22.

17. Stiell IG, Greenberg GH, McKnight RD, Nair RC, McDowell I, Worthington JR. A study to develop clinical decision rules for the use of radiography in acute ankle injuries. *Ann Emerg Med* 1992; **21**:386-90.

18. Magid D, Michelson JD, Ney DR, Fishman EK. Adult ankle fractures: comparison of plain films and interactive two- and three-dimensional CT scans. *Am J Roentgenol* 1989; **154**:1017-23.

19. Daffner, RH. Ankle trauma. *Radiol Clin North Am* 1990; **28**:395-421.

20. Pettrone FA, Gail M, Pee D, Fitzpatrick T, Van Herpe LB. Quantitative criteria for prediction of the results after displaced fracture of the ankle. *J Bone Joint Surg [Am]* 1983; **65A**:667-77.

21. Bone, RB. Fractures of the tibial plafond. The pilon fracture. *Orthop Clin North Am* 1987; **18**:95-104.

22. Mainwaring BL Daffner RH, Reimer BL. Pylon fractures of the ankle: a distinct clinical and radiologic entity, *Radiology* 1988; **168**:215-18.

23. Bourne RB. Pilon fractures of the distal tibia. *Clin Orthop* 1989; **240**:42-50.

24. Ovadia DN, Beals RK. Fractures of the tibial plafond. *J Bone Joint Surg [Am]* 1986; **68A**:543-51.

25. Ruedi TP, Allgower M. The operative treatment of intraarticular fractures of the lower end of the tibia. *Clin Orthop* 1979; **138**:477-95.

26. Zlatkin MB, Bjorkengren A, Sartoris DJ, Resnick D. Stress fractures of the distal tibia and calcaneus subsequent to acute fractures of the tibia and fibula. Am *J Roentgenol* 1987; **149**:329-32.

27. Steinbronn DJ, Bennett GL, Kay DB. The use of magnetic resonance imaging in the diagnosis of stress fractures of the foot and ankle: four case reports. *Foot Ankle* 1994; **15**:80-3.

28. Lee JK, Yao L. Stress fractures: MR imaging. *Radiology* 1988; **169**:217-20.

29. Brostrom L. Sprained ankles. Anatomic lesions in recent sprains. *Acta Chir Scand* 1964; **128**:483-95.

30. Trafton PG, Bray TJ, Simpson LA. Fractures and soft tissue injuries of the ankle. In: Browner BD, Jupiter JB, Levine AM, Trafton PG (eds). *Skeletal Trauma*. (WB Saunders: Philadelphia, 1992), 1871-1957.

31. Meyer JM, Hoffmeyer P, Savoy X. High resolution computed tomography in the chronically painful ankle sprain. *Foot Ankle* 1987; **8**:291-6.

32. Sauser DD, Nelson RC, Lavine MH, Wu CW. Acute injuries of the lateral ligaments of the ankle: comparison of stress radiography and arthrography. *Radiology* 1993; **148**:653-7.

33. Laurin CA, Ouellet R, Jacques R. Talar and subtalar tilt: an experimental investigation. *Can J Surg* 1968; **11**:270-9.

34. Rijke AM, Jones B, Vierhout PA. Stress examination of traumatized lateral ligaments of the ankle. *Clin Orthop* 1986; **210**:143-151.

35. Ala-Ketola L, Puranen J, Koivisto E, Puupera M. Arthrography in the diagnosis of ligament injuries and classification of ankle injuries. *Radiology* 1977; **125**:63-68.

36. Dory MA. Arthrography of the ankle joint in chronic instability. *Skeletal Radiol* 1986; **15**:291-4.

37. Evans GA, Frnyo SD. The stress-tenogram in the diagnosis of ruptures of the lateral ligament of the ankle. *J Bone Joint Surg [Br]* 1979; **61B**:347-51.

38. Erickson SJ, Smith JW, Ruiz ME, et al. MR imaging of the lateral collateral ligament of the ankle. *Am J Roentgenol* 1991; **156**:131-6.

39. Chandnani VP, Harper MT, Ficke JR, et al. Chronic ankle instability: evaluation with MR arthrography, MR imaging, and stress radiography. *Radiology* 1994; **192**:189-94.

40. Edwards GS, DeLee JC. Ankle diastasis without fracture. *Foot Ankle* 1984; **4**:305-12.

41. Manderson EL. The uncommon sprain: ligamentous diastasis of the ankle without fracture or bony deformity. *Orthop Rev* 1986; **15**:77-81.

42. Marymount JV, Lynch MA, Henning CE. Acute ligamentous diastasis of the ankle without fracture: evaluation by radionuclide imaging. *Am J Sports Med* 1986; **14**:407-9.

43. Lundeen RO. Medial impingement lesions of the tibial plafond. *J Foot Surg* 1987; **26**:37-40.

44. Salter RB, Harris WR. Injuries involving the epiphyseal plate. *J Bone Joint Surg [Am]* 1963; **45A**:587-621.

45. Rogers LF, Poznanski AK. Imaging of epiphyseal injuries. *Radiology* 1994; **191:**297–308.

46. Cone RO, Nguyen V, Fluornoy JG, Guerra J. Triplane fracture of the distal tibial epiphysis: radiographic and CT studies. *Radiology* 1984; **153:**763–7.

47. Cooperman DR, Spiegel PG, Laros GS. Tibial fractures involving the ankle in children. The so-called triplane epiphyseal fracture. *J Bone Joint Surg [Am]* 1978; **60A:**1040–6.

48. MacNealy GA, Rogers LF, Hernandez R, Poznanski AK. Injuries of the distal tibial epiphysis: systematic radiographic evaluation. *Am J Roentgenol* 1982; **138:**683–9.

49. Jaramillo D, Hoffer FA, Shapiro F, Rand F. MR Imaging of fractures of the growth plate. *Am J Roentgenol* 1990; **155:**1261–5.

50. Jaramillo D, Hoffer FA. Cartilaginous epiphysis and growth plate: normal and abnormal MR imaging findings. *Am J Roentgenol* 1992; **158:**1105–10.

4. INJURIES OF THE FOOT

FRACTURES OF THE TALUS

Osteochondral Fractures

Osteochondral (transchondral) fractures of the talar dome are also known as osteochondritis dissecans , a term that was coined before it was known that the condition is usually due to an inversion injury. The diagnosis is often not evident on radiographs at the time of injury, but is based on plain radiographs or advanced imaging at a later time when the patient presents with chronic ankle pain.[1]

The injury may be radiographically occult, and diagnosis is often delayed for this reason.[1] The frequency of osteochondral fractures is difficult to determine. They have been reported as accounting for only 1% of talar fractures.[2] A higher frequency is suggested by the study of Bosien et al,[3] who found osteochondral fractures in 4.1% of ankle sprains. Anderson et al[4] found osteochondral fractures in 14 of 30 patients referred for evaluation of chronic post-traumatic ankle pain.

The osteocartilaginous fragment loses its vascular supply when it is detached from the talar dome. The fragment may become revascularized and heal, or it may undergo avascular necrosis. When completely detached, the fragment may become an intra-articular loose body.

Mechanism of injury

Osteochondritis dissecans of the talus is usually caused by a single inversion injury.[1,4–6] A few cases are probably due to repetitive minor trauma or spontaneous osteonecrosis.[1,5] A case due to compressive force during weight training has been reported.[7]

The osteochondral fragment may be located either laterally or medially on the talar dome. Its location is thought to depend on the position of the foot at the time of injury.[4,8,9]

The lateral fracture occurs when the foot is dorsiflexed, and the medial lesion when it is plantar flexed. When the ankle is dorsiflexed, the talus is securely held in the mortise. If an inversion force is appplied, the talus rotates laterally, and the margin of the talar dome is impacted against the tibia (stage 1). Continued inversion creates a shear force on the talar dome, detaching a lateral fragment of cartilage and bone (stages 2–4). Stages 2–4 are associated with injury to the lateral collateral ligamentous complex.

When the foot is plantar flexed, the posterior aspect of the dome of the talus sits loosely in the mortise. When an inversion injury occurs, the talus rotates medially relative to the tibia, and the posterior aspect of the medial talar dome impacts against the tibia. The collateral ligaments become taut, and cause a compressive force on the medial talar dome (stage 1). The posterior fibers of the deltoid can rupture, causing posterior subluxation of the talus which may shear off an osteochondral fragment (stages 2–4).

Classification and treatment

Berndt and Harty[8] divided osteochondritis dissecans into four stages based on its radiographic appearance (Fig. 4.1). Their system has been found to be useful in determining prognosis and treatment.[1,4,5] It has since been expanded by Dipaolo et al[10] to include arthroscopic and MRI findings (Table 4.1). However, the appearance at arthroscopy does not necessarily correspond to the stage seen radiographically – patients with radiographic stage 4 lesions may show intact cartilage at arthroscopy,[11] presumably reflecting healing of the overlying cartilage.

Table 4.1. Staging System for Osteochondral Lesions. (Modified from Anderson et al,[4] Berndt and Harty,[8] and Dipaolo et al.[10] The radiographic staging is that of Berndt and Harty[8] as clarified by Anderson et al,[4] and the arthroscopic staging is that of Dipaolo et al.[10] The MRI staging has been modified from that of Dipaolo et al[10] and Anderson et al.[4]

	Radiographs	T2W-MRI	Arthroscopy
Stage 1	normal	marrow edema (diffuse high signal intensity)	normal, or irregularity and softening of cartilage
Stage 2	semicircular fragment	low-signal line surrounds fragment	articular cartilage breached, definable but nondisplaceable fragment
Stage 2A	subcortical lucency	high-signal fluid within fragment	
Stage 3	semicircular fragment	high-signal line surrounds fragment	displaceable fragment
Stage 4	loose body	defect talar dome; ± loose body	loose body

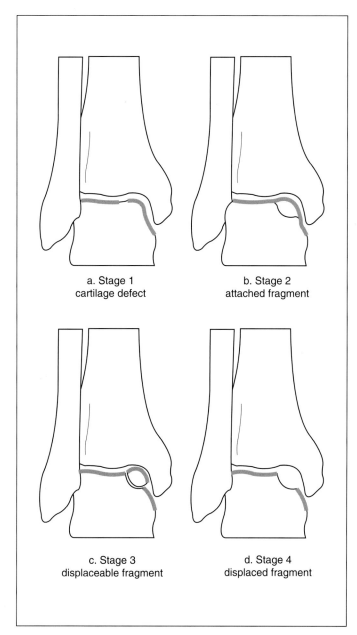

Fig. 4.1. Stages of osteochondritis dissecans. **a.** Stage 1. Impaction of talar dome. **b.** Stage 2. Fracture line without detachment of fragment **c.** Stage 3. Fragment detached but nondisplaced. **d.** Stage 4. Intra-articular loose body.

Radiographic findings

PLAIN RADIOGRAPHS

Plain radiographs of the ankle are normal in stage 1 osteochondritis dissecans.[4] Radiographs at stage 2 and greater (Fig. 4.2) often show a semicircular, sclerotic fracture line, located at either the lateral or medial margin of the talar dome. The fracture may have a cyst-like appearance. Detection of the osteochondral fragment is increased when the mortise view is obtained in both plantar and dorsiflexion.

An osteochondral fragment in the medial talar dome usually has a deep, semilunar configuration, while the lateral fragments tend to be thin slivers of bone. The medial fractures are most commonly located on the posterior aspect of the talar dome, while the lateral fractures are usually anterior, but analysis of CT images has shown that there is considerable variability in the position of the osteochondral fragment.[1]

CT

Polydirectional tomography or CT (Fig. 4.3) are more sensitive in the detection of osteochondritis dissecans than plain radiographs.[12-13] However, like plain radiographs, they will not detect a stage 1 lesion,[4] which can be seen on MRI. Plain radiographs or CT cannot differentiate between stage 2 and stage 3 lesions, and so arthrography (Fig. 4.4) or MRI are used to determine if an osteochondral fragment is loose or attached to the underlying bone. CT is more sensitive than MRI in detecting small intra-articular loose bodies.[4]

BONE SCAN

[99m]Technetium-methylene diphosphonate (MDP) bone scan is useful as a screening test[12] for chronic ankle pain. Although nonspecific, it pinpoints the location of the bony abnormality. Anderson et al[4] recommend that patients with chronic ankle pain and normal plain radiographs undergo bone scan – if the bone scan shows abnormal uptake, then MRI can be done to give the specific diagnosis. Bone scan may also predict the presence of an unstable fragment.

Mesgarzadeh and colleagues[15] graded uptake of [99m]technetium-MDP in osteochondritis dissecans of the knee, designating grade 0 as normal activity, grades 1 and 2 as localized increased uptake, grade 3 as intense uptake in a part of the femoral condyle, and grade 4 as intense uptake in the entire femoral condyle. He found that the presence of grade 3 or grade 4 uptake predicted a loose fragment with a sensitivity of 90% and specificity of 100%. However, his method has not yet been systematically applied to the ankle.

MRI

MRI is both sensitive and specific in detecting osteochondritis dissecans.[4,10,15-17] A crescentic fracture line of low signal intensity on all sequences (Fig. 4.5) is seen. The bone marrow within the fragment has variable signal characteristics. It may be of low-signal intensity on T1-weighted images if the fragment is sclerotic, or it may show the normal high signal of fatty marrow. The appearance varies from low to high signal on T2-weighted images as well.

Cystic areas may be present (stage 2A) and will show fluid intensity. T2-weighted MRI allows differentiation between attached and free osteochondral fragments (Table 4.1), although the pratical usefulness of this distinction has been questioned.[4] If the fragment is attached to the underlying bone by fibrous or bony union, a low-signal intensity rim is seen at the interface between the fragment and the talar dome. If the fragment is free, high-signal intensity surrounds the fragment, owing to the presence of joint fluid. If the fragment is partially attached, a partial rim of high signal is seen around it (Fig. 4.6).

MRI has been used to evaluate the cartilage overlying the talar dome.[10] However, the normal cartilage is thin, and defects within the cartilage are difficult to see, owing to limits of spatial resolution. Articular cartilage is better evaluated with CT arthrogram or arthrotomography, or with arthroscopy.

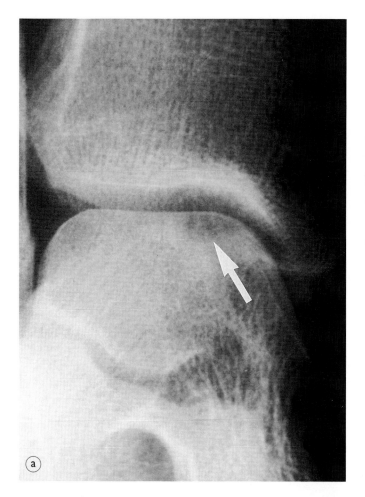

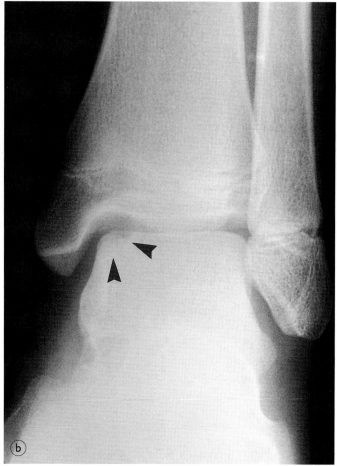

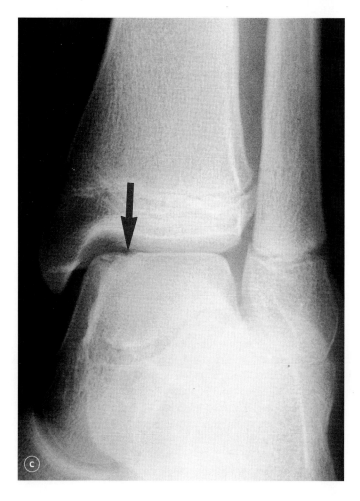

Fig. 4.2. Plain radiographic appearance of osteochondritis dissecans. **a.** 'Cyst-like' appearance. Mortise radiograph. There is a well-defined lucency in the medial talar dome. A rim of sclerotic bone surrounds the lucency. **b, c.** AP and mortise radiographs in a different patient show a medial lucency (arrowheads) surrounded by a rim of sclerosis. On mortise radiograph depression of the articular cortex (arrow) is evident.

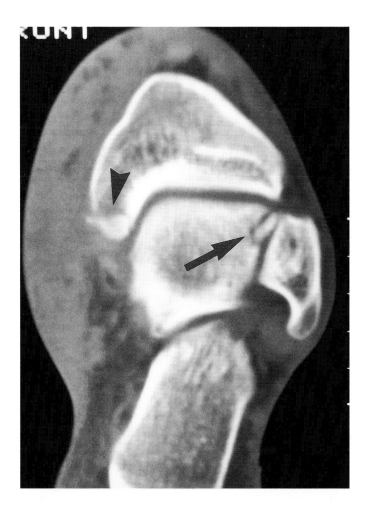

Fig. 4.3. Coronal noncontrast CT scan of osteochondritis dissecans. CT was done to evaluate calcaneal fracture of the opposite foot. It showed an unsuspected osteochondral fracture of the talus (arrow), as well as a medial malleolar fracture (arrowhead) evident on plain radiographs.

Fig. 4.4. Arthrogram and CT of osteochondritis dissecans. **a.** Mortise view. The osteochondral lesion on the lateral talar dome is obscured by overlying contrast. Contrast extravasation below the fibula (arrow) is due to rupture of the lateral collateral ligaments, which is usually present in osteochondritis dissecans. **b.** Coronal CT. Cartilage over the small lateral osteochondritis dissecans fragment (arrow) is intact, and no contrast extends between the fragment and the host bone, indicating that the fragment is not detached. Extravasation of contrast beneath the fibular tip is again seen.

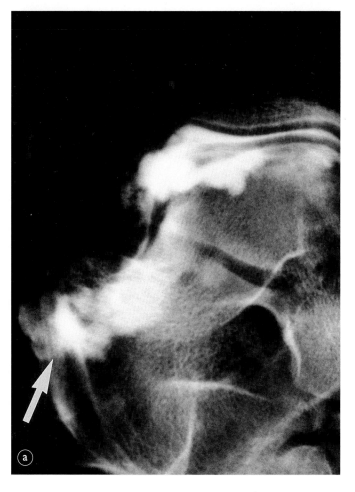

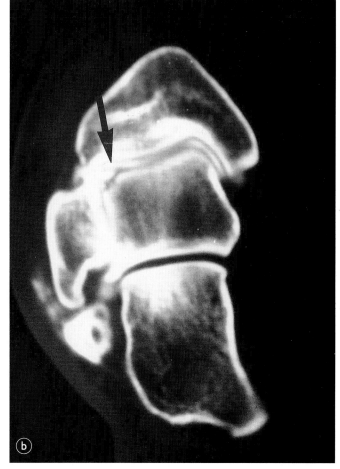

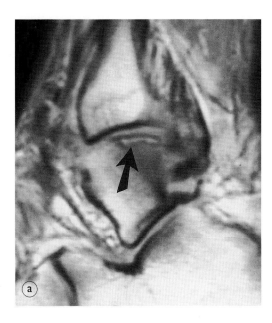

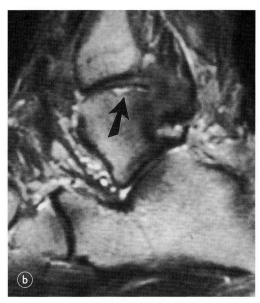

Fig. 4.5. MRI of osteochondritis dissecans in the lateral talar dome. The patient presented with chronic pain, and MRI was done to rule out tarsal sinus syndrome. **a.** Sagittal MRI (SE 2200/20) shows the low-signal-intensity line surrounding the osteochondritis dissecans fragment. **b.** Sagittal MRI (SE 2200/80). The signal intensity within the fragment is increased, but no fluid is seen surrounding the fragment. This is considered a stage 2 lesion.

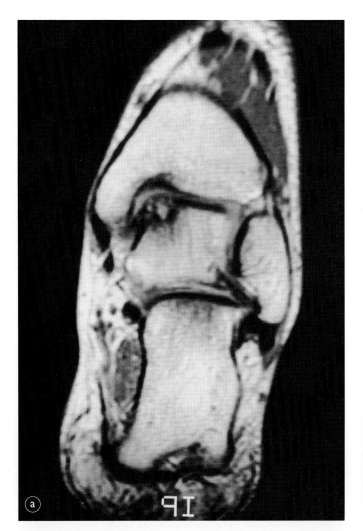

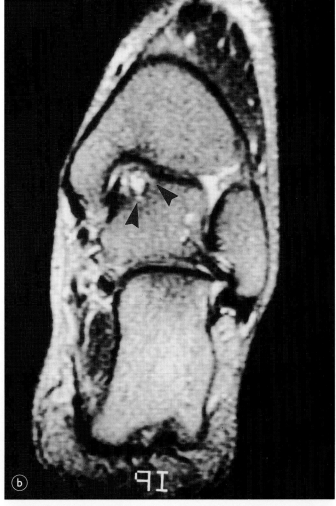

Fig. 4.6. MRI of partially attached osteochondritis dissecans fragment. **a.** Coronal MRI SE 2000/20. A bilobed osteochondritis dissecans fragment is seen in the medial talar dome. **b.** Coronal MRI SE 2000/80. There are small foci of high signal (arrowheads) adjacent to the fracture fragment, but the high signal does not completely surround the fragment. At arthroscopy, fragment was attached.

Differential diagnosis

In the acute stage, films should be scrutinized for other fractures that can mimic ankle sprain (see Chapter 3, Table 3.4). In the chronic phase, other causes of lateral ankle pain should be considered (see Chapter 7, Table 7.7).

Treatment

Stage 1 and stage 2 lesions often do well with conservative management. Stages 3 and 4 lesions, as well as lower grade lesions with persistent symptoms, can be treated with excision of the fragment and drilling of the underlying bone to stimulate development of fibrocartilage.[11] In general, osteochondritis dissecans of the ankle has a good prognosis,[5,14] although good results are less common in grades 3 and 4 injuries.[5] A 20-year study of 30 patients found that only one developed severe osteoarthritis of the ankle.[14]

Talar Neck Fractures

Approximately 50% of talar fractures involve the neck of the talus.[18] Talar neck fractures are often associated with other injuries, especially oblique or vertical fractures of the medial malleolus and fractures of the calcaneus.[19-20]

Mechanism of injury

Talar neck fractures can occur by three different mechanisms. The most common is a dorsally directed force on a braced foot and ankle.[20-21] It is usually caused by impaction of the foot against the floor pedal of a car in a head-on collision. It was originally described in aviators after plane crashes, hence the term 'aviator's astragalus'. Talar neck fractures can also be caused by inversion of the ankle, with impingement of the talar neck against the medial malleolus. The least common mechanism is a direct blow to the dorsum of the foot.[20-21]

Classification

The Hawkins classification[21] (Table 4.2) is generally used, because it predicts the risk of avascular necrosis and directs treatment. Hawkins originally described three types of fracture, and a fourth was added by Canale and Kelly.[22]

TYPE I FRACTURES

Type I fractures are nondisplaced. In these fractures, the risk of avascular necrosis is less than 10%. Note that even slight displacement of the fracture line indicates probable subluxation of the subtalar joint, and the fracture is considered a type II.

TYPE II FRACTURES

Type II fractures are displaced, and there is subluxation or dislocation of the subtalar joint. There is a 20–50% risk of avascular necrosis.[19] Symptomatic post-traumatic osteoarthritis of the subtalar joint occurs in about two-thirds of patients, with osteoarthritis of the ankle joints seen in one-third of patients.[19-20,22,23] There may be radiographic evidence of osteoarthritis in asymptomatic patients.

TYPE III FRACTURES

Type III fractures have subluxation or dislocation of both the tibiotalar and subtalar joints. The risk of avascular necrosis in

Table 4.2. Hawkins classification of talar neck fractures.

	Radiographic findings	Risk of avascular necrosis
Type I	nondisplaced fracture line	0–13%
Type II	fracture displaced, subtalar joint subluxed or dislocated	20–50%
Type III	dislocation subtalar and tibiotalar joints	69–100%
Type IV	disruption of talonavicular joint	high

these fractures is about 90%. About half of these fractures are open.[21] Type III fractures frequently have delayed union or malunion (usually varus alignment), with nonunion seen in about 10% of cases.[19-20] There is a high incidence of osteoarthritis, and the overall incidence of poor results ranges from 50–90%.[19-22]

TYPE IV FRACTURES

Type IV fractures have disruption of the talonavicular joint as well as the subtalar and and often the tibiotalar joints.[22] This fracture is rare. The risk of avascular necrosis approaches 100%, and may involve the head of the talus as well as the body.

Imaging

An ankle series is routinely obtained. The radiographs allow evaluation of associated medial malleolar fractures as well as the talar neck, subtalar, and tibiotalar joints (Figs 4.7–4.9). Anteroposterior and oblique radiographs of the foot are also useful. Type I fractures may be subtle radiographically, and they are sometimes missed on ankle series; foot radiographs are helpful in confirming the presence of fracture. It can be difficult to diagnose displacement of the talar neck, because the axis of the talar neck is variable, and it differs from that of the body in both the transverse and sagittal planes.[20]

By 6–8 weeks after the fracture, disuse osteoporosis develops in vascularized bone. Resorption of subcortical bone is seen in the talar dome, and is known as the Hawkins sign (Fig. 4.10). Hawkins[21] recognized that, if a patient develops this subcortical lucency, the talar dome is vascularized and avascular necrosis is therefore not a risk. Numerous authors have confirmed the usefulness of this sign, although its absence does not necessarily mean that avascular necrosis will develop. Generalized osteoporosis is also an indication of normal vascularity. MRI can be used in evaluating for avascular necrosis, and diagnostic images can usually be obtained despite the presence of metallic screws (see Chapter 5, Fig. 5.57). Avascular necrosis is discussed in detail in Chapter 5.

Treatment

Type I fractures are generally treated with immobilization and limitation of weight bearing. Types II–IV are usually treated with open reduction and internal fixation, although for some type II fractures, closed reduction can be achieved. Anatomic reduction is thought to be essential for good results. Protection of weight bearing reduces the risk of avascular necrosis.

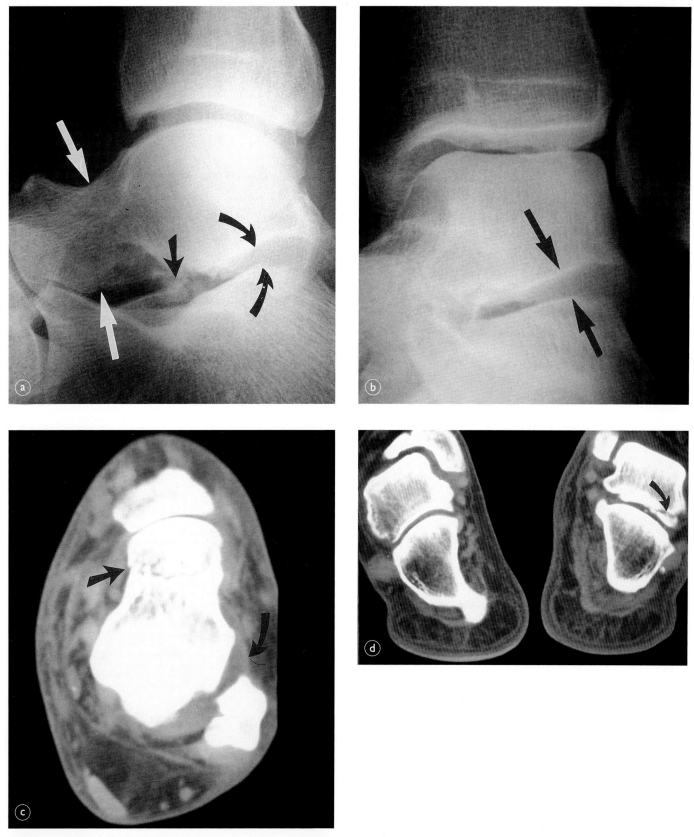

Fig. 4.7. Hawkins II fracture of the talar neck. **a.** Lateral radiograph. The fracture of the talar neck (white arrows) was almost invisible on the original radiographs. Small bone fragments were seen in the region of the lateral process of the talus (straight black arrow), and the posterior subtalar joint was seen to be slightly widened (curved arrows), with slight anterior subluxation of the calcaneus. **b.** Oblique radiograph. The subtle subluxation of the posterior subtalar joint, with loss of parallelism of the articular cortices (arrows), is better appreciated. **c.** Axial CT through the talar neck. The fracture of the talar neck is more easily seen (straight arrow). Note that the talofibular articulation is disrupted (curved arrow) due to rupture of the anterior talocalcaneal ligament. Although the talar neck fracture appears nondisplaced, the subluxation of the subtalar joint technically places this case as a type II fracture. The patient was treated in a cast, and did well. **d.** Coronal CT shows small fracture of the lateral process of the talus.

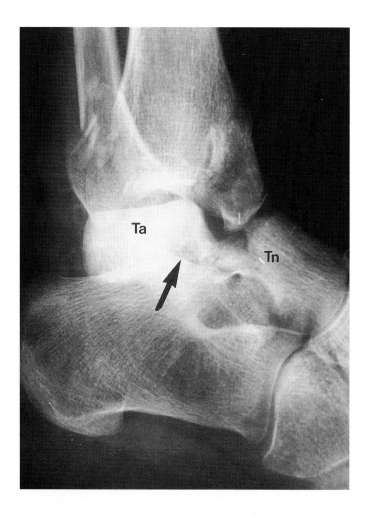

Fig. 4.8. Hawkins III fracture of talar neck. This radiograph shows the hindfoot in the lateral projection, but the ankle is seen frontally, due to the severe rotation at both the ankle joint dislocation and the fracture through the talar neck. The posterior facet of the calcaneus is clearly seen (arrow), but is dislocated from the talus. The ankle joint is discongruent, and there are fractures of the medial and lateral malleoli. (Ta – talar body, Tn – talar neck).

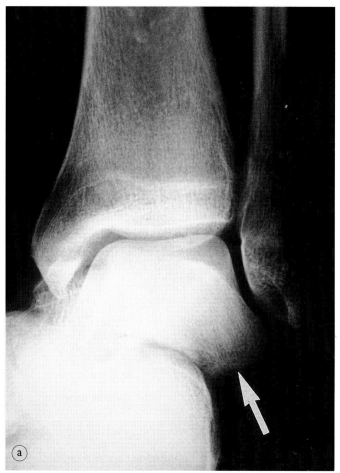

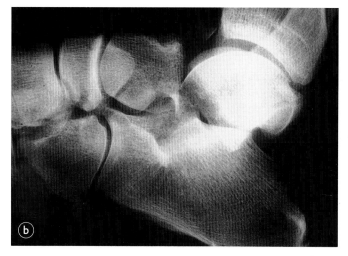

Fig. 4.9. Hawkins III fracture of talar neck. **a.** Mortise radiograph. The ankle joint appears intact on this view. Dislocation of the subtalar joint is seen (arrow points to the articular cortex of the talus, positioned lateral to the calcaneal articular surface.) **b.** Lateral radiograph. There is a displaced fracture of the talar neck, subluxation of the tibiotalar joint, and dislocation of the subtalar joint.

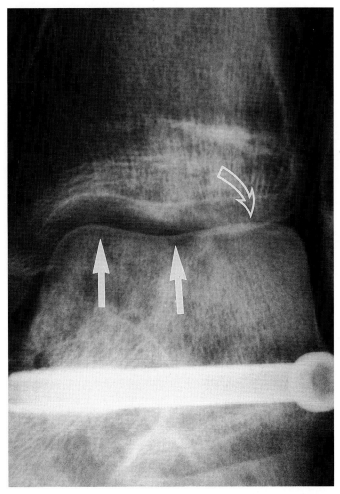
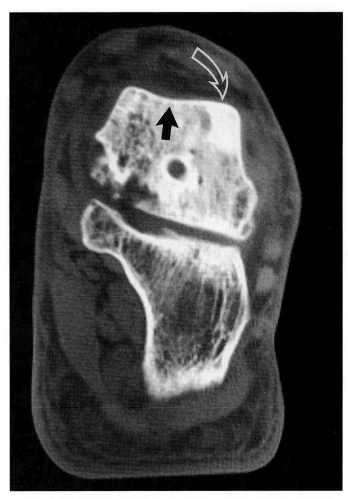

Fig. 4.10. Avascular necrosis with partial Hawkins sign, following Hawkins III fracture of the talar neck. **a.** Mortise radograph. A thin, lucent line (arrows) is present in the subcortical bone medially, but the line is absent laterally where mottled sclerosis is seen (open arrow). **b.** Coronal CT. The Hawkins sign (solid arrow) is again seen medially, with a sclerotic focus of bone necrosis laterally (open arrow).

Talar Body and Head Fractures

Fractures of the neck of the talus frequently extend into the talar body. Vertical fractures of the body may occur by the same mechanism as talar neck fractures (Fig. 4.11). Fractures of the talar head (Fig. 4.12) are usually associated either with capsular or ligamentous injuries, or with other fractures. Osteochondral fractures may occur at the posterior subtalar facet,[9] although they are rare in this location.

Lateral process fractures

The lateral process of the body of the talus extends beneath the lateral malleolus. It forms the anterolateral corner of the posterior subtalar facet. Fracture may be caused by avulsion by the anterior talofibular ligament in dorsiflexion and inversion,[24] or the lateral process may be sheared off by the calcaneus in an external rotation injury. A displaced fracture is easily seen on radiographs (Fig. 4.13), but nondisplaced fractures are often occult radiographically, and may be misdiagnosed as ankle sprain.

Physical examination will show acute local tenderness below the tip of the lateral malleolus. CT or MRI will reliably detect these fractures (Figs 4.7, 4.14, 4.15). Small or comminuted fragments are usually excised; larger fragments may be fixed

with a compression screw. Osteoarthritis of the subtalar joint can be a complication of this fracture.

Other Fractures of the Talus

Chip fractures are frequently seen at the anterior aspect of the talar neck, owing to avulsion of the ankle capsule (Fig. 4.16). Chip fractures also occur at the posterior process of the talus owing to plantar flexion injury, with compression of the posterior process (see Fig. 4.14). The flexor hallucis longus tendon may be injured in fractures of the posterior process. Tomograms or CT can be used to differentiate fractures of the posterior process of the talus from the os trigonum.

Stress fractures of the talus are uncommon, but they can occur in runners. They may also be seen as insufficiency fractures (see Chapter 5, Fig. 5.9).

TALAR DISLOCATIONS

Subtalar dislocations occur in motor vehicle accidents and falls, and they may be either in a medial or a lateral direction. The

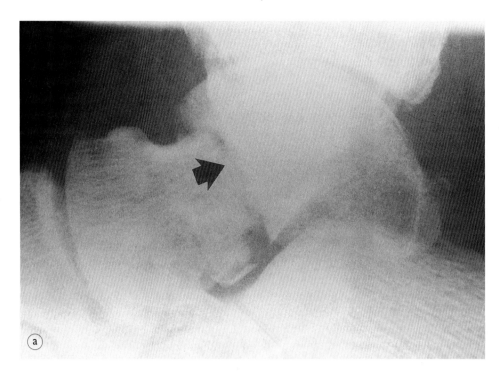

Fig. 4.11. Fracture of the body of the talus. **a.** Lateral radiograph. The coronally oriented fracture (arrow) is at the junction of the talar neck and body. **b.** Axial CT shows that the fracture line is primarily through the talar body. There is comminution of the fracture medially. **c.** Coronal CT demonstrates small, comminuted fragments medially and laterally, and involvement of the middle facet (arrow). The patient was treated in a cast, and had normal subtalar motion after the fracture healed.

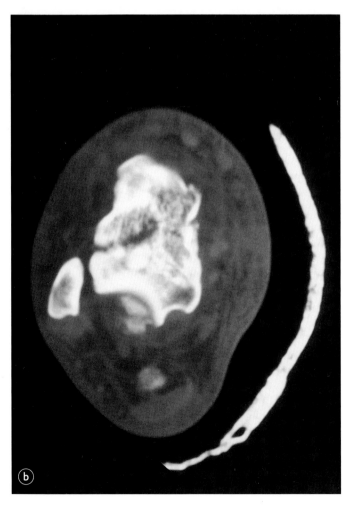

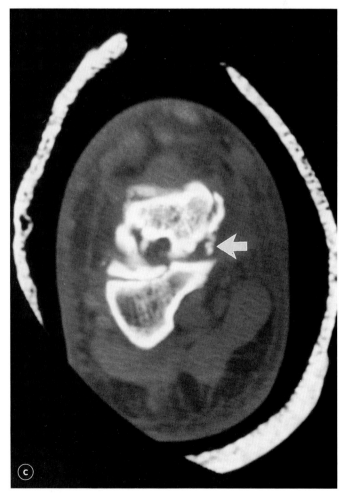

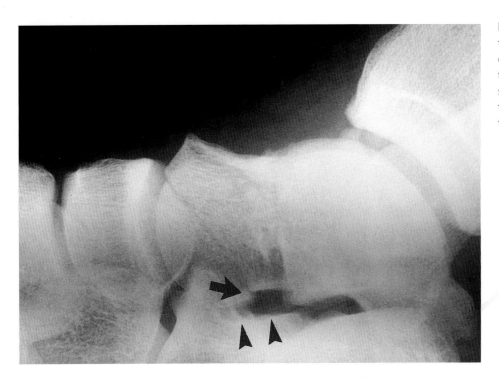

Fig. 4.12. Fracture of the head of the talus. Lateral radiograph. The fracture line courses obliquely through the talar head, from the talonavicular joint to the middle subtalar facet (arrow). Arrowheads point to articular surface of the sustentaculum tali.

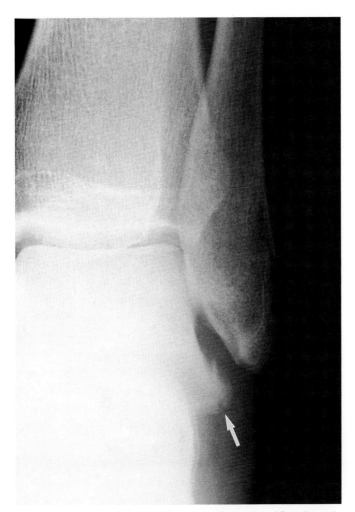

Fig. 4.13. Fracture of the lateral process of the talus. AP radiograph. A small, minimally displaced fragment is seen (arrow).

medial dislocations are sometimes referred to as basketball foot.[25] Lateral dislocations may result in tears of the posterior tibial tendon and injury to the posterior tibial vessels (Fig. 4.17). Complete dislocation of the talus from the ankle, the talonavicular joint and the subtalar joint rarely occurs (Fig. 4.18). Talonavicular dislocations are also uncommon (Fig. 4.19).

FRACTURES OF THE CALCANEUS

Fractures of the Posterior Facet

Approximately 75% of calcaneal fractures involve the posterior facet of the subtalar joint. The fractures are often bilateral, and are often associated with other fractures of the lower extremities as well as fractures of the pelvis and thoracolumbar junction of the spine. Complications of intra-articular calcaneal fractures include injury to the peroneal tendons, osteoarthritis of the subtalar joint, medial soft-tissue injury and chronic pain.[26–31] Owing to loss of height of the calcaneus, the lateral malleolus may impinge on the lateral aspect of the calcaneus.[31–32]

Mechanism of injury
Intra-articular calcaneal fractures are high velocity injuries, occuring when there is a sudden impact on the heel. They occur as the result of automobile accidents, or jumps or falls of 6 feet (2 m) or more when the person lands on his feet. The axial force drives the tuber of the talus like a wedge into the body of the calcaneus at the angle of Gissane, disrupting the posterior facet, depressing the central portion of the calcaneus, and often shattering the lateral calcaneal wall.

Classification
Essex-Lopresti[33] divided intra-articular calcaneal fractures into two major groups, the joint depression-type and the tongue-type

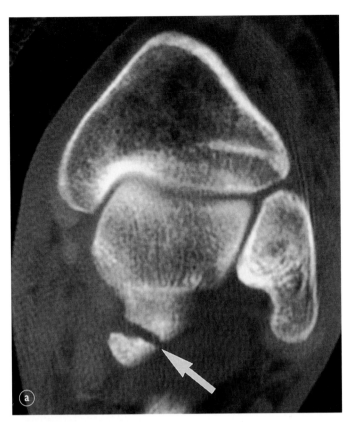
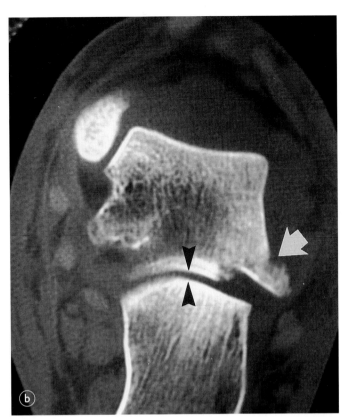

Fig. 4.14. Coronal CT of fractures of the lateral and posterior processes of the talus. **a.** Arrow points to the displaced fracture of the lateral process, with depression of the articular surface of the posterior facet. Arrowheads point to an uninvolved portion of the posterior facet. **b.** Image located more posteriorly shows a second fracture through the posterior process (arrow).

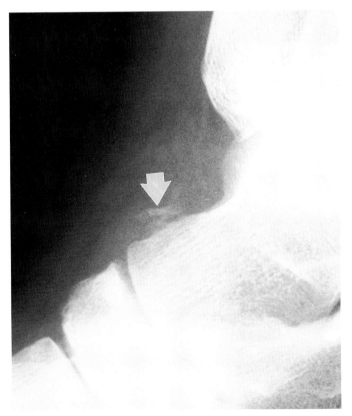

Fig. 4.15. Coronal MRI of chronic fracture of the lateral process. T2-weighted image, SE 2200/80. Patient had chronic pain, and MRI was performed to rule out tarsal sinus syndrome. High signal is seen in the marrow surrounding the low-signal intensity fracture line (arrow).

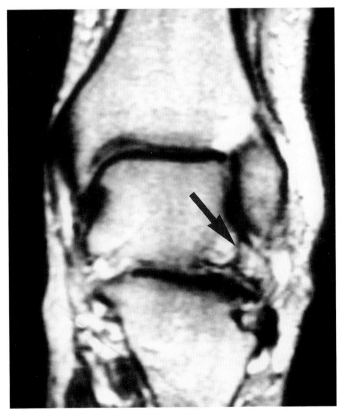

Fig. 4.16. Avulsion of the talar insertion of the ankle capsule. Lateral radiograph. This avulsion fracture (arrow) is typically a thin flake of cortical bone.

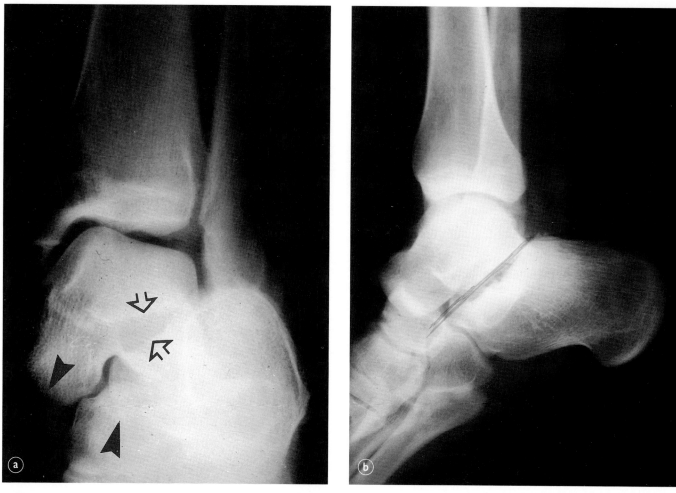

Fig. 4.17. Lateral subtalar dislocation. **a.** AP radiograph of the ankle. Arrowheads show the relative positions of the talar head and the corresponding articular surface of the navicular. Open arrows point to the articular surfaces of the posterior subtalar facet. **b.** Lateral radiograph. The head of the talus overlaps the navicular. There is posterior displacement of the calcaneus relative to the talus.

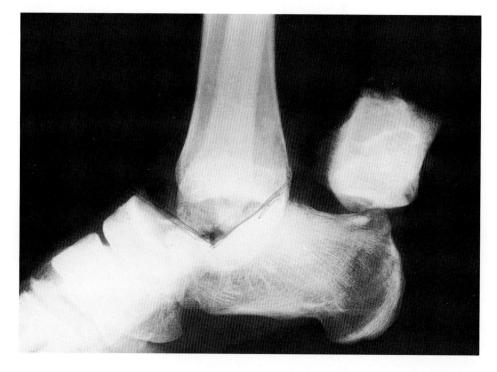

Fig. 4.18. Complete dislocation of the talus. Lateral radiograph. The talus is completely dislocated posteriorly, and the tibia rests on the calcaneus. The talus is intact, but appears shortened due to rotation.

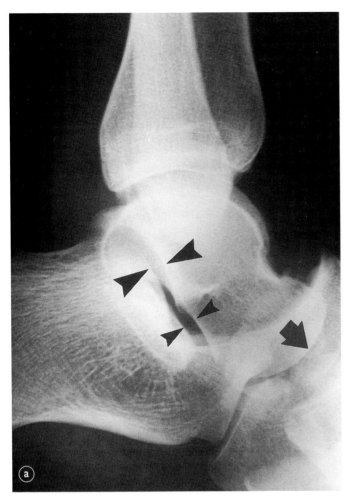 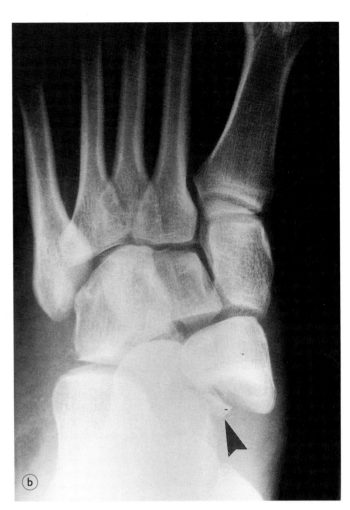

Fig. 4.19. Talonavicular dislocation. **a.** Lateral radiograph. The navicular is located dorsal to the talar head, and the silhouette of the talar head (arrow) overlaps the navicular. The subtalar joint is intact (large arrowheads show the apposing surfaces of the posterior facet, and small arrowheads the surfaces of the middle facet). **b.** Oblique radiograph. The navicular is medial to the head of the talus, and there is a small chip fracture of the navicular (arrowhead). There is also subluxation of the calcaneocuboid joint, and widening of the naviculocuneiform joints.

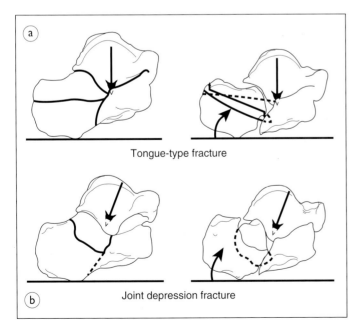

Fig. 4.20. Essex–Lopresti classification of intra-articular calcaneal fractures. **a.** Tongue-type. **b.** Joint depression-type.

Tongue-type fracture

Joint depression fracture

Table 4.3. Essex-Lopresti classification of calcaneal fractures

Extra-articular fractures (25%)
Intra-articular fractures (75%)
   A. Joint Depression
   intra-articular fracture with secondary fracture line located immediately behind the subtalar joint; there is resultant depression of the central fragment
   B. Tongue-type
   intra-articular fracture with secondary fracture line extending posteriorly in the horizontal plane to the tuberosity

(Fig. 4.20, Table 4.3). In both types, an oblique, sagittally oriented fracture line extends through the posterior facet, dividing the calcaneus into a medial fragment, which includes the sustentaculum tali and which moves with the talus, and a lateral fragment, which tends to become displaced laterally. In the joint depression-type of fracture, a second fracture line extends from

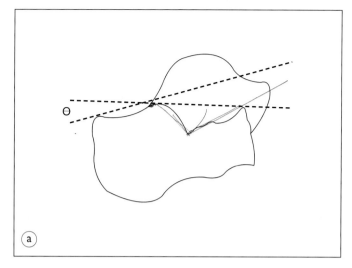

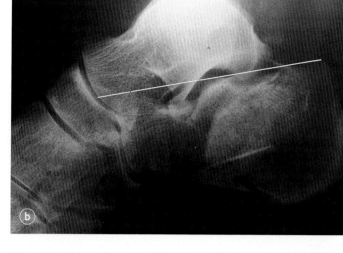

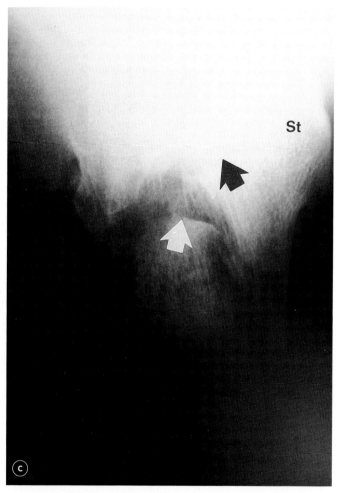

St

Fig. 4.21. Plain radiographs of joint depression-type calcaneal fracture. **a.** Diagram showing measurement of Boehler's angle. One line is drawn from the anterior process of the talus to the posterior margin of the posterior subtalar facet. A second line is drawn from the posterior margin of the posterior subtalar facet to the posterior process of the calcaneus. The angle between the lines should measure more than 20°. In most fractures of the posterior facet, Boehler's angle will be decreased. **b.** Lateral view. Marked disruption of the posterior facet is evident. The depressed portion of the posterior facet can be seen as a 'double density' superimposed on the body of the calcaneus. Boehler's angle is 0° —a single line extends from the anterior process of the calcaneus through the posterior aspect of the posterior facet to the posterior process. **c.** Axial view. The sustentaculum tali (St) is seen medially and provides orientation in evaluating this view. The white arrow points to the depressed lateral portion of the articular surface of the calcaneus. The black arrow points to the normally-positioned portion.

the main fracture line to just behind the joint, allowing depression of the posterior facet. In the tongue depression-type of fracture, the second line extends posteriorly to the tuberosity of the calcaneus. The joint depression-type is much more common.

Numerous classification systems for intra-articular calcaneal fractures have been proposed. CT scanning allows the most accurate evaluation of the fracture type.[34–38] Sanders[36] has classified intra-articular fractures on the basis of the number and location of articular fracture fragments seen on coronal CT scan.

In his system, the calcaneus is divided into three equal columns, the medial, central, and lateral columns. All nondisplaced fractures, regardless of the number of fracture lines, are considered type I. Type II fractures have two intra-articular fragments with displacement of the articular surface. Type III fractures have three intra-articular fragments, with a centrally depressed fragment analagous to the dye-punch fracture of the distal radius. Type IV fractures are severely comminuted. Fractures involving the medial column of the calcaneus have a worse prognosis

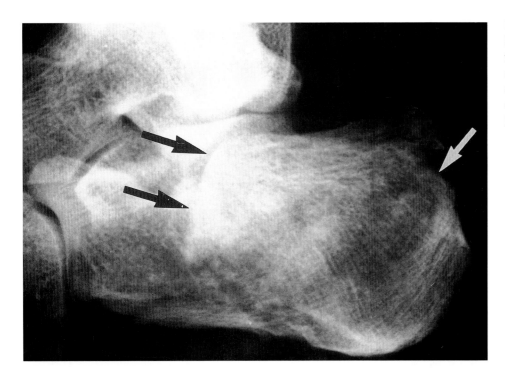

Fig. 4.22. Tongue-type calcaneal fracture. Lateral radiograph. A fracture line extends to the posterior process of the calcaneus (white arrow). Boehler's angle is markedly diminished. Black arrows point to a depressed portion of the posterior subtalar facet of the calcaneus.

because of the difficulty of obtaining adequate fixation of the medial fragment.

Imaging of Calcaneus Fractures

Plain radiographs

The fracture is most easily seen on a lateral radiograph of the ankle (Figs 4.21, 4.22). Boehler's angle is measured on this view and gives an approximate measure of the severity of articular depression. A routine ankle series is usually supplemented with axial views (see Fig. 4.21c; see also chapter 2) to show the disruption of the posterior facet. Unfortunately, axial views are difficult to obtain in the acutely injured patient, and if CT is planned this view is probably not needed.

CT

Plain radiographs offer a limited view of calcaneal fractures, and CT is routinely used for preoperative planning (Figs 4.23–4.25). CT often shows comminution that is not evident on plain radiographs, and it gives a more accurate determination of articular depression, as well as identifying any fragments within the joint that may prevent reduction of the fracture. CT is performed in both the axial plane and the direct coronal plane (with the patient's feet flat against the CT gantry). If the patient cannot tolerate the coronal scans, reformatted images can be obtained from axial scans, as discussed in Chapter 2. Sagittally reformatted images are sometimes helpful in complex fractures (see Fig. 4.25).

The classification system used by a radiologist to report the CT findings of an intra-articular fracture of the calcaneus will depend on the preference of the referring orthopedist. The classification system devised by Sanders[36] and described above is helpful in conveying the severity of the fracture. It is also helpful to describe the approximate percentage loss of height

---

Table 4.4. Important factors to include on CT reports of calcaneal fractures.

- approximate amount of widening and loss of height of calcaneus
- number of articular fragments, and location of intra-articular fracture lines
- amount of articular step-off (in mm), and size of depressed fragment
- presence of free fragments within the joint
- involvement of calcaneocuboid joint
- entrapment, subluxation, or other abnormality of peroneal tendons

---

and increase in mediolateral dimension in order to indicate the severity of the fracture deformity. Regardless of the classification system used, certain findings should always be mentioned (Table 4.4).

Injury to the peroneal tendons is common in calcaneal fractures because the fracture lines are often adjacent to the course of the tendons (Fig. 4.24). Rosenberg et al[29] studied the peroneal tendons in 24 cases of intra-articular calcaneal fractures and found there was lateral displacement of the tendons in 58%, impingement by bony fragments in 33%, subluxation or dislocation in 25%, hematomas surrounding the tendons in 21%, and entrapment of the tendons in 13%. Impingement of the tendons led to subsequent peroneal tenosynovitis, while hematoma surrounding the tendon proved to be clinically insignificant.

A single case of entrapment of the extensor digitorum brevis, abductor hallucis, and the medial neurovascular bundle has been described.[30] CT will frequently show fluid surrounding the flexor hallucis longus tendon and sometimes around the flexor

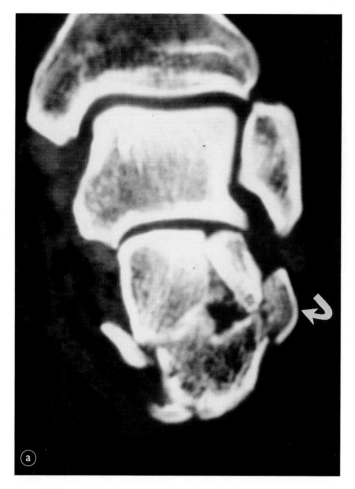

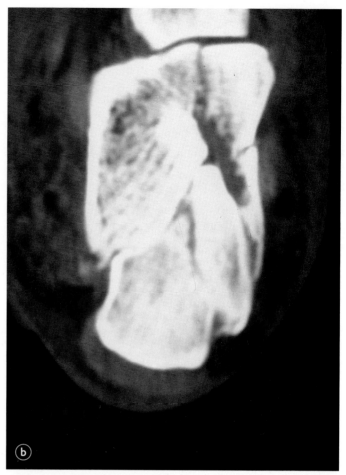

Fig. 4.23. CT of intra-articular calcaneal fracture. **a.** Coronal CT through the midportion of the posterior facet. The primary fracture line is the sagitally-oriented fracture through the facet, and is due to axial load. As the impaction of the bone continues, a secondary, comminuted, transverse fracture through the body of the calcaneus develops. Note that the peroneal tubercle (curved arrow) is displaced laterally. **b.** Axial CT. The fracture has a characteristic star-shaped pattern in the axial plane, with several fracture lines radiating outward from the primary sagittal fracture line.

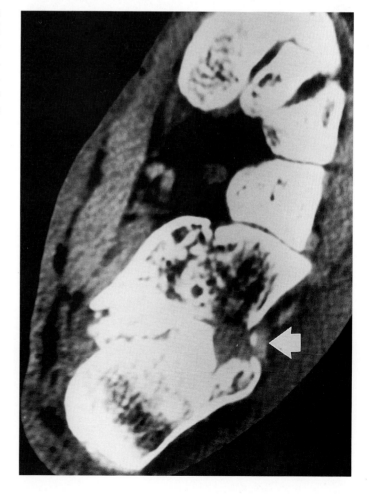

Fig. 4.24. Axial CT of calcaneal fracture. On this soft-tissue window, entrapment of the peroneal tendons (arrow) into the calcaneal fracture is seen.

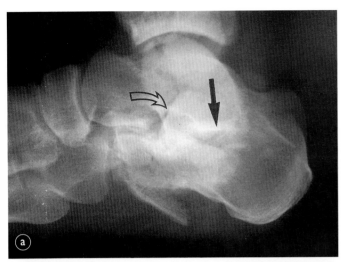

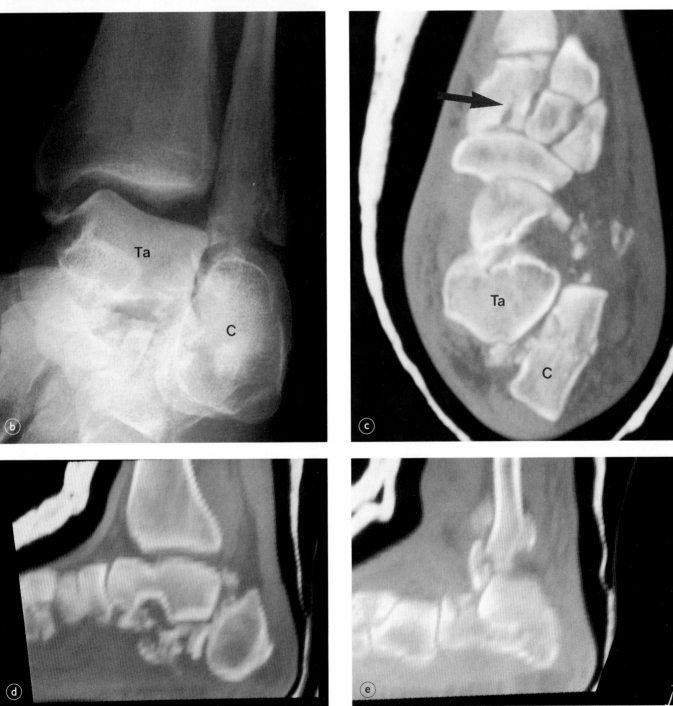

Fig. 4.25. Fracture-dislocation of the calcaneus. **a.** Lateral radiograph. A severe joint depression fracture of the calcaneus is evident, but the dislocation of the subtalar joint is not clearly seen (Closed arrow – articular cortex of talus. Open arow – articular cortex of calcaneus). **b.** Mortise radiograph. There is lateral dislocation of the calcaneus. A bimalleolar fracture of the ankle, most consistent with pronation-abduction injury, is also seen. **c.** Axial CT. The lateral dislocation of the calcaneus is more easily seen (Ta – talus, C – calcaneus). A fracture of the first cuneiform is also evident (arrow). **d.** Sagittally reformatted CT through the midportion of the ankle. The body of the talus is resting on several small calcaneal fragments, but the majority of the calcaneus is located more laterally and is not included in this section. **e.** Sagitally reformatted CT through the lateral aspect of the ankle. The calcaneal portion of the subtalar facet rests beneath the fractured lateral malleolus.

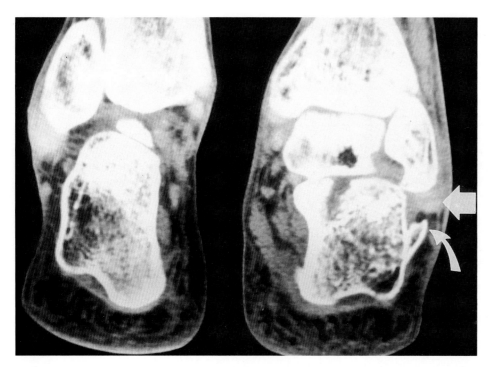

Fig. 4.26. Coronal CT 3 months after an intra-articular calcaneal fracture treated with closed reduction. Patient complained of continued pain, greatest with eversion of the foot. CT shows a lateral spur (curved arrow) formed by a healed, displaced bone fragment. The spur causes impingement of the peroneal tendons (straight arrow) as they course below the lateral malleolus. Impingement is most marked when the foot is everted.

digitorum longus tendon. The fluid is usually not a sign of injury to the tendon, although it should always be mentioned in the radiologist's report. Communication can exist between these tendon sheaths and the ankle and/or the subtalar joint, and therefore any condition causing fluid in the joint can also lead to fluid in the tendon sheaths.

CT scanning of nonacute calcaneal fractures can sometimes be useful in detecting causes of persistent pain. Chronic pain following calcaneal fractures is usually due to osteoarthritis of the subtalar joint. However, it can also be due to tenosynovitis or impingement of the peroneal tendons[29] (Fig. 4.26).

Treatment

The treatment of calcaneal fractures has vacillated between nonoperative and operative treatment for the past 50 years. Most authors would agree that minimally displaced fractures (less than 2 mm) without significant varus or loss of heel height should probably be treated nonoperatively, with early range of motion and delayed weight bearing. The dilemma arises with displaced fractures. Attempts to compare nonoperative and operative treatments has been difficult because of inconsistencies in classification and in qualification of a good outcome. In an attempt to summarize the literature on operative and nonoperative treatment, Paley[39] found that nonoperative treatment led to unsatisfactory results in 30–50% of patients, whereas operative treatment gave unsatisfactory results in 25–40% of patients. Sander's work[36,40] tends to indicate that results deteriorate as the number of articular fragments increase. However, Paley[39] suggests that there are a multitude of factors (including patient weight, increased time off work, heavy labor occupation, etc) that may be associated with an unsatisfactory outcome. Many contemporary surgeons feel that operative intervention is the treatment of choice for displaced fractures.[39,40] The goals of operative treatment are to restore articular congruity and heel height, to eliminate varus, and to narrow the width of the calcaneus.

Nonarticular Calcaneal Fractures

Rowe et al[41] divided calcaneal fractures into five types (Table 4.5, Fig. 4.27). His classification system is of little clinical utility and is seldom used by orthopedists. Most calcaneal fractures that do not involve the posterior facet are avulsion-type injuries.

Fracture of the tuberosity of the calcaneus

Beak-type fractures of the tuberosity of the calcaneus are due to avulsion by the Achilles tendon (Fig. 4.28). They usually occur in osteoporotic patients, and are caused by a dorsiflexion injury.

Table 4.5. Rowe classification of calcaneal fractures.

Type I (21%)
Fracture of anterior process, sustentaculum tali or medial tuberosity
Type II (3.8%)
Horizontal fracture of calcaneus posterior to subtalar joint, including avulsions of the Achilles tendon insertion
Type III (19.5%)
Oblique fracture not involving the subtalar joint
Type IV (24.7%)
Fracture involving the subtalar joint without significant depression of the posterior facet
Type V (31%)
Fracture of the subtalar joint with depression of the central calcaneus

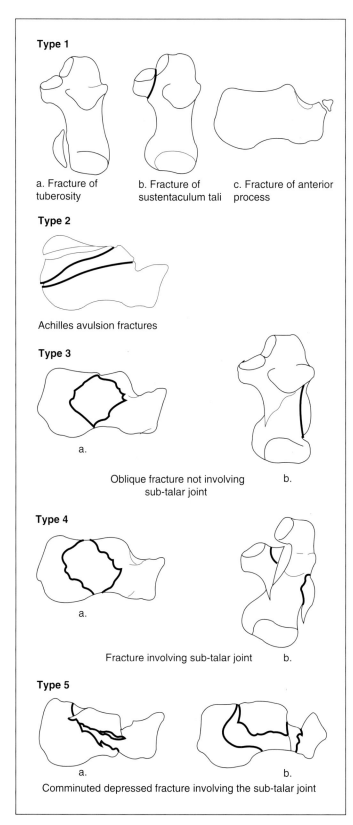

Fig. 4.27. Rowe's classification of calcaneal fractures.

Type 1

a. Fracture of tuberosity

b. Fracture of sustentaculum tali

c. Fracture of anterior process

Type 2

Achilles avulsion fractures

Type 3

a.

b.

Oblique fracture not involving sub-talar joint

Type 4

a.

b.

Fracture involving sub-talar joint

Type 5

a.

b.

Comminuted depressed fracture involving the sub-talar joint

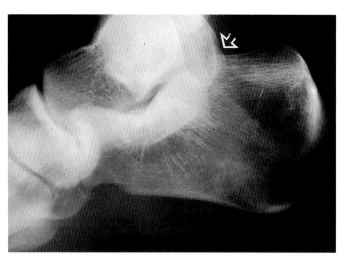

Fig. 4.28. Avulsion of the tuberosity of the calcaneus. Lateral radiograph. The Achilles tendon insertion is avulsed in this diabetic patient with osteoporosis. The fracture extends into the posterior margin of the posterior facet. Note a small compression fracture of the posterior process of the talus (open arrow).

They have been reported to be more common in patients with long-standing diabetes mellitus.[42] Patients who have normal bone density and a dorsiflexion injury of the heel usually rupture the Achilles tendon rather than fracturing the calcaneus.

Fractures of the medial tuberosity of the calcaneus are uncommon (Fig. 4.29). They can occur as a result of avulsion injury of the abductor hallucis muscle, owing to forced dorsiflexion of the forefoot.[43]

Fracture of the anterior process of the calcaneus

The bifurcate ligament connects the anterior process of the calcaneus to the navicular and cuboid. In an inversion injury, the bifurcate ligament can avulse the anterior process. In an eversion injury, the anterior process can be crushed between the navicular and the adjacent portion of the calcaneus. These fractures are almost always nondisplaced, and they are difficult to see on radiographs (Fig. 4.30). Coned-down views at different obliquities are helpful to confirm a fracture suspected on routine foot radiographs. An accessory ossicle, the os calcis secundarium, can occur in the location of the anterior process, and mimic a fracture (see Chapter 1).

Fracture of the extensor digitorum brevis origin

The extensor digitorum brevis originates on the anterolateral aspect of the calcaneus.[44,45] A thin flake of bone at its origin can be avulsed during an inversion injury . The fracture is most readily seen on anteroposterior radiographs of the ankle (Fig. 4.31), although it can sometimes be identified on anteroposterior radiographs of the foot.

Stress fractures

Stress fractures of the calcaneus are usually insufficiency fractures associated with osteoporosis, although they have also been seen as fatigue fractures in military recruits.[46] Radiographically, they are usually seen as lines of sclerosis perpendicular to the major trabeculae of the posterior process of the calcaneus (Fig. 4.32). Rarely, the insufficiency fracture occurs centrally (Fig. 4.33).

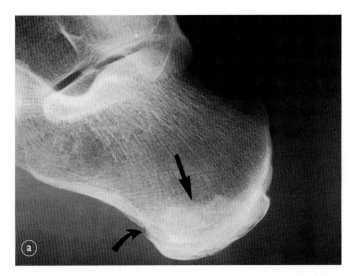

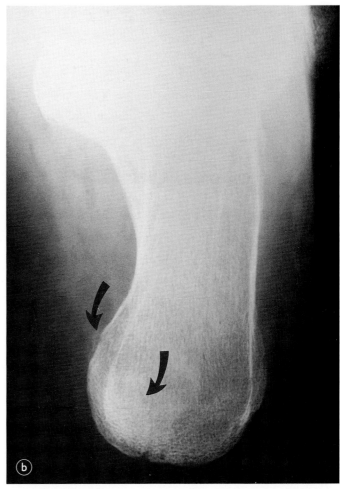

Fig. 4.29. Fracture of medial aspect of calcaneal tuberosity. **a.** Lateral view. A subtle cortical break is seen (curved arrow), but the most prominent evidence of fracture is the 'double density' (straight arrow) formed by superimposition of the fracture fragments. **b.** Axial view. The nondisplaced fracture line is faintly seen (curved arrows).

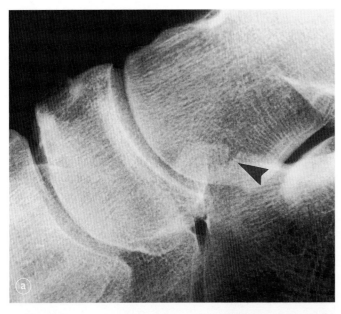

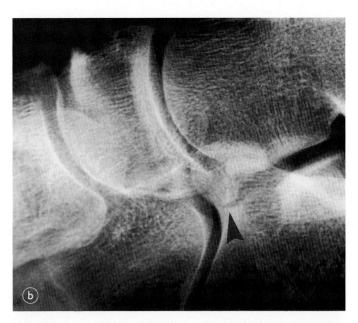

Fig. 4.30. Fractures of the anterior process of the calcaneus. **a.** Lateral radiograph at time of injury. The anterior process of the talus overlaps the head of the talus and the medial aspect of the navicular, so careful attention to this area is need to detect fractures. In this case, the fracture line is slightly separated superiorly (arrowhead). **b.** Lateral radiograph in another patient. Initial radiographs were interpreted as negative. On repeat radiograph 10 days later, the fracture is easily seen (arrowhead) due to bone resorption at the fracture line.

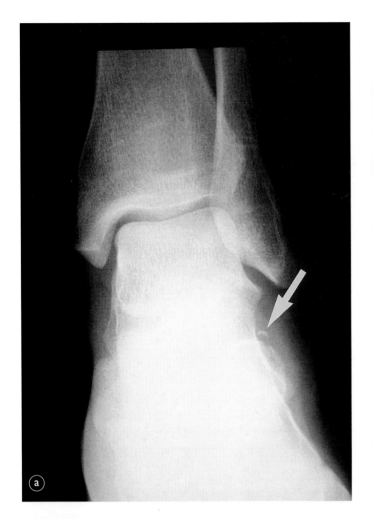

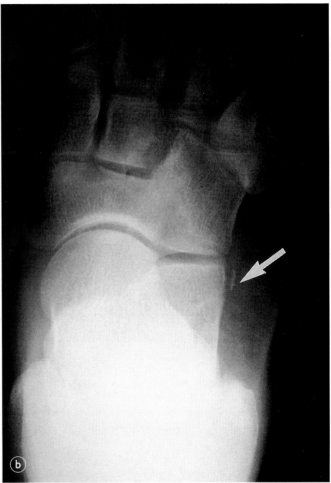

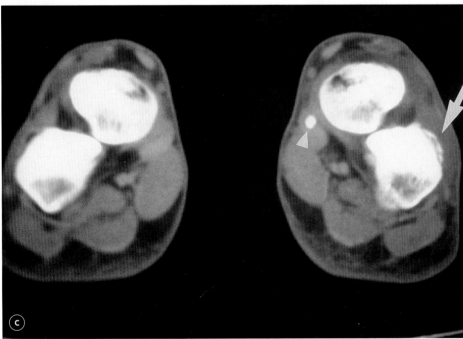

Fig. 4.31. Avulsion of extensor digitorum brevis origin. **a.** AP radiograph of the ankle. A flake of bone (arrow) is seen at the lateral aspect of the calcaneus. **b.** AP radiograph of the foot in another patient. A similar flake-like avulsion is seen (arrow). **c.** Coronal CT in another patient, obtained after fracture was missed on plain radiographs. The fracture is easily identified (arrow). Soft-tissue windows showed edema of the extensor digitorum brevis muscle. An accessory navicular is noted medially (arrowhead).

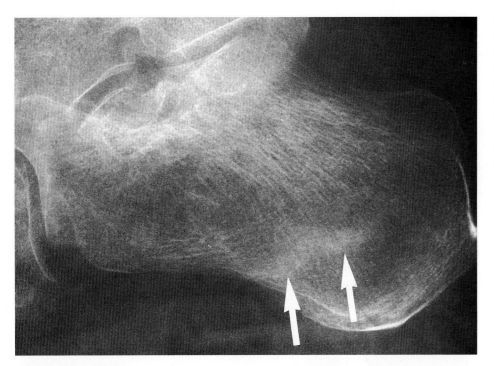

Fig. 4.32. Insufficiency fracture of calcaneus. Lateral radiograph. Patient had pain after stepping off a curb. White arrows point to a thick, ill-defined sclerotic line perpendicular to the orientation of the major trabeculae in this region, and roughly parallel to the plantar surface of the foot. The orientation of the fracture line reflects the axial compressive force causing the fracture. Bones are severely osteoporotic.

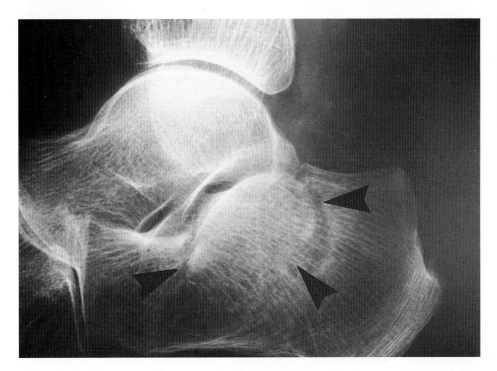

Fig. 4.33. Central insufficiency fracture of the calcaneus. Lateral radiograph. The posterior facet is depressed slightly. Arrowheads show the semilunar fracture line. There was no history of trauma in this elderly patient, who complained of sudden onset of heel pain.

NAVICULAR FRACTURES

Stress Fractures

Stress fracture of the tarsal navicular, which is associated with running and jumping, commonly occurs as a fatigue fracture in athletes. The patients present with ill-defined midfoot soreness, and diagnosis may be delayed owing to the lack of findings on plain radiographs.[47]

Stress fractures of the navicular arise in the central one-third of the bone, originating on the dorsal surface. The fracture line is sagitally oriented. The majority of fractures are not complete.[48]

Bipartite naviculars have been reported, and if diagnosis of fracture is in doubt, ^{99m}technetium bone scan is recommended to differentiate fracture from a bipartite bone.

Early fractures may be treated with immobilization and nonweight-bearing, and gradual resumption of activity.[47,49] If the injury has progressed to a complete fracture and conservative management fails, screw fixation can be performed. Bone grafting is sometimes used for nonunion.[47]

Complications of navicular stress fractures include nonunion, avascular necrosis (especially in the lateral fragment of bone), and secondary osteoarthritis of the talonavicular joint.

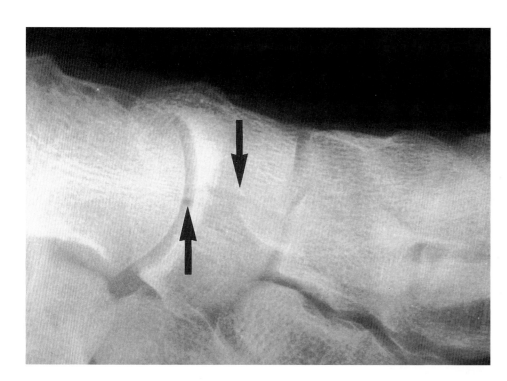

Fig. 4.34. Stress fracture of the navicular. Oblique radiograph. The nondisplaced fracture is shown by arrows.

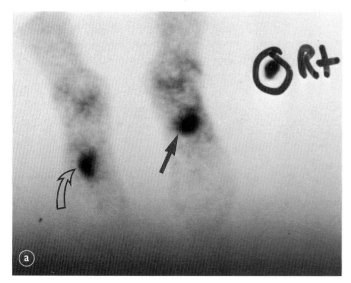

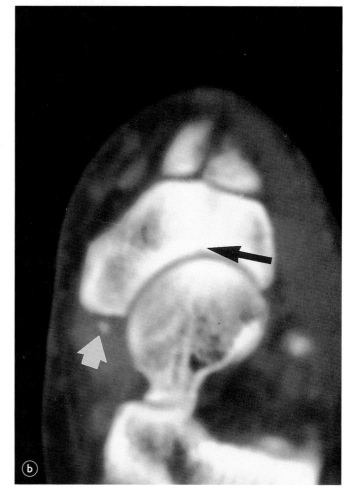

Fig. 4.35. Stress fracture of the navicular in a runner. Plain radiographs were negative. **a.** 99mTechnetium-bone scan, feet on detector view. There is abnormal uptake, owing to stress fracture of the right navicular (solid arrow). Patient also had a stress fracture of the left third metatarsal (open arrow). **b.** Axial CT. The midportion of the navicular is sclerotic, and a faint fracture line is seen (black arrow). Incidental note is made of a small type I accessory navicular bone (white arrow).

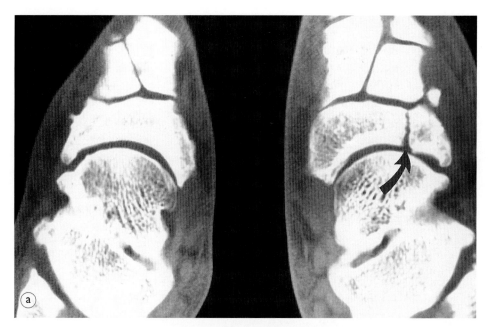

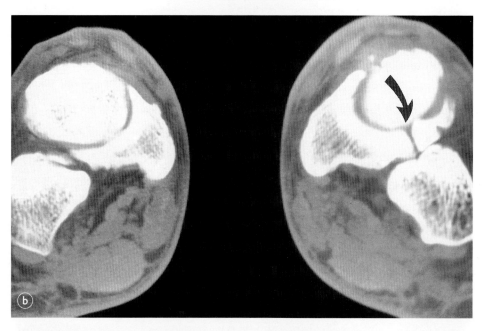

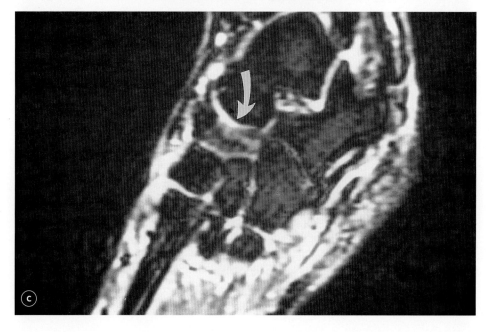

Fig. 4.36. Chronic stress fracture of the navicular. **a.** Axial CT. Fracture fragments are slightly separated (arrow) and have sclerotic margins. **b.** Coronal CT. Fracture (arrow) extends completely through the navicular. **c.** Sagittal MRI, STIR 2366.7/40/155. Edema (arrow) is seen in the navicular. Fracture was missed on axial and coronal images because image planes were poorly chosen, and did not correspond to the long and short axes of the foot.

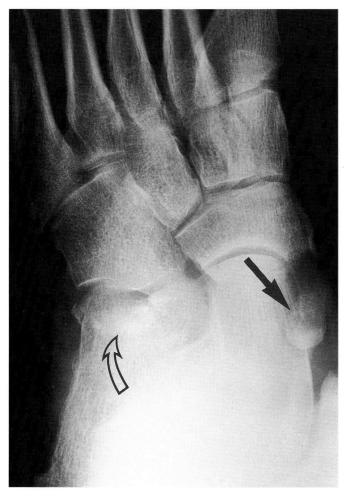

Fig. 4.37. Nutcracker injury. Oblique radiograph. There has been avulsion of the tuberosity of the navicular (black arrow) by the posterior tibial tendon, and a comminuted impaction fracture of the anterior margin of the calcaneus at the calcaneocuboid joint (open arrow).

Imaging of navicular stress fractures

Plain radiographs sometimes show a nondisplaced, sagitally oriented fracture line in the middle third of the navicular (Fig. 4.34), but they are often normal or show only sclerosis of the navicular. [99m]Technetium bone scans are useful to detect the fracture early, when radiographs are commonly negative.[47] Bone scan will show increased flow and increased activity on both immediate and delayed images, owing to reparative new bone formation. The entire navicular will often show increased radionuclide activity (Fig. 4.35), and osteonecrosis of the navicular should be considered in the differential diagnosis. In subtle fractures, tomograms or CT are helpful in showing the lucent fracture line or a sclerotic band of callus formation (Figs 4.35, 4.36) and in differentiating partial from complete fracture.[48,50] They can also be used to monitor fracture healing.[50] MRI can also show the fracture line.[51]

Intra-articular Navicular Fractures

Intra-articular fractures of the navicular are uncommon and are usually associated with other injuries. Dislocation of the talo-navicular joint is usually present (see Fig. 4.19).

Avulsion Fractures and Fractures of the Accessory Navicular

Avulsion fractures are seen dorsally, when they are caused by capsular avulsion, or medially. Medially, the tuberosity of the navicular may be avulsed by the posterior tibial tendon in an eversion injury. Avulsions of the navicular tuberosity may be associated with fractures of the anterior calcaneus or the cuboid, or injury to the calcaneocuboid joint – the 'nutcracker' injury[52] (Fig. 4.37). This injury is due to eversion of the midfoot. Howie et al[53] found this combination in seven out of 14 avulsions of the navicular tuberosity.

A type 2 accessory navicular ossicle (also known as os tibiale externum, see Chapter 1), which is united to the remainder of the navicular by a synchondrosis, can be avulsed by the posterior tibial tendon. This injury may not be evident radiographically, but it can be suspected in a patient with a type 2 accessory navicular and pain at the synchondrosis. The injury is evident on CT scan (Fig. 4.38) or MRI (see Fig. 7.22). A type 1 accessory navicular may also fracture in association with injury of the posterior tibial tendon.

Avulsions of the dorsal aspect of the navicular are usually small cortical avulsions, which present as 'ankle sprain'.

CUNEIFORM FRACTURES

Fractures of the cuneiforms are rare as isolated injuries (Fig. 4.39). They usually occur with dislocations at the Lisfranc or Chopart joints. CT (see Fig. 4.26) is very helpful in elucidating complex injuries.

CUBOID FRACTURES

The cuboid may be compressed in an eversion injury.[52,53] It is rarely injured in isolation (Fig. 4.40). Stress fractures may occur.

FRACTURES AND DISLOCATIONS OF THE TARSOMETATARSAL JOINTS

The tarsometatarsal joint, or joint of Lisfranc, is infrequently injured, and most dislocations at this level are due to neuropathic disease rather than a single episode of trauma. A traumatic dislocation usually occurs because of a fall with the foot in hyperplantar flexion (e.g. going down stairs or stepping off a curb), or as a result of a motor vehicle accident.[54] Fractures of the second metatarsal or the cuneiforms are commonly associated with Lisfranc dislocations.

The primary stabilizer of the Lisfranc joint is the recessed position of the second metatarsal relative to the first and third metatarsals. The second metatarsal is tightly held between the first and third cuneiform, and this mortise and tendon configuration prevents mediolateral motion of the second metatarsal. The second to fifth metatarsal bases are attached to the adjacent metatarsals by strong intermetatarsal ligaments. There is no ligament between the bases of the first and second metatarsals. Instead, this region is stabilized by the Lisfranc ligament, which extends obliquely from the medial cuneiform to the base of the

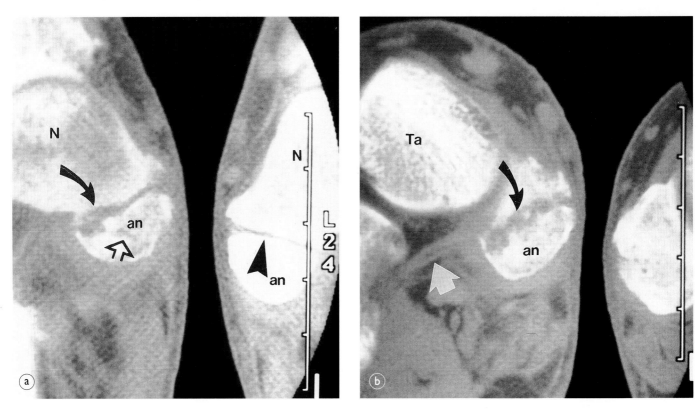

Fig. 4.38. Avulsion of the accessory navicular. **a.** Axial CT. Patient has accessory navicular (an) bilaterally. On the left, there is a normal synchondrosis (arrowhead) with the navicular (N). On the right, the synchondrosis is widened and irregular (curved arrow), and there is a nondisplaced fracture (open arrow) through the accessory navicular. **b.** Coronal CT. Widening and irregularity of the synchondrosis (curved arrow) are again seen. Note that the accessory navicular is located medial to the head of the talus (Ta). White arrow points to the normal calcaneonavicular ligament, inserting on the navicular in the region of the synchondrosis.

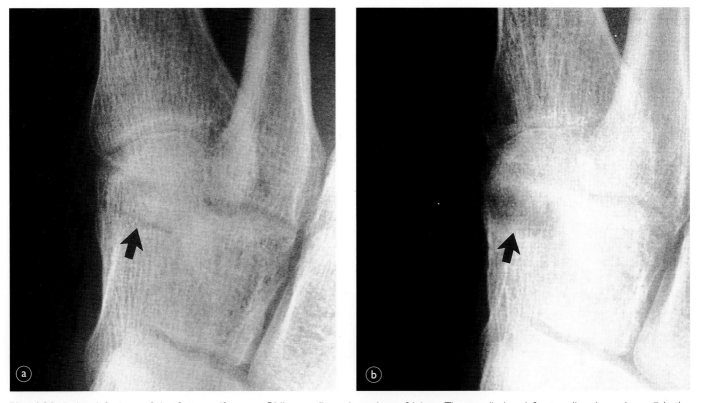

Fig. 4.39. Isolated fracture of the first cuneiform. **a.** Oblique radiograph at time of injury. The nondisplaced fracture line (arrow) parallels the base of the first metatarsal, and was not recognised. Patient had severe, continued foot pain. **b.** Oblique radiograph 1 month later. There is bone resorption along the fracture line. A lytic tumor was questioned at this time, and CT was performed, confirming the presence of a fracture and ruling out tumor.

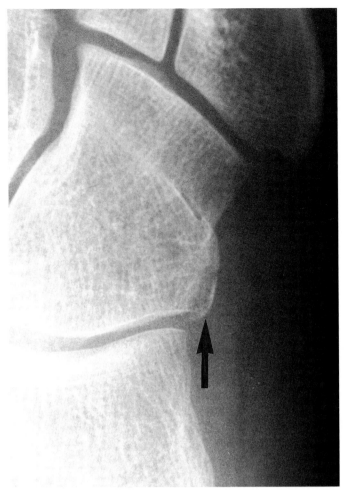

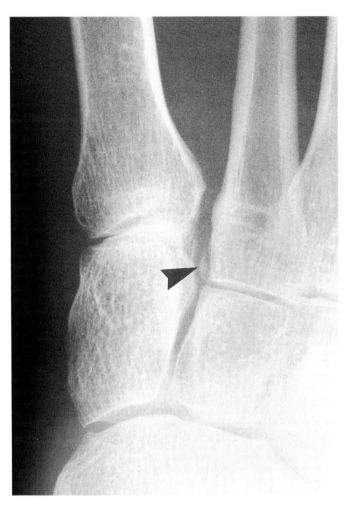

Fig. 4.40. Chip fracture of the cuboid. Oblique radiograph. There is a small chip of the lateral cortex of the cuboid (arrow), probably due to abduction injury at the calcaneocuboid joint.

Fig. 4.41. Lisfranc joint injury. AP radiograph. Patient had pain in the foot after a tennis game. There is a subtle flake-like avulsion of the attachment of the Lisfranc ligament to the base of the second metatarsal (arrowhead).

second metatarsal. A fracture of the attachment of this ligament, or lateral subluxation of the base of the second metatarsal indicating ligamentous rupture, implies a significant compromise of the stability of the Lisfranc joint[55] (Figs 4.42, 4.43).

Dislocations of the Lisfranc joint are divided into two major types.[56] A homolateral dislocation is a lateral dislocation of the first through fifth metatarsals. A divergent dislocation is one where the first metatarsal is displaced medially, and the second through fifth metatarsals are displaced laterally. The first metatarsal may also remain in a normal position, and this is termed a partial or isloated dislocation. Rarely, isolated dislocations involve the fourth and fifth rays only.

Imaging of Lisfranc Injuries

Careful attention to the attachment of the Lisfranc ligament to the second metatarsal is needed to discern limited injuries to the Lisfranc joint (see Figs 4.41, 4.42). The normal anatomic relation-

ships of the Lisfranc joint must be carefully analysed. On the anteroposterior view of the normal foot, the medial cortex of the base of the second metatarsal should always line up exactly with the medial cortex of the second cuneiform.[57–59] On the oblique radiograph, the lateral margin of the third metatarsal should line up with the lateral margin of the third cuneiform, and the medial margin of the fourth metatarsal should line up with the medial margin of the cuboid. The base of the fifth metatarsal should project beyond the cuboid. On the lateral view, the base of the second metatarsal can be recognized because of its recessed position. Its dorsal surface should align with the dorsal surface of the second cuneiform.

In suspected injuries of the Lisfranc joint and in injuries limited to the second ray, weight-bearing or stress views should be obtained. Flattening of the longitudinal arch has been associated with a poorer prognosis in these fractures.[55]

CT scanning has been used to assess the extent of injury better, and it is helpful in detecting superoinferior subluxation, which can be difficult to see on plain radiographs.[60]

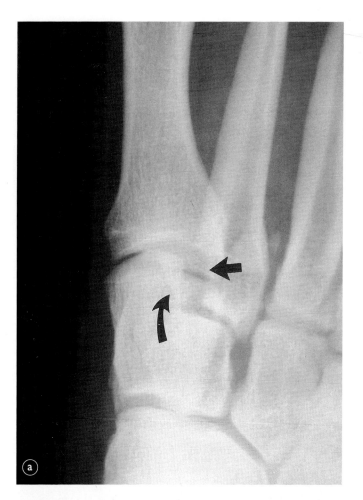

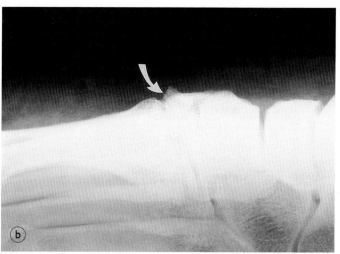

Fig. 4.42. Lisfranc joint injury. **a.** Oblique radiograph. There is an avulsion of the medial base of the second metatarsal, at the attachment of the Lisfranc ligament. The avulsed fragment (curved arrow) is difficult to see on this view because it overlies the first cuneiform. However, the corresponding defect in the base of the second metatarsal (straight arrow) is evident. **b.** Lateral radiograph. The avulsed fragment (curved arrow) is rotated 45° and displaced posteriorly.

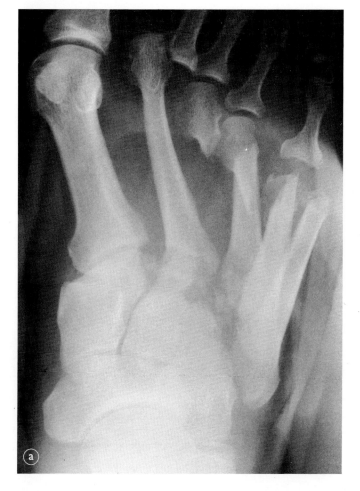

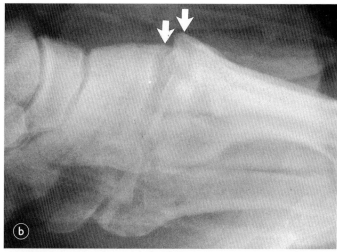

Fig. 4.43. Lisfranc fracture-dislocation caused by motorcycle accident. **a.** AP radiograph. There is lateral dislocation of the second through fifth tarsometatarsal joints and fragmentation of the bases of the second and third metatarsal bases. Extensive injury is also present at the metatarsophalangeal joints, with dislocation of the second and fifth metatarsophalangeal joints, and displaced fractures of the third through fifth metatarsal necks. **b.** Lateral radiograph. There is dorsal dislocation of the second tarsometatarsal joint. Arrows point to the relative positions of the dorsal surfaces of the second cuneiform and second metatarsal base.

Treatment of Lisfranc Injuries

Injuries limited to subluxation or fracture of the second metatarsal, or both, can often be treated with closed reduction and casting, but internal fixation is often needed.[54-57] It is difficult to immobilize this area with a cast. Disabling midfoot pain can occur as a late complication, and its incidence is reduced with internal fixation.[57]

METATARSAL FRACTURES

Metatarsal Neck Fractures

Fracture of the metatarsal neck is a fairly common injury. Often two or more adjacent metatarsal necks will be fractured (Fig. 4.43). There is usually rotation of the metatarsal head, and this is a helpful sign in subtle fractures.

Stress Fractures of the Metatarsals

Stress fractures of the metatarsals, usually the second through fourth metatarsals, are a common problem. When occurring as a fatigue fracture of normal bone, they are referred to as 'march fractures' because they are a frequent occurrence in military recruits. Metatarsal stress fractures also develop as insufficiency fractures due to osteoporosis. A stress fracture of the second metatarsal involving the Lisfranc joint has been described in dancers.[61] Most stress fractures of the metatarsals, however, are in the shaft or neck.

Stress fractures are usually initially negative on plain radiographs. A complete or incomplete fracture line is sometimes evident (Fig. 4.44). Later, periosteal reaction develops (Fig. 4.45). Before the radiographs are positive, the diagnosis can be suspected clinically in a patient with acute onset of pain over a metatarsal and pinpoint tenderness to palpation. The patient usually admits to increased physical activity prior to the onset of pain but denies a specific trauma.

Three-phase [99m]technetium bone scans are highly sensitive in the diagnosis (Fig. 4.45). When the patient's history is considered together with the location of the scintigraphic findings, the bone scan is highly specific. The diagnosis can be made on MRI[51] (Fig. 4.46), but given the cost differential and the efficacy of bone scan in this location, MRI is not advocated as a diagnostic method of choice.

Fifth Metatarsal Fractures

Three distinct types of fractures commonly occur at the base of the fifth metatarsal.[62] The Jones fracture is a transverse fracture of the metadiaphysis[63] (Fig. 4.47) caused by an acute injury, most likely adduction of the forefoot with a plantar flexed ankle. Stress fractures may also occur at this location or slightly more distally (Fig. 4.48). The third type of fracture is a fracture of the tuberosity (Fig. 4.49), which is often wrongly called a Jones

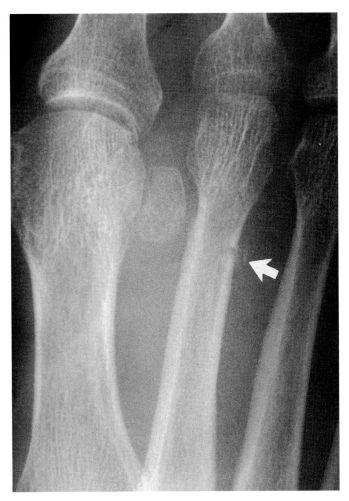

Fig. 4.44. Stress fracture of the second metatarsal neck. AP radiograph. An ill-defined, lucent line (arrow) traverses the metatarsal neck. Hazy periosteal new bone is evident adjacent to the fracture.

fracture. This fracture is usually considered to be due to avulsion by the peroneus brevis tendon, although it has been suggested that the avulsion is caused by the lateral plantar aponeurosis.[64] Fractures of the tuberosity of the fifth metatarsal are transversely oriented, which distinguishes them from the vertically oriented accessory center of ossification that is found at the same location. The os vesalianum (see Chapter 1) is an accessory ossicle that occurs in this location.

INJURIES OF THE FIRST METATARSOPHALANGEAL JOINT

Adductor Hallucis Avulsion

A fracture of the lateral aspect of the base of the proximal phalanx indicates avulsion of the adductor hallucis insertion (Fig. 4.50). The fracture is often displaced by several millimeters, and it requires surgical fixation to prevent development of varus deformity of the great toe.[65] It is a rare injury.

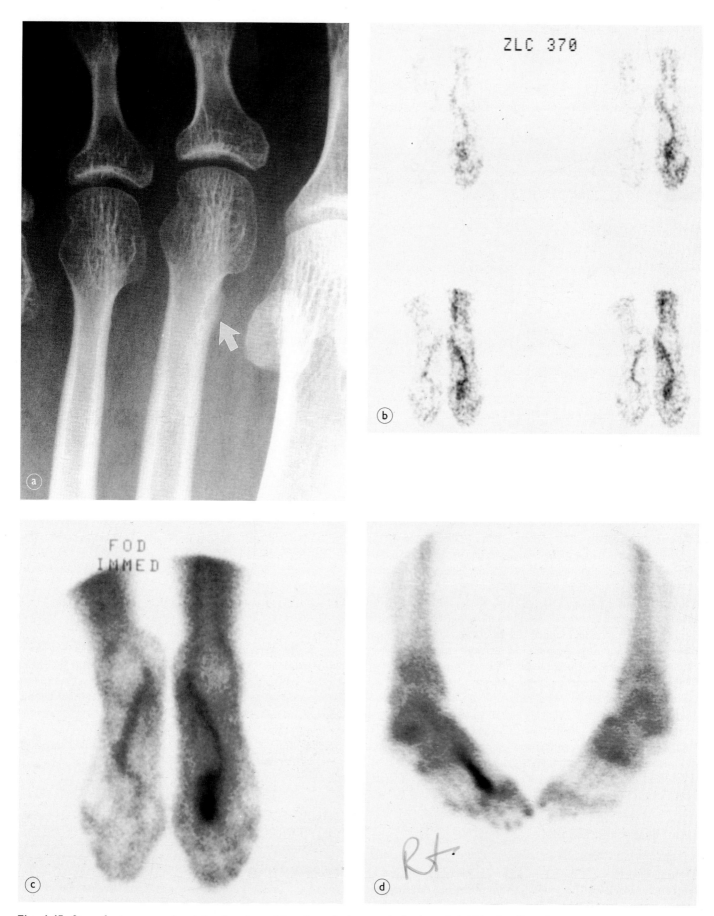

Fig. 4.45. Stress fracture second metatarsal neck. **a.** AP radiograph shows only focal cortical thickening (arrow) due to appositional periosteal new bone. **b.** ⁹⁹ᵐTechnetium bone scan, select images from radionuclide angiogram, foot on detector view. Increased flow to the right second metatarsal is seen. **c.** Blood pool image, same projection. Hyperemia is evident around the second metatarsal neck. **d.** Three hour image, anterior oblique projection, shows markedly increased radionuclide uptake in the 2nd metatarsal.

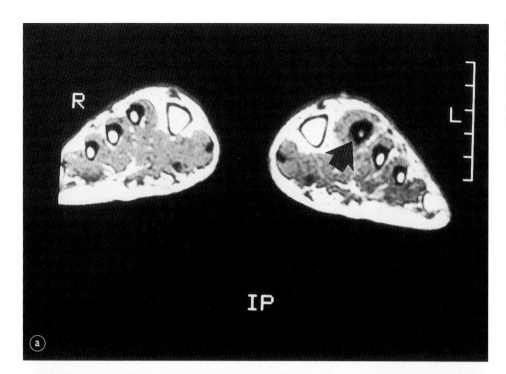

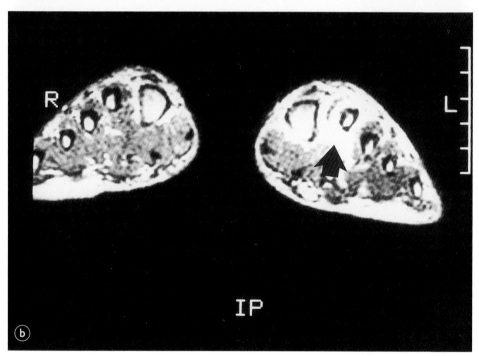

Fig. 4.46. MRI showing stress fracture of the second metatarsal. **a.** Coronal SE 2000/20. the cortex of the left 2nd metatarsal (arrow) is thickened. **b.** Coronal SE 2000/80. High signal intensity reflecting soft-tissue edema (arrow) is seen surrounding the metatarsal.

Sesamoid Fractures

The sesamoids of the first metatarsal are uncommonly fractured. An acute fracture may occur because of a direct blow. Fatigue stress fractures occur in runners and dancers.[66] It is sometimes difficult to differentiate between bipartite or multipartite sesamoids and sesamoid fracture (Figs 4.51, 4.52). Tenderness over the sesamoid may be due to sesamoiditis as well as fracture. Tomography or CT will often show fracture lines that are not apparent on plain radiographs.

Sesamoid dislocations may be caused by rupture of the plantar capsule, either in isolation or in conjunction with dislocation of the first metatarsophalangeal joint.[66,67]

Sprains

Forced hyperextension of the first metatarsophalangeal joint may cause a tear of the plantar capsule known as 'turf toe'. Valgus injury may cause injury to the medial collateral ligaments and a traumatic hallux valgus deformity.

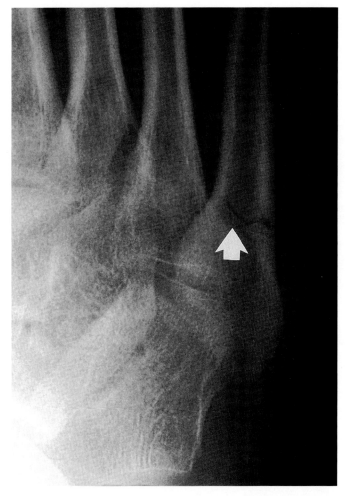

Fig. 4.47. Jones fracture of the base of the fifth metatarsal. AP radiograph. The fracture originally suffered and described by Dr Jones was due to an injury while dancing.

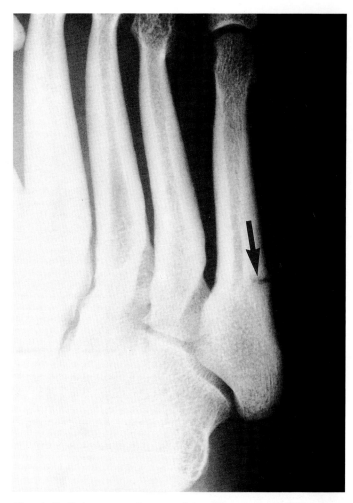

Fig. 4.48. Fatigue stress fracture of the fifth metatarsal. This fracture is in the same location as the Jones fracture, but unlike the Jones fracture, which is due to a single episode of trauma, it is due to repeated stress. Note that in this case the fracture line is incomplete (arrow).

INJURIES OF THE LESSER TOES

Plantar Plate Injury

The plantar plate of the metatarsophalangeal joints is formed by the plantar aponeurosis and the plantar capsule. It supports the undersurface of the metatarsal head and prevents hyperextension of the metatarsophalangeal joint.[68] Rupture of the plantar plate, most commonly of the second toe, may present with pain (lesser metatarsalgia), hammer toe deformity, or both. Subluxation or dislocation of the metatarsophalangeal joint may develop.[69] Women wearing high-heeled, narrow-toed shoes are predisposed to injure the plantar plate.

Injuries of the plantar plate have been imaged with arthrography,[68,70] and more recently MRI[68] (Figs 4.53, 4.54). In addition to disruption of the plate itself, secondary signs of rupture include synovitis of the joint, hyperextension of the joint, and fluid in the flexor tendon sheath.

Differential diagnosis includes stress fracture, degenerative and inflammatory arthritis, Morton's neuroma, and Freiberg's infraction.[68,71,72]

Phalangeal Fractures

Phalangeal fractures are fairly common, and they often occur as the result of a stubbed toe. Generally, they are radiographically obvious but they may be visible on only a single view (Figs 4.55, 4.56). Treatment is usually limited to 'buddy taping' the fractured toe to the adjacent toe. An exception is made for unstable fractures of the first proximal phalanx, which are treated with Kirschner wire or lag screw fixation (see Fig. 4.50).

Fractures involving the PIP joints may also be fixed internally.

FRACTURES OF ACCESSORY OSSICLES

Fractures of the accessory navicular are discussed above, with fractures of the navicular. Other accessory ossicles can also

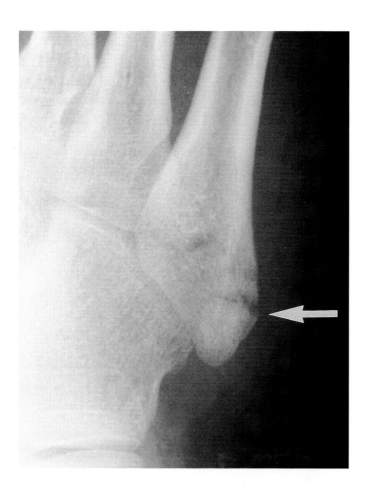

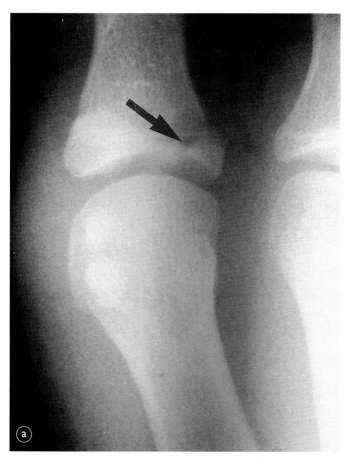

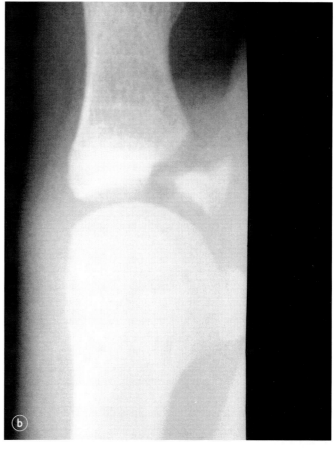

Fig. 4.49. Fracture of the tuberosity of the base of the fifth metatarsal. Oblique radiograph. In this case, the fracture spares the tarsometatarsal joint and enters the intermetatarsal joint. In other cases it may enter the TMT joint. The fracture is rarely displaced.

Fig. 4.50. Avulsion of adductor hallucis insertion. **a.** AP radiograph. The avulsion fracture (arrow) appears minimally displaced. **b.** Oblique radiograph. The significant displacement of the fragment is evident in this view.

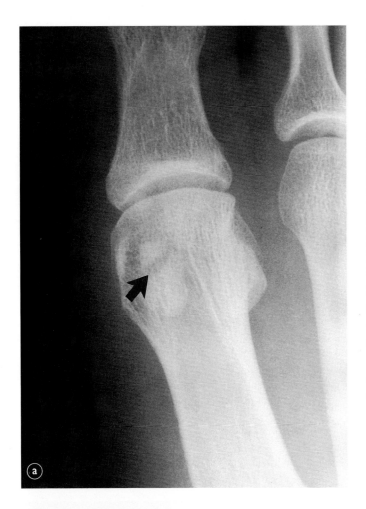

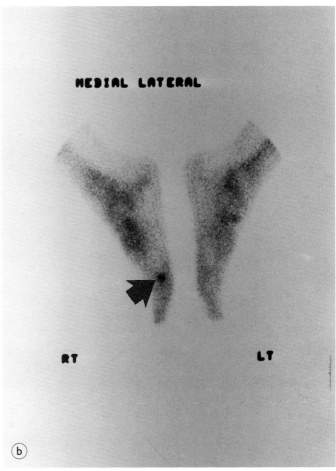

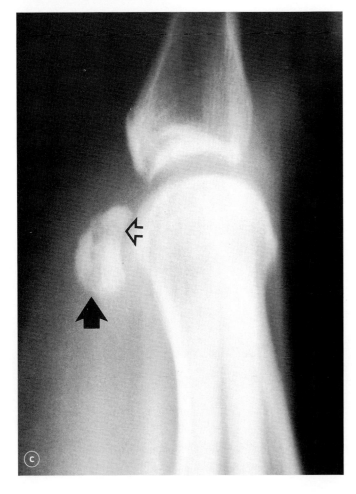

Fig. 4.51. Fracture of the medial sesamoid of the first toe. **a.** AP radiograph. The medial sesamoid appears bipartite (arrow). However, radiograph several years previously showed a unipartite sesamoid. **b.** 99mTechnetium-MDP bone scan shows focally increased uptake in the sesamoid (arrow) on this delayed image. Increased blood flow and blood pool activity were also present. **c.** Lateral tomogram shows a fracture in the axial plane, not evident on plain radiographs (solid arrow). The oblique coronal fracture line seen on radiographs is indistinct (open arrow) because of its oblique plane.

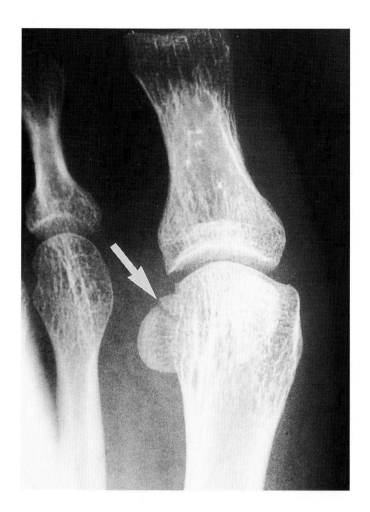

Fig. 4.52. Fracture of lateral sesamoid of first metatarsal. AP radiograph. The lateral sesamoid is less commonly multipartite than is the medial. Other signs indicating that a fracture rather than a bipartite sesamoid is present are that the two fragments have irregular, noncorticated apposing margins, and acutely angled rather than rounded corners. A bipartite sesamoid also tends to be slightly larger than a fractured, unipartite sesamoid.

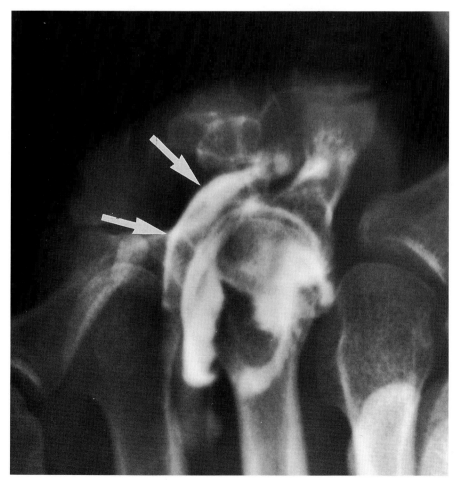

Fig. 4.53. Arthrogram showing rupture of the plantar plate of the third metatarsophalangeal joint. Oblique radiograph. Contrast filling the flexor tendon sheath (arrows) is diagnostic of rupture of the plantar plate. (From Yao et al,[68] with permission.)

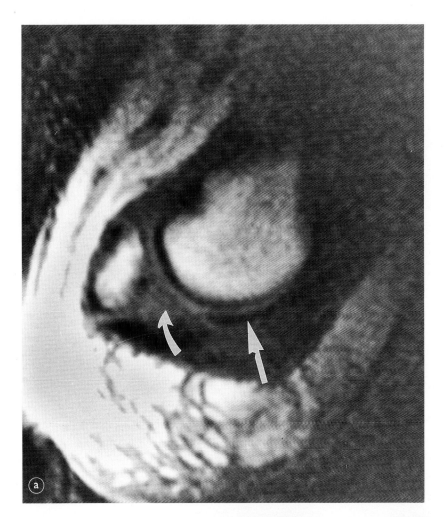

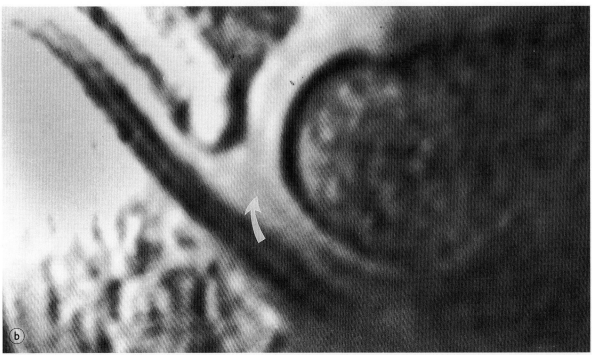

Fig. 4.54. MRI of plantar plate rupture. **a.** Sagittal T1-weighted MRI (SE 500/20). The proximal plantar plate (straight arrow) is seen as a black line which is absent distally (curved arrow). **b.** Oblique sagittal reformation of GRE GRASS MRI (33/10/10). There is a high-signal defect in the distal plantar plate (curved arrow). (From Yao et al,[68] with permission.)

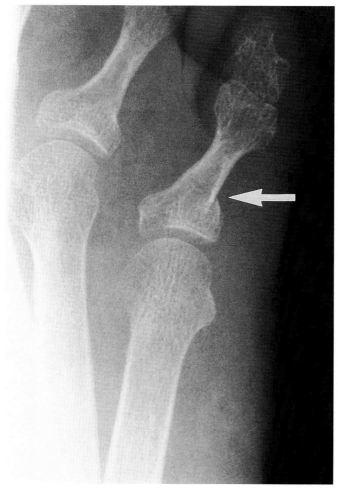

Fig. 4.55. Fracture of the fifth proximal phalanx. AP radiograph. The fracture line is difficult to see, but a break in the lateral cortex is evident (arrow), and there is valgus alignment at the fracture site.

fracture. It must be remembered that accessory ossicles are often multipartite. Fractures can be distinguished from multipartite ossicles when the fragments are irregular and poorly marginated.

FOOT FRACTURES IN CHILDREN

Fractures of the growth plate are discussed in Chapter 3. They occur in the foot less commonly than the ankle, but they may be seen in the metatarsals or phalanges. Greenstick (incomplete) fractures are also seen.

Salter–Harris fractures of the distal phalanx of the first toe (Fig. 4.57) merit special consideration. These fractures are generally due to plantar flexion of the toe ('stubbed toe'). There is apex posterior angulation at the fracture site, and the bone protrudes through the germinal matrix of the nail to create an open fracture. Seeding of the fracture through this open wound leads to osteomyelitis.[73]

The epiphysis of the first proximal phalanx may be bipartite, and this normal variant should be distinguished from Salter–Harris fractures.[74] The vertically oriented accessory center of ossification at the base of the fifth metatarsal must also be distinguished from tuberosity fractures, which are transversely oriented.

The 'bunk-bed' fracture is a fracture of the base of the first metatarsal extending through the epiphysis.[74,75] As its name implies, it is caused by a fall or jump from a height. There may be an associated injury to the ligaments between the first cuneiform and the first metatarsal epiphysis.[75]

Toddlers may develop stress fractures of the calcaneus or cuboid which are not radiographically evident. Diagnosis can be made by bone scan,[75,76] combined with history of trauma. Osteomyelitis has a similar appearance on bone scan, and if the diagnosis is in doubt an MRI can be performed to confirm the presence of a fracture line.

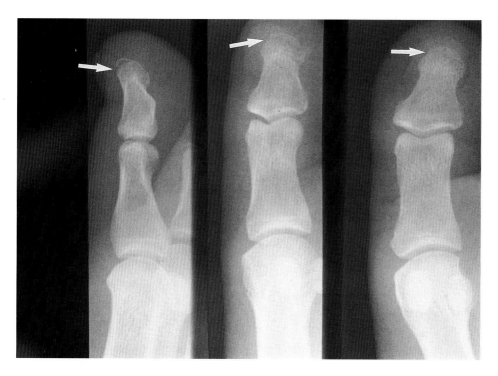

Fig. 4.56. Ungual tuft fracture of the first toe. Lateral, oblique, and AP radiographs. The nondisplaced fracture of the ungual tuft (arrow) is best seen on the lateral view.

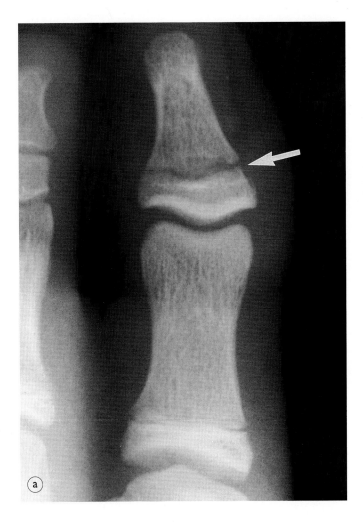

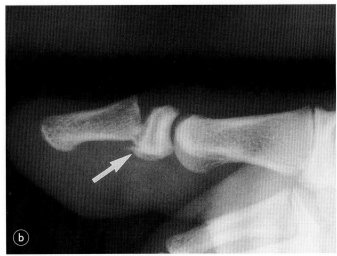

Fig. 4.57. Salter-Harris type II fracture of the first distal phalanx, secondary to 'stubbed toe'. **a.** AP radiograph shows widening of the physis (arrow). **b.** Lateral radiograph shows apex dorsal angulation at the fracture site. A small metaphyseal fragment (arrow) is present at the plantar aspect of the phalanx.

REFERENCES

1. Loomer R, Fisher C, Lloyd-Smith R, Sisler J, Cooney T. Osteochondral lesions of the talus. *Am J Sports Med* 1993; **21:**13–9.

2. Flick AB, Gould N. Osteochondritis dissecans of the talus (transchondral fractures of the talus): review of the literature and new surgical approach for medial dome lesions. *Foot Ankle* 1985; **5:**165–85.

3. Bosien WR, Staples OS, Russell SW. Residual disability following acute ankle sprains. *J Bone Joint Surg [Am]* 1955; **37A:**1237–43.

4. Anderson IF, Crichton KJ, Grattan-Smith T, et al. Osteochondral fractures of the dome of the talus. *J Bone Joint Surg [Am]* 1989; **70A:**1143–52.

5. Pettine KA, Morrey BF. Osteochondral fractures of the talus: a long-term follow-up. *J Bone Joint Surg [Br]* 1987; **69B:**89–92.

6. Canale T, Belding RH. Osteochondral lesions of the talus. *J Bone Joint Surg [Am]* 1980; **62A:**97–102.

7. Mannis CI. Transchondral fracture of the dome of the talus sustained during weight training. *Am J Sports Med* 1983; **11:**354–6.

8. Berndt AL, Harty M. Transchondral fractures (osteochondritis dissecans) of the talus. *J Bone Joint Surg [Am]* 1959; **41A:**988–1020.

9. Shea MP, Manoli A. Osteochondral lesions of the talar dome. *Foot Ankle* 1993; **14:**48–55.

10. Dipaola JD, Nelson DW, Colville MR. Characterizing osteochondral lesions by magnetic resonance imaging. *J Arthroscopy Rel Surg* 1991; **7:**101–4.

11. Pritsch M, Horoshovski H, Farine I. Arthroscopic treatment of osteochondral lesions of the talus. *J Bone Joint Surg [Am]* 1986; **68A:** 862–5.

12. Burkus JK, Sella EJ, Southwick WO. Occult injuries of the talus diagnosed by bone scan and tomography. *Foot Ankle* 1984; **4:**316–24.

13. Zinman C, Reis ND. Osteochondritis dissecans of the talus: use of the high resolution computed tomography scanner. *Acta Orthop Scand* 1982; **53:**697–700.

14. Bauer M, Jonsson K, Linden B. Osteochondritis dissecans of the ankle: a twenty year follow-up study. *J Bone Joint Surg [Br]* 1987; **69B:**93–6.

15. Mesgarzadeh M, Sapega AA, Bonakdarpour A, et al. Osteochondritis dissecans: analysis of mechanical stability with radiography, scintigraphy, and MR imaging. *Radiology* 1987; **165:**775–80.

16. De Smet AA, Fisher DR, Burnstein MI, Graf BK, Lange RH. Value of MR imaging in staging osteochondral lesions of the talus (osteochondritis dissecans): results in 14 patients. *Am J Roentgenol* 1990; **154:**555–8.

17. Yulish BS, Mulopulos GP, Goodfellow DB, et al. MR Imaging of

osteochondral lesions of talus. *J Comput Assist Tomog* 1987; **11:**296–301.

18. Kenwright J, Taylor RG. Major injuries of the talus. *J Bone Joint Surg [Br]* 1970; **52B:**36–48.

19. Lorentzen JE, Christensen SB, Krosgoe O, Sneppen O. Fractures of the neck of the talus. *Acta Orthop Scand* 1977; **48:**115–20.

20. Daniels TR, Smith JW. Talar neck fractures. *Foot Ankle* 1993; **14:**225–34.

21. Hawkins LG. Fractures of the neck of the talus. *J Bone Joint Surg [Am]* 1970; **52A:**991–1002.

22. Canale JB, Kelly FB. Fractures of the neck of the talus: Long-term evaluation of seventy-one cases. *J Bone Joint Surg [Am]* 1978; **60A:**143–56.

23. Peterson L, Goldie IF, Irstam L. Fracture of the neck of the talus. A clinical study. *Acta Orthop Scand* 1977; **48:**696–706.

24. Mukherjee S, Pringle RM, Baxter AD. Fracture of the lateral process of the talus: a report of thirteen cases. *J Bone Joint Surg [Br]* 1974; **56B:**263–73.

25. El-Khoury GY, Yousefzadeh DK, Mulligan GM, Moore TE. Subtalar dislocation. *Skeletal Radiol* 1982; **8:**99–103.

26. Miller WE. Pain and impairment considerations following treatment of disruptive os calcis fractures. *Clin Orthop* 1983; **177:**82–6.

27. James ETR, Hunter GA. The dilemma of painful old os calcis fractures. *Clin Orthop* 1983; **177:**112–5.

28. McLaughlin HL. Treatment of late complications after os calcis fractures. *Clin Orthop* 1963; **30:**111–5.

29. Rosenberg ZS, Feldman F, Singson RD, Price GJ. Peroneal tendon injury associated with calcaneal fractures: CT findings. *Am J Roentgenol* 1987; **149:**125–9.

30. Mallik AR, Chase MD, Lee PC, Whitelaw GP. Calcaneal fracture-dislocation with entrapment of the medial neurovascular bundle: a Case report. *Foot Ankle* 1993; **14:**411–3.

31. Bradley SA, Davies AM. Computed tomographic assessment of old calcaneal fractures. *Br J Radiol* 1990; **63:**926–33.

32. Saint-Isister JF. Calcaneo-fibular abutment following crush fracture of the calcaneus. *J Bone Joint Surg [Br]* 1974; **56B:**274–8.

33. Essex-Lopresti P. Fractures of the os calcis. The mechanism, reduction technique and results in fractures of the os calcis. *Br J Surg* 1952; **39:**395–419.

34. Gilmer PW, Herzenberg J, Frank JL, et al. Computerized tomographic analysis of acute calcaneal fractures. *Foot Ankle* 1986; **6:**184–93.

35. Crosby LA, Fitzgibbons T. Computerized tomography scanning of acute intra-articular fractures of the calcaneus: a new classification system. *J Bone Joint Surg [Am]* 1990; **72A:**852–9.

36. Sanders R, Hansen ST Jr, McReynolds IS. Trauma to the calcaneus and its tendon. In: Jahss MH (ed). *Disorders of the Foot and Ankle*, 2nd edn. (WB Saunders: Philadelphia, 1991), 2326–54.

37. Giachino AA, Uhthoff HK. Current concepts review – intra-articular fractures of the calcaneus. *J Bone Joint Surg [Am]* 1989; **71A:**784–7.

38. Eastwood DM, Gregg PJ, Atkins RM. Intra-articular fractures of the calcaneum: Part I: Pathological anatomy and classification. *J Bone Joint Surg [Br]* 1993; **75B:**183–8.

39. Paley D. Fractures of the calcaneus. In: Gould JS (ed). *Operative Foot Surgery*, 2nd edn. (WB Saunders: Philadelphia, 1994, 429–31.

40. Sanders R, Fortin P, DiPasqueale T, Walling A. Operative treatment in 120 displaced intra-articular calcaneus fractures – results using a prognostic computed tomography scan classification. *Clin Orthop* 1993; **290:**87–95.

41. Rowe CR, Sakellarides HT, Freeman PA, Sorbie C. Fractures of the os calcis: a long-term follow-up study of 146 patients. *JAMA* 1963; **184:**920–3.

42. Kathol MH, El-Khoury GY, Moore TE, Marsh JL. Calcaneal insufficiency avulsion fractures in patients with diabetes mellitus. *Radiology* 1991; **180:**725–9.

43. Pelletier JP, Kanat IO. Avulsion fracture of the calcaneus at the origin of the abductor hallucis muscle. *J Foot Surg* 1990; **29:**268–71.

44. Norfray JF, Rogers LF, Adamo GP, et al. Common calcaneal avulsion fracture. *Am J Roentgenol* 1980; **134:**119–23.

45. Renfrew DL, El-Khoury GY. Anterior process fractures of the calcaneus. *Skeletal Radiol* 1985; **14:**121–5.

46. Darby RE. Stress fractures of the os calcis. *JAMA* 1967; **200:**1183–4.

47. Torg JS, Pavlov H, Cooley LH et al. Stress fracture of the tarsal navicular. *J Bone Joint Surg [Am]* 1982; **64A:**700–12.

48. Kiss ZS, Khan KM, Fuller PJ. Stress fractures of the tarsal navicular bone: CT findings in 55 cases. *Am J Roentgenol* 1993; **160:**111–5.

49. Khan KM, Fuller PJ, Brukner PD, et al. Outcome of conservative and surgical management of navicular stress fracture in athletes. *Am J Sports Med* 1992; **6:**657–66.

50. Pavlov I, Torg JS, Freiberger HH. Tarsal navicular stress fractures: radiographic evaluation. *Radiology* 1983; **148:**641–5.

51. Steinbronn DJ, Bennett GL, Kay DB. The use of magnetic resonance imaging in the diagnosis of stress fractures of the foot and ankle: four case reports. *Foot Ankle* 1994; **15:**80–3.

52. Hermel MB, Gershon-Cohen J. The nutcracker fracture of the cuboid caused by indirect violence. *Radiology* 1953; **60:**850–4.

53. Howie CR, Hooper G, Hughes SPF. Occult midtarsal subluxation. *Clin Orthop* 1986; **208:**206–9.

54. Hardcastle PH, Reschauer R, Kutscha–Lissberg E, Schoffman W. Injuries to the tarsometatarsal joint: Incidence, classification and treatment. *J Bone Joint Surg [Br]* 1982; **64B:**349–56.

55. Faciszewki T, Burks RT, Manaster BJ. Subtle injuries of the Lisfranc joint. *J Bone Joint Surg [Am]* 1990; **72A:** 1519–22.

56. Myerson MS, Fisher RT, Burgess AR, Kenzora JE. Fracture dislocations of the tarsometatarsal joints: end results correlated with pathology and treatment. *Foot Ankle* 1986; **6:**225–42.

57. Arntz CT, Hansen ST. Dislocations and fracture dislocations of the tarsometatarsal joints. *Orthop Clin North Am* 1987; **18:**105–14.

58. Norfray JF, Geline RA, Steinberg RI, Galinski AW, Gilula LA. Subtleties of Lisfranc fracture-dislocations. *Am J Roentgenol* 1981; **137:**1151-6.

59. Stein RE. Radiological aspects of the tarsometatarsal joints. *Foot Ankle* 1983; **3:**286–9.

60. Goiney RC, Connell DG, Nichols DM. CT evaluation of tarsometatarsal fracture-dislocation injuries. *Am J Roentgenol* 1985; **144:**985–90.

61. Micheli LJ, Sohn RS, Solomon R. Stress fractures of the second metatarsal involving Lisfranc's joint in ballet dancers: a new overuse injury of the foot. *J Bone Joint Surg [Am]* 1985; **67A:** 1372–5.

62. Lawrence SJ, Botte MJ. Jones' fractures and related fractures of the fifth metatarsal. *Foot Ankle* 1993; **14:**358–65.

63. Jones R. Fracture of the base of the fifth metatarsal bone by indirect violence. *Ann Surg* 1902; **35:**697–700.

64. Richli WR, Rosenthal DI. Avulsion fracture of the fifth metatarsal: Experimental study of pathomechanics. *Am J Roentgenol* 1984; **143:**889–93.

65. Hansen ST. Foot injuries. In: Browner BD, Jupiter JB, Levine AM, Trafton PG (eds). *Skeletal Trauma.* (WB Saunders: Philadelphia, 1992), 1959-91.

66. Taylor JA, Sartoris DJ, Huang GS, Resnick DL. Painful conditions affecting the first metatarsal sesamoid bones. *Radiographics* 1993; **13:**817–30.

67. Jahss MH. The sesamoids of the hallux. *Clin Orthop* 1981; **157:**88–97.

68. Yao L, Do HM, Cracchiolo A, Farahani K. Plantar plate of the foot: findings on conventional arthrography and MR imaging. *Am J Roentgenol* 1994; **163:**641–4.

69. Coughlin MJ. Subluxation and dislocation of the second metatarsophalangeal joint. *Orthop Clin North Am* 1989; **20:**535–51.

70. Karpman RR, McCollum MS III. Arthrography of the metatarsophalangeal joint. *Foot Ankle* 1988; **9:**125–9.

71. Gould JS. Metatarsalgia. *Orthop Clin North Am* 1989; **20:**553–62.

72. Thompson FM, Hamilton WG. Problems of the second metatarsophalangeal joint. *Orthopedics* 1987; **10:**83–9.

73. Pinckney LE, Currarino G, Kennedy LA. The stubbed great toe: a cause of occult compound fracture and infection. *Radiology* 1981; **138:**375–7.

74. Karasick D. Fractures and dislocations of the foot. *Semin Roentgenol* 1994; **29:**152–75.

75. Johnson GF. Pediatric Lisfranc injury. 'Bunk bed' fracture. *Am J Roentgenol* 1981; **137:**1041–4.

75. Moss EH, Carty H. Scintigraphy in the diagnosis of occult fractures of the calcaneus. *Skeletal Radiol* 1990; **19:**575–7.

76. Blumberg K, Patterson RJ. The toddler's cuboid fracture. *Radiology* 1991; **179:**93–4.

5. ARTHRITIS
JULIA R CRIM, RICHARD H GOLD
AND ANDREA CRACCHIOLO III

A precise diagnosis of the type of arthritis present in a patient can usually be made on the basis of careful analysis of the plain radiographs. A number of criteria are used to make the radiographic diagnosis:

- whether the arthritis is monoarticular or polyarticular (Table 5.1);

Table 5.1. Monoarticular arthritides.

Almost always monoarticular	infection
	pigmented villonodular synovitis
	synovial chondromatosis
Usually monoarticular	neuropathic joint
	avascular necrosis
Sometimes monoarticular	osteoarthritis
	early rheumatoid arthritis

- which joints are involved;
- whether certain radiographic features are present – decreased bone density, altered alignment, osteophytes, erosions, subchondral cyst formation, periosteal new bone, cartilage loss, joint effusions, and soft-tissue calcifications (Table 5.2).

It should be remembered that the presence of one or more of the radiographic features listed above does not necessarily imply the presence of arthritis. For instance, the altered alignment seen in hallux valgus (bunion deformity) is usually due to mechanical factors; osteoporosis may be due to age, disuse, or reflex sympathetic dystrophy as well as other causes; and there are many causes of periosteal new bone. The entire radiologic picture must be considered to make the diagnosis. Radiographs of the contralateral foot, the hand and wrist, or the spine are often useful in making a differential diagnosis, since various arthritides tend to have charateristic sites of involvement in these regions. When the radiographic diagnosis is in doubt, laboratory data and history almost always allow distinction between two arthritides that have an overlapping appearance

Table 5.2. Radiographic characteristics of arthritis.

Characteristic	Type of arthritis						
	Degenerative joint disease	Rheumatoid arthritis	Reiter's*	Charcot	Infection	Gout	HADD
Joint narrowing – uniform	–	+++	+++	–	+++	–	–
Joint narrowing – nonuniform	+++	–	–	+++	–	+	+
Subluxations	++	++	+	+++	–	–	–
Osteophytes	+++	–	–	+++	–	+	–
Erosions	–	+++	+++	+	+++	++	–
Cysts	++	++	–	++	++	++	–
Osteoporosis	–	++	+	–	++	–	–
Effusions	–	+++	++	+++	+++	+++	++
Periosteal new bone	–	–	+++	+++	++	+	–
Soft tissue calcification	–	–	–	++	–	+	+++

Key: – this finding is generally absent
+ this finding is sometimes present
++ this finding is often present
+++ this finding is almost always present
*same features are found in psoriatic arthritis and, less commonly, in ankylosing spondylitis

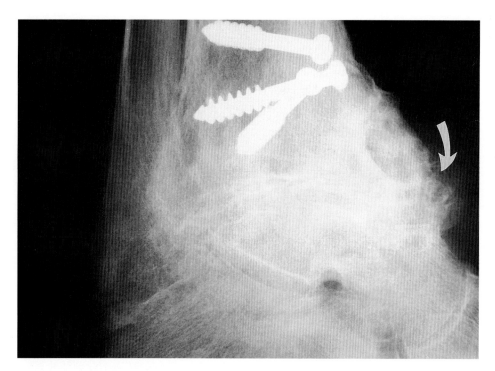

Fig. 5.1. Severe post-traumatic osteoarthritis of the ankle. Mortise view radiograph. Three screws remain in place from prior fixation of ankle fracture. The subarticular bone is sclerotic. The joint space is severely narrowed, the talar dome is flattened, and large osteophytes anteriorly (arrows) result in an almost immobile joint.

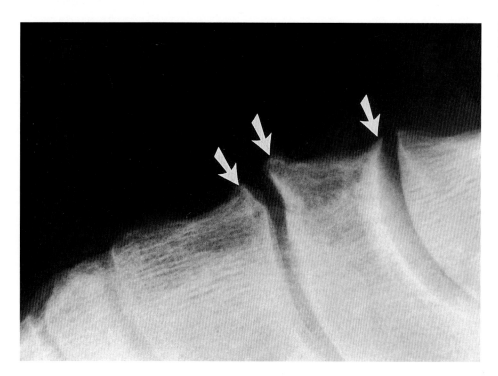

Fig. 5.2. Osteoarthritis of the midfoot. Lateral radiograph. There are small dorsal osteophytes (arrows) at the talonavicular and naviculocuneiform articulations.

radiographically. In order to utilize the radiograph as an independent diagnostic test, however, it is best for the radiologist to review radiographs before receiving clinical information about the patient.

The American Rheumatism Association has divided arthritis and rheumatism into thirteen categories based on etiology.[1] For radiographic analysis, arthritis is usually divided into four main categories:

- degenerative;
- inflammatory;
- metabolic; and
- miscellaneous.

The inflammatory arthritides include rheumatoid arthritis, the seronegative spondyloarthropathies, and infectious arthritis, as well as the articular manifestations of connective tissue diseases such as progressive systemic sclerosis. Metabolic arthritides include those due to crystal deposition, hyperparathyroidism, hemodialysis, and acromegaly. Miscellaneous entities include neuropathic joint disease, pigmented villonodular synovitis, sarcoid and avascular necrosis. Infectious arthritis is discussed

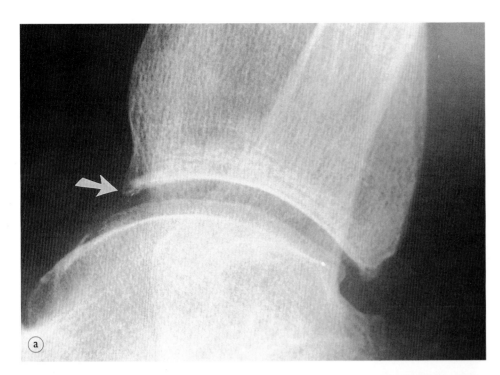

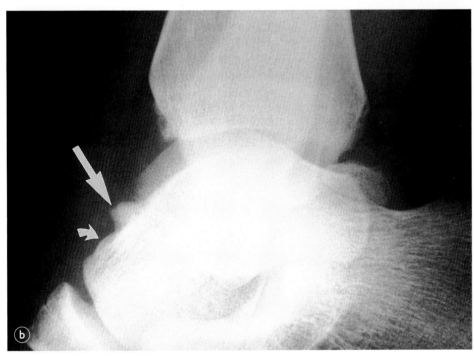

Fig. 5.3. Osteophytes which can cause dorsal impingement of the ankle. **a.** Lateral radiograph shows osteophyte (arrow) at anterior aspect of tibial articular surface as well as small posterior osteophytes. The attachment of the joint capsule is located slightly more superiorly, away from the articular surface; a spur at the capsular insertion can also develop, but is not thought to be significant. **b.** Lateral radiograph shows large osteophyte (arrow) at talar neck in a different patient, with pes cavus and dorsiflexion impingement at ankle. The dorsal ridge of the talus (curved arrow) is located slightly distal to the osteophyte, and is a normal finding which can be quite prominent.

with osteomyelitis in Chapter 6, while arthritides associated with hyperparathyroidism, hemodialysis, and acromegaly are discussed in Chapter 12.

DEGENERATIVE ARTHRITIS

The suffix -itis implies inflammation, and degenerative changes in a joint are not inflammatory in nature. For this reason, some authors employ the term osteoarthrosis rather than osteoarthri-

tis. Since the terms degenerative arthritis and osteoarthritis are both well-entrenched terms, they are probably preferable, despite their inaccuracy.

Pathogenesis

Degenerative arthritis is the result of wearing away of cartilage. The damage to cartilage is most severe where the mechanical stress on the joint is greatest, and therefore cartilage loss is not

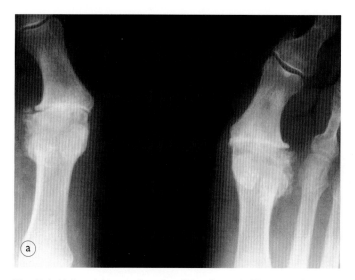

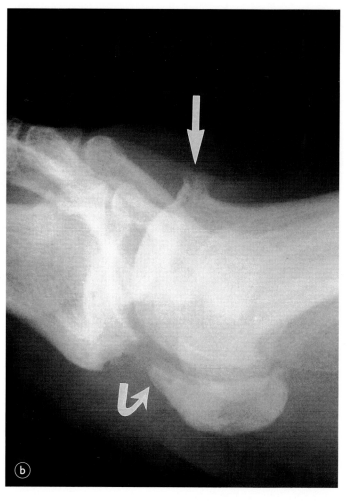

Fig. 5.4. Hallux rigidus. **a.** Standing AP radiograph. There is a flattened contour of the first metatarsal heads bilaterally, which predisposes a patient to hallux rigidus. Joint spaces of the first metatarsophalangeal joints are narrowed, and prominent lateral osteophytes are present. **b.** Standing lateral radiograph. Dorsal osteophyte (straight arrow) limits dorsiflexion of the metatarsophalangeal joint. Note also the osteoarthritis between the sesamoids of and the head of the first metatarsal; curved arrow points to a sesamoid osteophyte.

uniform across the entire joint. Both cartilage and bone undergo a reparative response.[2] Cartilage proliferates at the periphery of the joint and then ossifies, forming osteophytes. Beneath the articular cartilage, reactive new bone is laid down, resulting in subchondral sclerosis. Stresses on the joint create microfractures of the subchondral bone, resulting in flattening of the articular surface. Subchondral radiolucencies may develop. They contain fluid or fibrous tissue, and are commonly called subchondral cysts, although, unlike true cysts, they do not have an epithelial lining. The term 'geode' has also been used to describe these subchondral lucencies, as an analogy to the cavities found in geode rocks. Loose bodies, sometimes called joint mice, develop from articular cartilage that breaks off into the joint. If the cartilage fragment ossifies, the loose body can be seen on plain radiographs.

Degenerative arthritis may be classified as either primary or secondary. Primary generalized osteoarthritis is 'normal' joint wear, primarily in the interphalangeal joints and first carpometacarpal joints of the hands in elderly patients. Secondary arthritis is joint degeneration resulting from or superimposed on another underlying condition. For example, fractures that result in articular incongruity lead to secondary osteoarthritis. Secondary osteoarthritis can occur in a joint initially damaged by inflammatory arthritis.

Distribution of Osteoarthritis

The foot is subjected to a high level of mechanical stress, but osteoarthritis of the foot is less frequent than might be expected. Secondary osteoarthritis is most commonly seen in the first metatarsophalangeal joint. It is also seen in the ankle and subtalar joints, where it can be a result of fracture, sprain, or chronic overuse (Fig. 5.1). Osteoarthritis of the midfoot is usually mild (Fig. 5.2), although severe osteoarthritis can develop as a result of chronic rupture of the posterior tibial tendon.

Anterior Ankle Impingement

Osteoarthritis of the ankle may lead to anterior ankle impingement. Patients with anterior impingement have chronic ankle pain and limited dorsiflexion, with difficulty climbing stairs, walking uphill, or running.[3–5] The condition may be seen in any athlete, especially those such as dancers and basketball players,[5] whose sport involves jumping. Osteophytes are seen at the anterior margin of the tibia or the anterior talar neck or both (Fig. 5.3). The presence of spurs does not necessarily indicate symptomatic impingement, even in athletes.[6] Anterior ankle impingement may also occur because of soft tissue abnormalities (see Chapter 8).

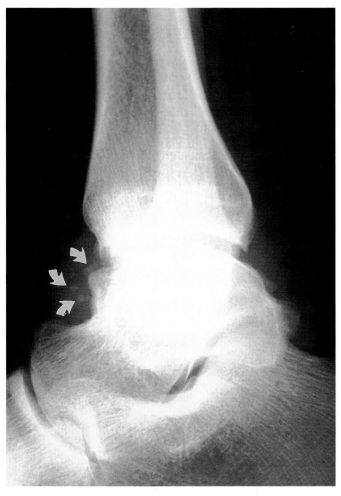

Fig. 5.5. Intra-articular loose bodies. Lateral radiograph. Several small osseous loose bodies (arrows) are present anteriorly within the ankle joint in this patient with post-traumatic osteoarthritis.

Impingement between the lateral process of the talus and the fibular tip may be caused by osteoarthritis,[7] and this will limit eversion and inversion of the hindfoot.

Hallux Rigidus

Osteoarthritis limited to the metatarsophalangeal joint of the great toe may restrict joint motion, a condition known as hallux rigidus (Fig. 5.4). After hallux valgus, it is the second most common abnormality of the first metatarsophalangeal joint.[8] Hallux rigidus causes pain with walking because it restricts dorsiflexion of the hallux. The pain is exacerbated by sports such as tennis and basketball in which there is a strong push-off of the forefoot.[8] People with a relatively flat first metatarsal head, which limits medial and lateral motion, are prone to develop this condition.[9] It may also be caused by repetitive trauma, especially in patients with a pronated foot, hyperextension of the first metatarsal, or an abnormally long first metatarsal.[9]

Radiographic Findings

Nonuniform joint space loss is the first radiographic finding of osteoarthritis. Osteophytes form at the margin of the joint, and subsequently sclerosis of the subarticular bone develops (see Figs 5.1–5.4). Subchondral cysts can occur in the foot and ankle, but are less comon than in other joints such as the knee and hip. Intra-articular loose bodies may develop (Fig. 5.5). Chondrocalcinosis due to osteoarthritis is rare in the foot and ankle.

Erosive osteoarthritis

Erosive or inflammatory osteoarthritis occurs primarily in middle-aged women and affects the interphalangeal joints. It is generally seen in the hands, and is rare in the foot (Fig. 5.6). Erosions

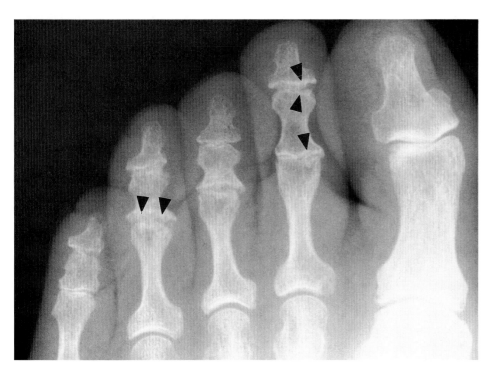

Fig. 5.6. Erosive osteoarthritis. AP radiograph of the toes. Small, centrally located erosions are present at multiple interphalangeal joints. Several of these are marked with arrowheads. This patient also had severe involvement of the interphalangeal joints of the hands.

occur in the central portion of the joint, a feature that differentiates them from the marginal erosions seen at the bases of the phalanges in psoriatic arthritis. Fusion of a joint may occur.

Differential diagnosis

Early neuropathic joint destruction appears similar to osteoarthritis but has a more rapid progression, and joint subluxation is more severe. Rheumatoid arthritis, like osteoarthritis, may feature subchondral cysts, but in rheumatoid arthritis, joint space loss is uniform, and osteophytes and bony sclerosis are absent. Subchondral cysts and sometimes osteophytes are present in gout, but gouty cysts are often para-articular rather than intra-articular, and unlike degenerative arthritis the joint space is preserved until late in the course of the disease. Calcium pyrophosphate dihydrate deposition disease (CPPD) tends to involve the talonavicular and tibiotalar joints, and has similar radiographic features to osteoarthritis; both CPPD and osteoarthritis may exhibit chondrocalcinosis, but chondrocalcinosis is a much more prominent feature of CPPD. Characteristic findings of chondrocalcinosis in the wrist, knee or pubic symphysis suggest CPPD.

Treatment

Treatment of osteoarthritis is usually aimed at symptomatic relief, using nonsteroidal anti-inflammatory medications. Intra-articular injection of steroids may be used. Bone spurs that are causing impingement of a joint can be surgically excised. Severe osteoarthritis, especially of the first metatarsophalangeal joint, may require surgical fusion or in some cases a double stem silicone implant.[10]

INFLAMMATORY ARTHROPATHIES

Rheumatoid Arthritis

Rheumatoid arthritis is an inflammatory arthritis with a predilection for the small joints of the hands and feet. It is two to four times more common in women than men. The first symptoms and signs tend to present between the ages of 25 and 55. Rheumatoid arthritis may cause systemic abnormalities, such as pleuritis and pleural effusions, pulmonary nodules, and interstitial fibrosis.

Pathogenesis

The etiology of rheumatoid arthritis is still unknown. There is an hereditary predisposition and a known association with the HLA-DR4 histocompatibility antigen. The target tissue is the synovium of joints, bursae, and tendon sheaths. The synovium becomes inflamed, hyperemic, and hypertrophied. A granulation tissue known as pannus develops. In the joints, pannus erodes the underlying cartilage and bone, while in tendon sheaths it can lead to tendon rupture. Joint effusions of patients with relatively acute disease contain large numbers of white blood cells.

Criteria for diagnosis

The relationship between clinical tests for rheumatoid factor and rheumatoid arthritis is variable. The presence of rheumatoid

Table 5.3. 1987 revised criteria for rheumatoid arthritis. (From Arnett et al.[12])

Morning stiffness for at least 1 hr for 6 weeks or more
Swelling of 3 or more joints for 6 weeks or more
Swelling of wrist, MCP or PIP joints for 6 weeks or more
Symmetrical swelling
Hand X-ray changes
Subcutaneous nodules
Rheumatoid factor
The presence of any four of these seven criteria yields 93% sensitivity and 90% specificity.

factor (RF) does not necessarily indicate rheumatoid arthritis, as RF can be positive in a low titer in elderly patients who do not have rheumatoid arthritis. Patients with rheumatoid arthritis generally will have a positive serum RF with a titer of 1:320 or greater,[11] but RF can be absent early in the course of the disease. There is also a variant form of the disease, seronegative

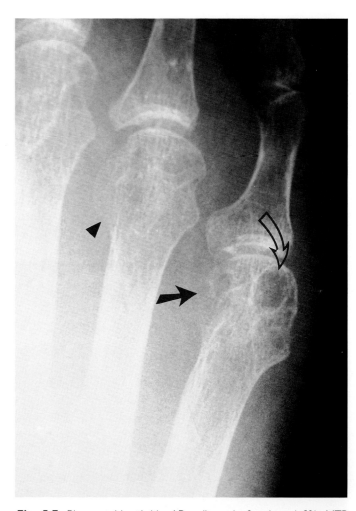

Fig. 5.7. Rheumatoid arthritis. AP radiograph, fourth and fifth MTP joints. Juxta-articular osteoporosis is seen. There is destruction of the medial cortex of the fifth metatarsal head due to extensive erosions (solid arrow). A subchondral cyst is also seen (open arrow). A very early erosion is present in the bare area of the fourth metatarsal head (arrowhead).

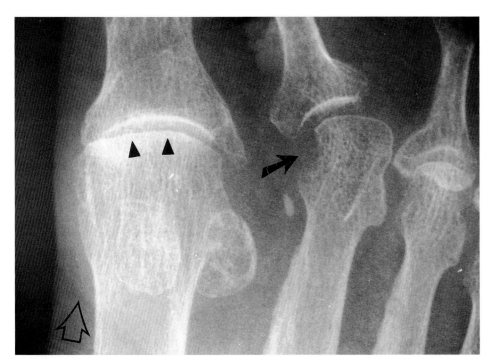

Fig. 5.8. Rheumatoid arthritis. AP radiograph of first through third metatarsophalangeal joints. There is a large marginal erosion of the second metatarsal head (solid arrow). The joint is subluxed. No distinct erosions are evident in the first metatarsophalangeal joint, but the joint space is narrowed and the articular cortex of the first metatarsal head appears thin and serrated (arrowheads), compared to the smooth, normal-appearing cortex of the base of the proximal phalanx. Soft-tissue prominence medially (open arrow) is due to bursitis.

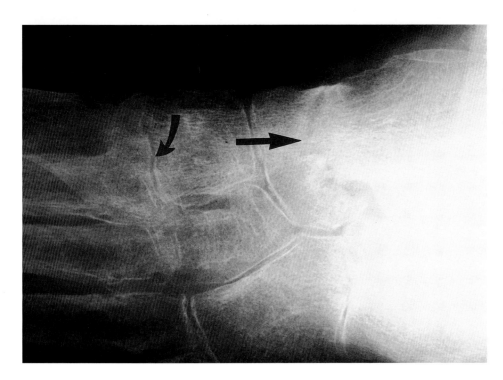

Fig. 5.9. Rheumatoid arthritis of the hind and midfoot. Oblique radiograph. There is marked osteoporosis. Joint space narrowing is evident throughout. Curved arrow points to narrowed tarsometatarsal joint. There is an insufficiency fracture of the neck of the talus (straight arrow).

rheumatoid arthritis,[11] in which seropositivity fails to develop. Seronegative rheumatoid arthritis usually has a milder course than seropositive arthritis, but it cannot be distinguished from seropositive cases by radiographic criteria.

The current diagnositc criteria of the American College of Rheumatology are based on the American Rheumatism Association (ARA) 1987 revised criteria[12] (Table 5.3). Although these criteria refer only to the presence of characteristic radiographic changes in the hand, changes in the feet may precede those in the hands.[13–16] Thould and Simon[13] studied hand and foot radiographs in 105 patients who met ARA criteria for rheumatoid arthritis. Of these patients, 91% had abnormal radiographs. The patients with negative radiographs of both the hand and the foot all had early disease. Sixteen percent of patients had abnormal foot radiographs and normal hand radiographs, but no patients had normal foot radiographs in the presence of positive findings in the hands. Brook and Corbett[14] found that, of 94 patients with early rheumatoid arthritis, 36% had their first erosions in the feet, compared to 16% with the first erosions in the hands. The remainder of the patients had simultaneous development of erosions in the hands and feet.

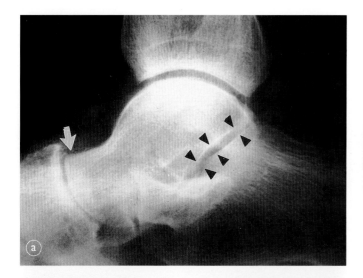

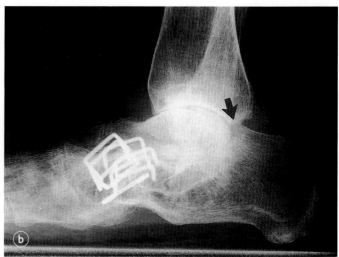

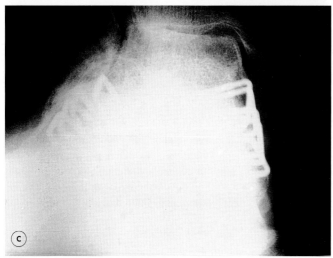

Fig. 5.10. Hindfoot deformities in a patient with longstanding rheumatoid arthritis. **a.** Standing lateral radiograph prior to surgery shows plantar subluxation of the head of the talus (arrow) due to posterior tibial tendon rupture (see Chapter 7). The posterior subtalar joint (arrowheads) appears normal at this time. Flatfoot deformity was treated with triple arthrodesis. **b.** Standing lateral radiograph 6 years later. The posterior subtalar joint can no longer be discerned, because of the severe articular destruction. There is anterior subluxation of the talus relative to the calcaneus, and collapse of the hindfoot. The posterior malleolus of the tibia (arrow) is resting on the calcaneus. Joint narrowing due to rheumatoid arthritis is also seen in the tibiotalar joint. **c.** Standing AP radiograph of the ankle at the same time as (b). Valgus deformity of the hindfoot is present, caused partly by arthritis of the ankle, and partly by subtalar joint disease.

Robust rheumatoid arthritis

Robust rheumatoid arthritis is a form of the disease in which patients are not as impaired functionally as the typical rheumatoid patient, and bone density is relatively well preserved.[17] Radiographically, these patients often have the cystic variant of rheumatoid arthritis.[18]

Distribution of rheumatoid arthritis

Although patients with rheumatoid arthritis develop bilaterally symmetric involvement of both feet and hands, early in the course of the disease as many as 28% of patients may have involvement of one side only.[13] The fourth or fifth metatarsophalangeal joint is almost always the first joint of the foot to be involved (Fig. 5.7). The remainder of the metatarsophalangeal joints eventually are also frequently involved (Fig. 5.8). When rheumatoid arthritis affects the first metatarsophalangeal joint, it usually causes erosions of the sesamoids as well. Except for the interphalangeal joint of the great toe, which may undergo early erosion, the interphalangeal joints tend to be spared.

Involvement of the ankle, hindfoot and midfoot is common (Figs 5.9, 5.10). A study of 99 patients with rheumatoid arthritis found that 93 had had symptoms involving the foot and ankle.[19] Severe involvement of the heel is less common than with seronegative spondyloarthropathies.

Soft-tissue abnormalities

The inflammatory process of rheumatoid arthritis involves not only joint synovium, but the synovium of tendon sheaths and bursae, leading to tenosynovitis, tendon rupture, and bursitis. The most commonly ruptured tendon in the foot is the posterior tibial, but other tendons are affected as well (see Chapter 7). Tenosynovitis of the extrinsic flexor tendons can cause tarsal tunnel syndrome (see Chapter 8). The pre-Achilles bursa is commonly involved with rheumatoid arthritis (Fig. 5.11). Synovial diverticulae may develop, reflecting the marked proliferation of synovial fluid and pannus.[20]

Deformities of the foot

Foot deformities are very common in rheumatoid arthritis. Imbalance of the intrinsic muscles of the foot causes widening of the forefoot, claw toe deformities and hallux valgus[19,21] (Figs

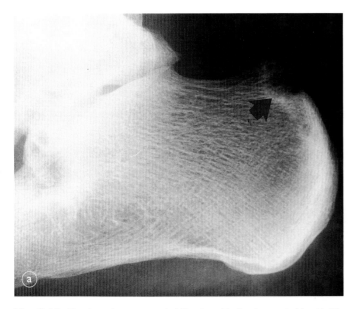

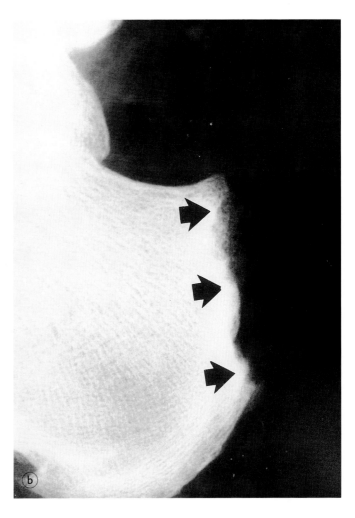

Fig. 5.11. Erosion due to pre-Achilles bursitis in rheumatoid arthritis. **a.** Lateral radiograph. There is a small erosion (arrow) of the superior margin of the posterior process of the calcaneus. **b.** Lateral radiograph in another patient with more severe involvement of the pre-Achilles bursa. Erosions (arrows) are seen extending along posterior aspect of the calcaneus to the insertion of the Achilles tendon.

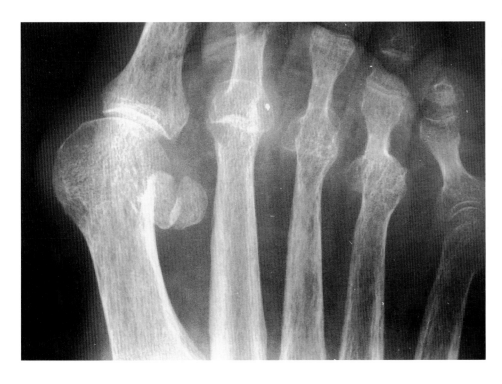

Fig. 5.12. Deformities of the toes due to rheumatoid arthritis. Standing AP radiograph of metatarsophalangeal joints. There is hallux valgus deformity. The second through fourth metatarsal heads are dislocated. Marginal erosions are seen on the metatarsal heads.

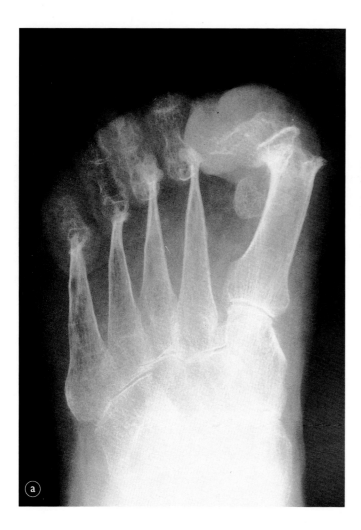

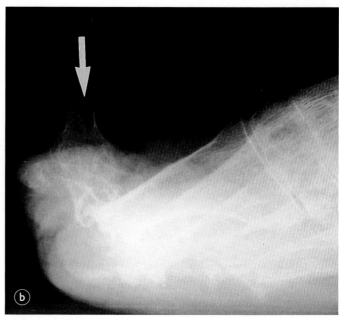

Fig. 5.13. Deformities of the toes due to rheumatoid arthritis. **a.** Standing AP radiograph of forefoot. There is severe destruction of all of the metatarsal heads, 'whittling' of the metatarsal shafts, and dislocations of the metatarsophalangeal joints. **b.** Standing lateral radiograph in the same patient shows 'cock-up' deformities of the toes. Arrow points to position of the tip of the first toe.

5.12, 5.13). Flatfoot deformity results both from arthritis of the hindfoot and from tibialis posterior tendon rupture (see Fig. 5.10).

Radiographic findings

Plain radiographs Rheumatoid arthritis may involve any joint of the foot and ankle (Figs 5.7–5.15). It tends to be bilaterally symmetric in distribution, although early in its course arthritis may be limited to one extremity. Rheumatoid arthritis usually causes juxta-articular osteoporosis; this occurs because of inflammatory hyperemia, disuse, and corticosteroid therapy. Osteoporosis becomes uniform and severe in long-standing rheumatoid arthritis, and can lead to insufficiency fractures (see Fig. 5.9). Robust rheumatoid arthritis is a well-described variant in which patients tend to maintain their bone density,[17,18] and therefore a lack of osteoporosis does not exclude rheumatoid arthritis (see Fig. 5.14).

The fourth and fifth metatarsal heads are usually the first joints affected in the foot (see Fig. 5.7). Erosions of the articular bone initially occur on the metatarsal head at the margin of the joint, in the 'bare area' that is not covered by cartilage. Joint effusions are present, but are not usually evident radiographically in the forefoot. Cartilage destruction is manifest radiographically as uniform loss of joint space. As the arthritis

progresses, joint destruction and ligamentous and tendinous abnormalities lead to subluxation and dislocation of the toes (see Figs 5.12, 5.13). Fibular deviation and 'cocking up' of the digits may be seen, but bony ankylosis is rare in the forefoot. The endstage of rheumatoid arthritis (or other inflammatory arthritis) in which there is severe bone destruction and deformities is known as 'arthritis mutilans' (see Fig. 5.13).

In the hindfoot and midfoot, erosions tend to be less prominent radiographically than in the forefoot, but uniform joint space narrowing is seen (see Fig. 5.9). Flatfoot deformity may develop (see Fig. 5.10). Bony ankylosis occasionally occurs late in the course of the disease.

Cystic rheumatoid arthritis Subchondral cysts rather than erosions may predominate[18, 22–24] (see Fig 5.15). This variant is known as cystic rheumatoid arthritis. Gubler et al[18] found that, out of 770 consecutive patients with rheumatoid arthritis, 70 had radiographs that showed subchondral cysts but no bone erosions. Patients with cystic rheumatoid arthritis often present clinically with robust rheumatoid arthritis (i.e. patients remain robust in health and are less likely to be functionally impaired). In these patients, bone density is preserved. The distribution of cysts is the same as that of erosions. Patients may have coexistent cysts and erosions.[22–24]

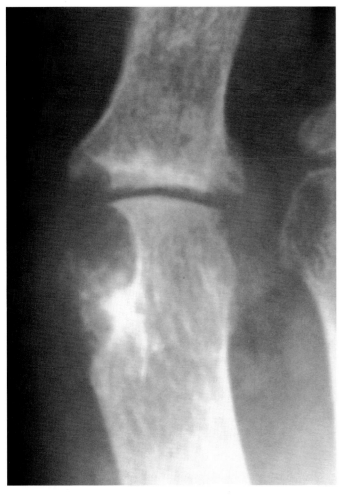

Fig. 5.14. Robust rheumatoid arthritis. AP radiograph of first MTP joint. Bone density is well-preserved. The joint space narrowing is a diagnostic clue that this is a case of rheumatoid arthritis, rather than gout, where the joint space is preserved until late in the course of the disease.

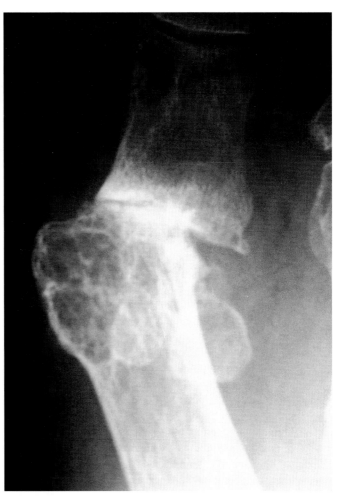

Fig. 5.15. Cystic rheumatoid arthritis. AP radiograph of first MTP joint. A large cyst occupies the medial aspect of the first metatarsal head.

Seronegative rheumatoid arthritis Efforts have been made to differentiate radiographically between seronegative and seropositive rheumatoid arthritis.[25-26] In general, seropositive disease has more severe findings, but in any one patient there are no reliable radiographic criteria that can differentiate between seropositive and seronegative disease.[25]

Plain radiographic findings of soft-tissue abnormalities Examination of plain radiographs should include scrutiny for findings that suggest bursitis or tendon abnormalities. Pre-Achilles bursitis causes erosion of the calcaneus above the calcaneal tuberosity (see Fig. 5.11), and inflammation of the plantar fascia causes erosion of the plantar aspect of the calcaneus. Rupture of the Achilles tendon results in blurring of the pre-Achilles fat pad (see Chapter 7). Rupture of the posterior tibial tendon causes a flatfoot deformity, hindfoot valgus, and medial and plantar drift of the head of the talus (see Fig. 5.10; see also Chapter 7).

Assessing progression of disease Serial radiographs can be used to assess progression of rheumatoid arthritis, but apparent changes in the radiographs should be viewed critically. Erosions may appear worse because of changes in patient position between two radiographs. In addition, erosions may appear more prominent, and become more sharply demarcated, as they heal.[27] Although a healed erosion may be manifest by a sclerotic rim, rheumatoid erosions rarely resolve. Moreover, radiographs may reveal progressive changes despite a clinical response to therapy.[28]

Pre-operative assessment Only a few basic radiographs are needed to assess the foot for a surgical procedure.[29] All films should be taken with the patient weight bearing, and should include:

- an anteroposterior view of the foot (see Fig. 5.13a). This will assess the forefoot area, the midfoot joints (infrequently showing significant involvement) and, if technique is good, will also show the talonavicular and calcaneocuboid joints;

- a lateral view of the foot, which should include the ankle (see Figs 5.10, 5.13). This is the most useful view in assessing the hindfoot joints, especially the talonavicular and calcaneocuboid joints, and the relationship between the hindfoot and the midfoot, as discussed in Chapter 10. In rheumatoid arthritis, valgus deformity of the hindfoot develops, with pronation of the midfoot and forefoot. The talus, which is devoid of any tendon insertions, rotates medially and plantarward, while the calcaneus drifts into valgus bringing with it the remainder of the hindfoot, midfoot and forefoot. The deformity may be due either to articular abnormalities or to posterior tibial dysfunction;

- an anteroposterior view of the ankle (see Fig. 5.10). Although the ankle joint is less frequently involved than the forefoot and hindfoot, it is at times very difficult to detect ankle abnormalities clinically, and it can be difficult to distinguish the valgus deformity produced by hindfoot abnormalities from a deformity that might be present, either entirely or in part, at the ankle joint. Moreover, the ankle joint may deteriorate even after a successful fusion of the hindfoot.[30] This may be more likely to occur if there is a malalignment of the tibiotalar joint preoperatively (even an angulation of as little as 5–10°), or other evidence of joint abnormality.

RADIONUCLIDE STUDIES

[99m]Technetium-MDP bone scans may be positive in all three phases of the scan before the disease is evident on plain radiographs.[16] The first and second phases of the bone scan are positive because of the soft-tissue hyperemia associated with pannus formation, and the positive third phase is caused by a combination of reparative osteoblastic activity and increased capillary permeability. In cases of persistent arthralgias and negative plain radiographs, a diagnosis of rheumatoid arthritis can be strongly suspected when the bone scan shows characteristic sites of bilaterally symmetric joint involvement.

White blood cells accumulate in the joint in active rheumatoid arthritis, and white blood cell radionuclide scans may therefore be positive. Although the technique remains investigational, an assessment of disease activity may be possible by studying the localization of white cells labelled with either [99m]technetium or [111]indium.[31,32]

MRI AND CT

Both MRI and CT are useful for detecting tendon abnormalities (see Chapter 7) associated with rheumatoid arthritis. MRI, especially with gadolinium enhancement, has been used to assess the severity of joint involvement, depicting erosions that are not evident on plain radiographs.[33–35] Like white-blood-cell scanning, it is a research tool in evaluating disease activity.[34]

Differential diagnosis

Robust rheumatoid arthritis is not infrequently confused with gout on radiographs. Both demonstrate preserved bone density and well-marginated erosions or subchondral cysts, and both may involve the metatarsophalangeal joints. Rheumatoid nodules tend to appear identical on radiographs to uncalcified gouty tophi. Joint space narrowing is an early finding in rheumatoid arthritis, but a late finding in gout. Another differentiating feature is that the erosions of rheumatoid arthritis are more likely to be

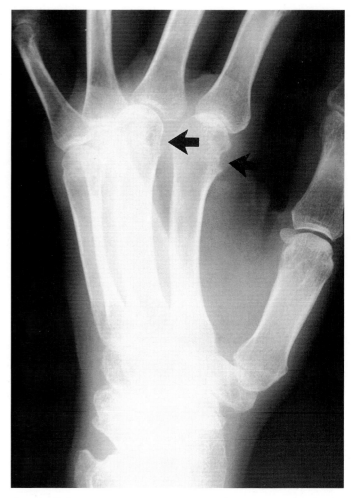

Fig. 5.16. Rheumatoid arthritis of the hand. Oblique radiograph. In the hand, the first erosions of rheumatoid arthritis typically occur at the volar and radial aspect of the second and third metacarpal heads (arrows), and are best seen on the oblique view of the hands.

on the plantar aspect of the joint whereas those of gout are more likely to be dorsal in location.

If there is uncertainty as to whether gout or rheumatoid arthritis is present, it is useful to obtain radiographs of the contralateral foot or the hands. Rheumatoid arthritis, unlike gout, is generally bilaterally symmetric. The characteristic distribution of rheumatoid arthritis in the hands also aids in diagnosis (Fig. 5.16).

Early in the course of rheumatoid arthritis, only a single joint may be affected, mimicking infectious arthritis. Both rheumatoid arthritis and infection may manifest a red, swollen, painful joint, and both will be positive on three-phase bone scan and on indium-labeled white blood cell scan. Joint aspiration and culture will provide the correct diagnosis.

An important feature distinguishing rheumatoid arthritis from the seronegative spondyloarthropathies is the paucity of periosteal new bone formation in rheumatoid arthritis. Periosteal new bone can be seen associated with insufficiency fractures in patients with rheumatoid arthritis, but this should not lead to misdiagnosis of a seronegative arthropathy because the periosteal reaction from insufficiency fractures occurs along the shaft of the bone, whereas periosteal new bone seen in the seronegative arthritides tends to occur at ligamentous and capsular insertions. One common site of periosteal new bone in patients with rheumatoid arthritis is the plantar surface of the calcaneus, where a spur may form at the site of an inflamed plantar aponeurosis. However, the spur tends to be smaller and not as exuberant as the plantar spurs associated with the seronegative spondyloarthropathies.

Treatment

Medical treatments for rheumatoid arthritis include nonsteroidal anti-inflammatory drugs, steroids, gold, methotrexate, D-penicillamine, hydroxychloroquine and sulfasalazine.

Physical modalities available through physical and occupational therapy are frequently helpful. Shoe modifications, as well as the use of shoes with a wider and deeper toe box are very helpful in treating the rheumatoid patient with a painful foot.[36]

Early surgical treatment is best directed toward any tendon abnormality that does not promptly respond to nonoperative treatment. A proliferative tenosynovitis, which can affect any of the tendons that cross the ankle and hindfoot, may result in tendon rupture or dysfunction. A synovectomy and decompression of the tendon can preserve function and prevent rupture. If possible, tendon ruptures should be repaired.

When severe joint deformities occur, surgical treatment may be necessary. The metatarsal heads can be resected, with or without silastic joint replacements.[10,38,39] Arthrodesis can be used to alleviate pain and correct deformity in the hindfoot (see Fig. 5.10).[37,40]

Patients with rheumatoid arthritis may have poor wound healing related to steroid and methotrexate medication. The poor wound healing predisposes the patient to osteomyelitis. Although the arthrodesis rate is very high, nonunions, delayed unions, or malunion do occur.[37] Postoperative neurovascular complications are rare.

Juvenile Chronic Arthritis

Juvenile chronic arthritis consists of a heterogeneous group of arthropathies that may be classified into the following subgroups:

- seronegative chronic arthritis (Still's disease), which accounts for approximately 70% of cases;
- juvenile-onset adult type (seropositive) rheumatoid arthritis, which accounts for about 10% of cases;
- juvenile-onset ankylosing spondylitis, which accounts for about 10% of cases; and
- smaller subgroups of patients with juvenile-onset psoriatic arthritis, Reiter's syndrome. and the arthritis of inflammatory bowel disease.[41,42]

This discussion will concentrate on seronegative chronic arthritis, the largest of the subgroups.

Clinical features

Seronegative chronic arthritis, or Still's disease, is defined as persistent arthritis of one or more joints of at least 6 weeks' duration with onset before 16 years of age.[43,44] Girls are affected far more than boys. Three types of disease are distinguished, according to the number of joints involved and the presence or absence of systemic symptoms during the first 6 months of the disease:

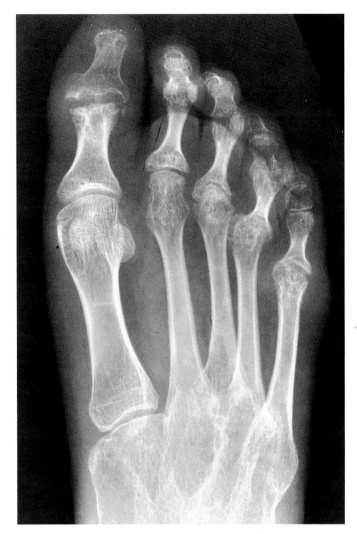

Fig. 5.17. Adult patient with Still's disease. The second through fifth metatarsophalangeal joints and the interphalangeal joint of the great toe are severely eroded. The bases of the second and third proximal phalanges are overgrown. The fifth MTP joint is subluxed. The second through fifth metatarsals have fused with the tarsal bones which have also fused with each other.

- classic systemic disease, which is usually observed below the age of 5 years, and manifests fever, rash, hepatosplenomegaly, lymphadenopathy, pericarditis, leukocytosis, and mild arthritis;
- monoarticular or pauciarticular disease, which is seen in young children, and is generally confined to four or fewer large joints, such as the knee, ankle, elbow, or wrist. Systemic disease is usually absent, except for iridocyclitis, which may lead to blindness; and
- polyarticular disease, which usually presents with symmetric involvement of the metacarpophalangeal and interphalangeal joints of the hands and the metatarsophalangeal and interphalangeal joints of the feet, and also involves the wrist, ankles, intertarsal joints, hips, knees, and cervical spine. It is often accompanied by rash, splenomegaly, lymphadenopathy, carditis, fever, and leukocytosis. Tenosynovitis may lead to periosteal new bone formation of the short tubular bones of the hands and feet.

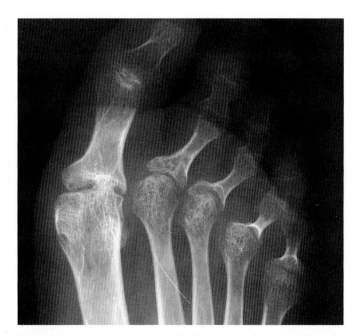

Fig. 5.18. Adult patient with Still's disease. Standing AP radiograph. Erosions of the metatarsophalangeal joints are accompanied by fibular deviation of the second, third, and fourth toes.

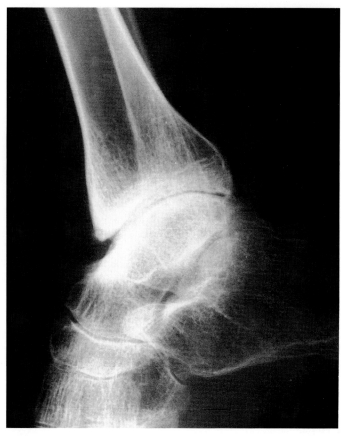

Fig. 5.19. Still's disease affecting the tibiotalar joint. Lateral radiograph. There is severe erosion of the tibiotalar joint, and the intertarsal joints are narrowed.

Fig. 5.20. Still's disease in an adolescent. Lateral radiograph. The tarsals are completely fused.

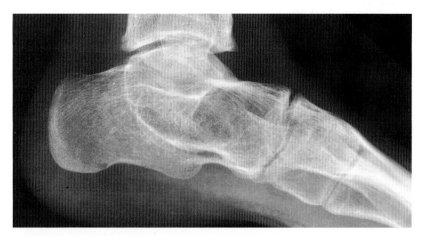

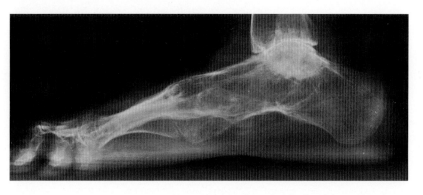

Fig. 5.21. Adult patient with Still's disease. Standing lateral radiograph. Claw toe deformities are present. There is extensive bony fusion, and the tibiotalar joint is severly eroded. Severe osteoporosis reflects chronic immobility.

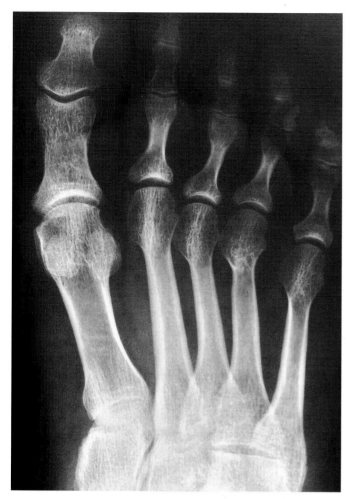

Fig. 5.22. Adult patient with Still's disease. Standing AP radiograph. The only abnormality is shortening of the third metatarsal due to premature fusion of its epiphysis.

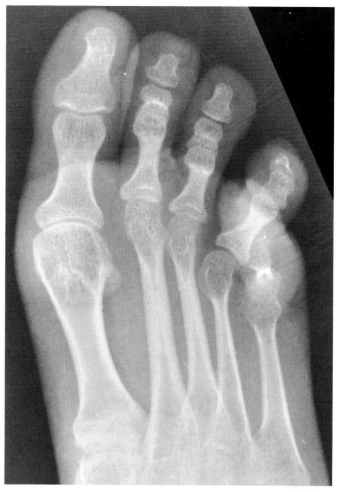

Fig. 5.23. Still's disease in an adolescent. Standing AP radiograph. The fourth and fifth metatarsals are shortened owing to premature fusion of their epiphyses. The third and fourth toes are deviated in a fibular direction. The fourth toe is overlapped by the fifth toe, whose proximal phalanx is cocked up.

In any of the subtypes of Still's disease, hyperemia of the inflamed joints and underlying bone results in epiphyseal overgrowth. Premature fusion of the epiphysis may occur, resulting in shortening of the involved bone.[45]

Radiographic findings

The earliest radiographic findings are soft-tissue swelling and osteoporosis. Periostitis of the metatarsals takes the form of linear periosteal new bone that is a frequent and often striking early finding. It may be limited to the part of the bone adjacent to a capsular attachment of an inflamed joint, or it may extend along the shaft of a bone, particularly at the insertion of an inflamed tendon sheath. The new bone may eventually become incorporated into the cortex to thicken it and broaden the shaft of the bone. Alternatively, resorption of the endosteal surface of the cortex may proceed concomitantly with new bone formation, and an enlarged bone with a thin cortex and widened medullary space may result.

Bone erosion is a relatively late manifestation, beginning at the joint margin where there is no protective articular cartilage,

and progressing along the articular surface (Figs 5.17–5.19). In young children, the relatively thick articular cartilage tends to protect the underlying bone from erosions, but as increasing maturation of bone causes the cartilage to thin in later childhood, erosions become more likely.[46]

By adulthood, the shafts of the tubular bones may undergo concentric atrophy owing to immobility and chronic absence of muscle stress. Bony ankylosis of the tarsal bones is a common finding. The entire mass of tarsal bones may fuse, and the tarsometatarsal joints may also undergo bony ankylosis (Figs 5.20, 5.21). Shortening of the tubular bones due to premature fusion of epiphyses may affect the metatarsals (Figs 5.22–5.24), especially the fourth metatarsal. Premature fusion of epiphyses may also occur in all the bones distal to an inflamed ankle or knee, so that even when the small pedal joints are spared, the bones of the foot may be smaller than normal. Encountering such disturbances in an adult with arthritis implies that it began in early childhood.[47]

The pressure of the metatarsal heads on the articular surface of the proximal phalangeal epiphyses may inhibit their central

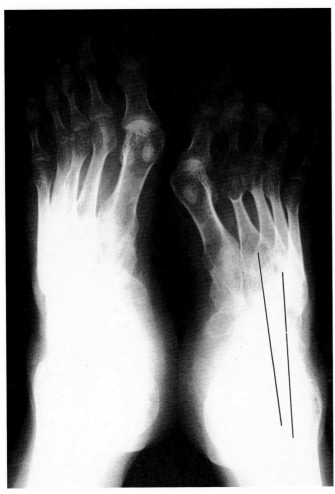

Fig. 5.24. Adult patient with Still's disease. Standing AP radiograph. A decrease in the talocalcaneal angle (black lines show relative axes of the right talus and calcaneus) indicates varus deformity of the hindfoot bilaterally. Bilateral hallux valgus deformities are noted. The feet are both small, but the right is smaller. Metatarsal shortening is evident, most severe in the right second metatarsal.

development and may cause peripheral overgrowth of the bases of the proximal phalanges. Foot deformities include claw toes (see Fig. 5.21), hammer toes, fibular deviation of the toes (Figs 5.18, 5.23), hindfoot varus or valgus (Fig. 5.24), pes cavus, and hallux valgus (Fig. 5.24).[46,47] At the tibiotalar joint, the distal tibial epiphysis may be slanted, owing to asymmetric overgrowth of the epiphysis.

Differential diagnosis
Juvenile onset of seronegative spondyloarthropathies should be considered, as well as other connective tissue diseases and nonrheumatologic conditions which are summarized in Table 5.4.

Treatment
Medical treatment is similar to treatment for adult rheumatoid arthritis. Surgical treatment is rarely needed.

Table 5.4. Differential diagnosis of juvenile rheumatoid arthritis. (Modified from Cassidy et al.[44])

Other connective tissue diseases	SLE
	dermatomyositis
	vasculitis
	scleroderma
Seronegative spondyloarthropathies	
Infectious arthritis	
Congenital anomalies	
Nonrheumatic conditions	RSDS
	post-traumatic arthritis
	osteochondritis dissecans
Hematologic diseases	hemophilia
	leukemia and lymphoma
	sickle cell anemia
Neoplastic diseases	malignant and benign tumors
	histiocytosis X
Arthromyalgia	growing pains
	psychogenic rheumatism

THE INFLAMMATORY SPONDYLOARTHROPATHIES

There are three major inflammatory spondyloarthropathies:
- ankylosing spondylitis;
- Reiter's syndrome; and
- psoriatic arthritis.

A spondyloarthropathy can also develop in association with inflammatory bowel disease.

The inflammatory spondyloarthropathies are often referred to as the seronegative inflammatory arthritides, because rheumatoid factor is absent. This latter term is somewhat confusing because, as discussed above, rheumatoid arthritis itself can be seronegative.

The inflammatory spondyloarthropathies primarily involve the sacroiliac joints and spine. Of the three, Reiter's syndrome is the most likely to demonstrate abnormalities of the foot, but when ankylosing spondylitis and psoriatic arthritis involve the foot, the findings are identical to those of Reiter's syndrome. Therefore, for the purposes of this chapter, the radiographic findings in the foot are discussed together, after a brief description of the features of each of these entities.

Ankylosing Spondylitis

Ankylosing spondylitis is an autoimmune disorder, more common in men than women. It usually has its onset between the ages of 15 and 36 years. Ninety percent of patients have the HLA-B27 antigen.[48] In addition to the arthritis, systemic abnormalities may develop, including heart disease (especially aortic insufficiency), pulmonary fibrosis and pleuritis, and amyloidosis.[48] Radiographically, ankylosing spondylitis is characterized by symmetric erosive arthritis of the sacroiliac joints which progresses to fusion, and by bony ankylosis of the spine (Fig. 5.25). It commonly affects the large joints of the skeleton

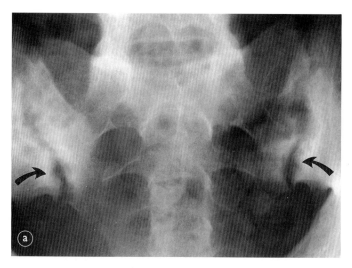

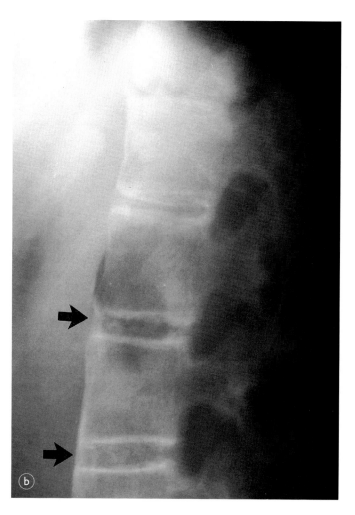

Fig. 5.25. Ankylosing spondylitis. **a.** PA radiograph of sacroiliac joints. The sacroiliac joints (arrows) are widened and irregular, and the articular cortex is poorly defined, especially on the iliac side of the joint. **b.** Lateral radiograph of the upper lumbar spine. The anterior contour of the vertebral bodies is straightened, and the vertebrae are fused by thin syndesmophytes (arrows) that do not extend beyond the contour of the vertebral body.

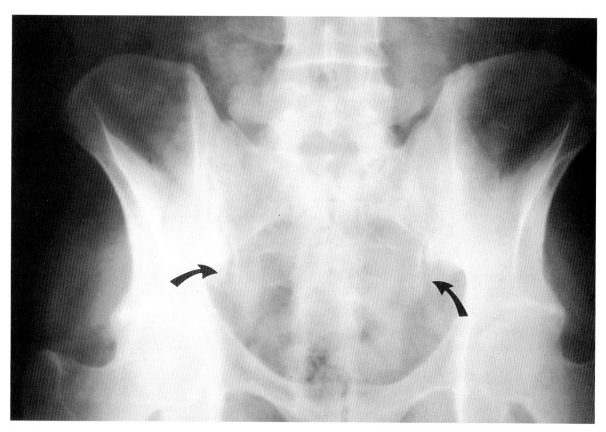

Fig. 5.26. Reiter's disease. PA radiograph of sacroiliac joints. There is asymmetric erosive arthritis of the sacroiliac joints.

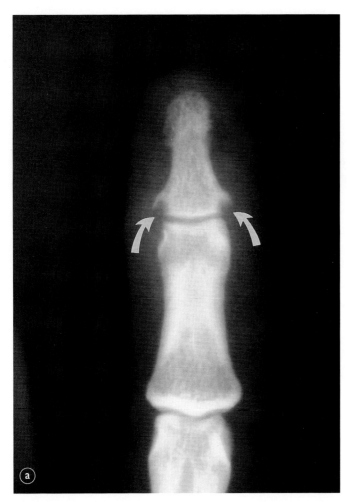 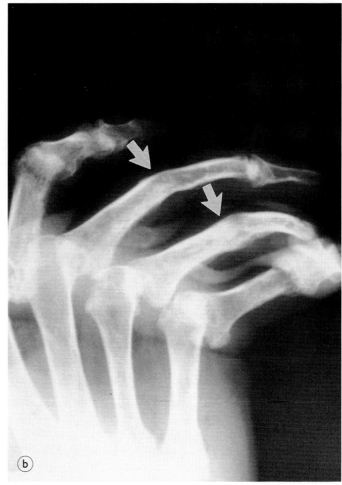

Fig. 5.27. Psoriatic arthritis in the hands. **a.** PA radiograph of the index finger in early psoriatic arthritis. There are typical 'Mickey Mouse ear' erosions (arrows) at the distal interphalangeal joint. **b.** PA radiograph of fingers in advanced psoriatic arthritis. Subluxations of the metacarpophalangeal joints are present, and may be seen in rheumatoid arthritis as well as psoriatic arthritis. However, fusion of the proximal interphalangeal joints (arrows) is very unlikely in rheumatoid arthritis, and is characteristic of psoriatic arthritis. Psoriatic arthritis tends to involve the distal interphalangeal joints to a greater extent than the metacarpophalangeal joints, whereas the converse is true of rheumatoid arthritis.

(especially the shoulder, hip, and knee) and is not common in the foot and ankle. However, heel pain may be an early complaint, and bilateral symmetrical heel pain in a young man should alert the physician to the possibility of ankylosing spondylitis.

Reiter's Disease

Reiter's disease is a spondyloarthropathy that occurs in association with sexually transmitted or diarrheal infections, and is much more common in men than women. There is a clinical triad of findings: urethritis (cystitis in women), arthritis, and conjunctivitis,[49] although not all patients demonstrate all three findings. Balanitis, a skin rash (keratoderma blenorrhagicum), buccal erosions, peripheral neuropathy, cardiac valve abnormalities and palpitations, and pulmonary fibrosis and pleurisy may also occur.[50] Like ankylosing spondylitis, Reiter's disease has a high association with HLA-B27.

Arthritis is seen most frequently in the sacroiliac joints, where it tends to be bilateral but asymmetric (Fig. 5.26). In the spine, bulky syndesmophytes (osteophytes uniting adjacent vertebral bodies) form. The foot, especially the calcaneus, is commonly involved, and the patient's primary complaint is often heel pain.

Psoriatic Arthritis

This spondyloarthropathy is associated with psoriasis, and may precede the development of skin lesions.[51] The arthritis is very similar to that of Reiter's syndrome, but unlike Reiter's syndrome it tends to affect the hands (Fig. 5.27) more than the feet.

Radiographic Findings in the Spondyloarthropathies

There are two types of radiographic abnormalities in the spondyloarthropathies: those due to joint abnormalities, and those due

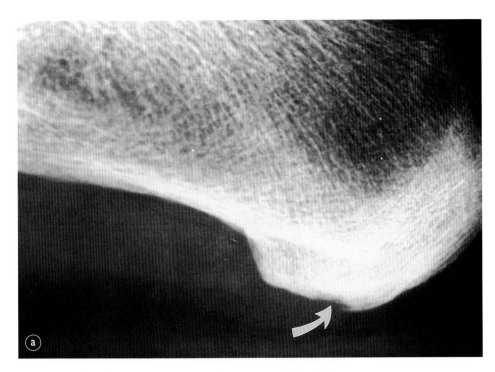

Fig. 5.28. Early Reiter's Syndrome involving the calcaneus. **a.** Lateral radiograph. The patient presented with heel pain, and an MRI was requested. Careful inspection of the lateral radiograph shows an early erosion at the origin of the plantar aponeurosis (curved arrow). **b.** Coronal MRI, T1-weighted, SE 600/20. There is edema of the plantar fascia and the origins of the flexor digitorum brevis and abductor hallucis muscles (arrows), shown on MRI by enlargement of the muscles and blurring of the soft-tissue planes. A small erosion is present in the calcaneus (curved arrow). Edema within the calcaneus is evident as an area of low signal intensity adjacent to the erosion. **c.** Sagittal MRI, T2-weighted, FSE 4000/105. Edema at the origin of the plantar fascia has a high signal intensity. Bone marrow edema is masked on this FSE image by the signal from the adjacent fatty marrow.

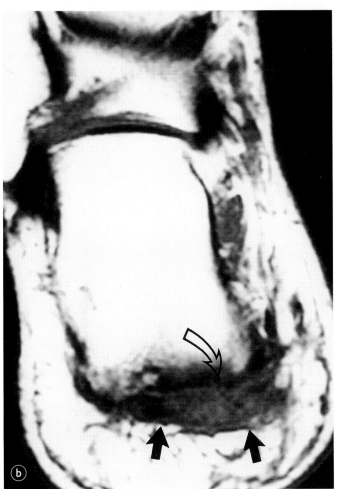

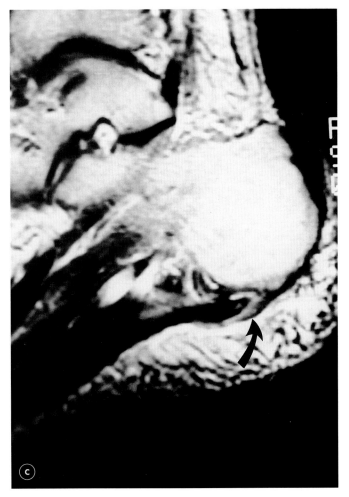

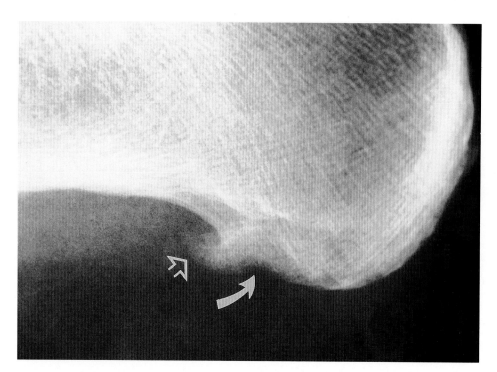

Fig. 5.29. Advanced enthesopathic changes of the calcaneus due to psoriatic arthritis. Lateral radiograph. There is a cortical erosion (curved arrow), and fluffy periosteal new bone formation (open arrow) has developed adjacent to the erosion. Compare the findings in these two patients to the well-marginated enthesophytes associated with DISH (Fig. 5.50).

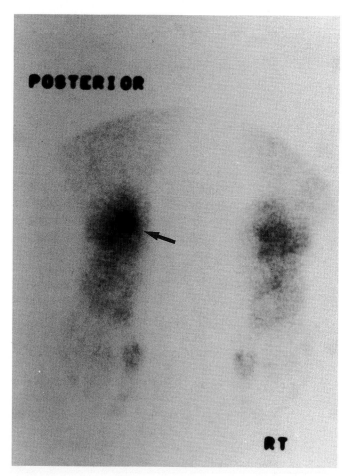

Fig. 5.30. Reiter's syndrome detected on bone scan. Plain radiographs were normal. Foot on detector projection obtained 3 hours after injection of 15 mCi of ^{99m}technetium MDP. There is markedly increased radionuclide activity (arrow) at the origin of the left plantar aponeurosis, with less prominent uptake in the same location in the right foot. Uptake can also be seen in a calcaneal spur associated with plantar fasciitis (see Chapter 8).

to enthesopathy. An enthesis is the bony insertion of a tendon or ligament; an enthesopathy is an abnormality of a tendinous or ligamentous insertion.

Inflammatory enthesopathic changes in the hindfoot are characteristic of the spondyloarthropathies. Most occur on the plantar aspect of the calcaneus at the origin of the plantar fascia (Figs 5.28–5.30) or on the posterior process of the calcaneus at the Achilles tendon insertion.[52] Initially, a small focus of cortical bone resorption is seen at the enthesis. As the inflammation progresses, reparative periosteal new bone develops, forming a poorly-marginated, irregular, 'fluffy' spur. Periosteal reaction can also involve the malleoli. At the time of presentation, radiographs are often normal, and the diagnosis can be suggested in the presence of a positive radionuclide bone scan[53] (see Fig. 5.30) or MRI (see Fig. 5.28).

In the forefoot, many of the radiographic changes are similar to those of rheumatoid arthritis, with the development of erosions of the metatarsophalangeal and interphalangeal joints (Fig. 5.31). An important distinguishing feature, which tends to be absent in rheumatoid arthritis, is the presence of exuberant periosteal new bone (Figs 5.31–5.33) at entheses. Another hallmark of the seronegative arthritides is bony fusion of a digit. The 'pencil in cup' deformity (Fig. 5.34) is a characteristic finding. A diffusely enlarged digit, called a 'sausage digit' may develop because of tendon sheath inflammation. Tendon ruptures may occur, especially of the posterior tibial tendon. Acro-osteolysis may occur.

Treatment of Foot Abnormalities in the Spondyloarthropathies

The foot deformities seen in the inflammatory spondyloarthropathies, in contrast to the deformities caused by rheumatoid arthritis, rarely require surgical correction. Although the patients may have pain and residual deformity, the foot and ankle symptoms are usually controlled by medications, physical therapy, and shoe modifications. Symptomatic relief of heel pain

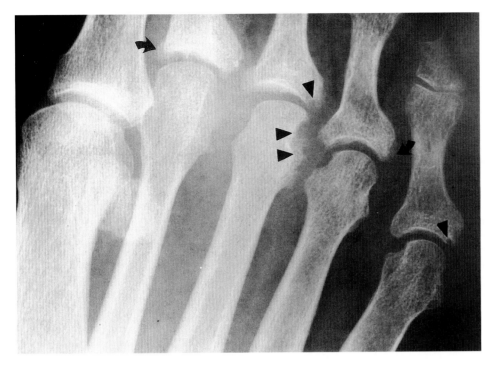

Fig. 5.31. Psoriatic arthritis of the metatarsophalangeal joints. The appearance is similar to rheumatoid arthritis, with multiple marginal erosions (arrowheads). However, periosteal new bone formation (arrow) can be seen at the joint margins. Note the increased density in the soft tissues surrounding the second and third metatarsophalangeal joints, probably caused by joint effusions.

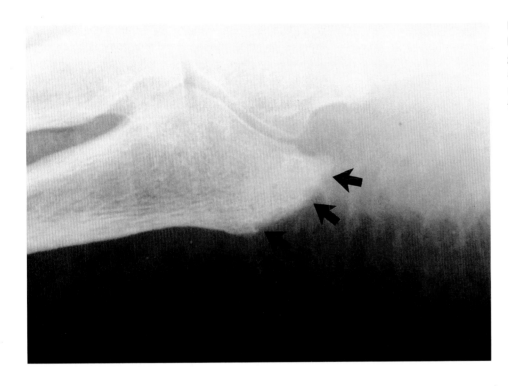

Fig. 5.32. Psoriatic arthritis involving the base of the fifth metatarsal. Oblique radiograph. Multiple small erosions (arrows), accompanied by delicate wisps of periosteal new bone, are present at the insertion of the peroneus brevis tendon.

can be achieved with a cushioned heel, and injection of a corticosteroid and local anesthetic. However, injections should not be placed near the Achilles tendon.

COLLAGEN VASCULAR DISEASES

Progressive Systemic Sclerosis (Scleroderma)

Progressive systemic sclerosis (PSS), commonly called by the less appropriate name of scleroderma, is characterized by excessive fibrosis throughout the body, particularly the skin. It is three times more common in women than men. The mean age of

onset is 40 years. Although in some patients the disease remains confined to the skin, in many it progresses to death from renal or cardiac failure, intestinal malabsorption, or pulmonary insufficiency. PSS can be divided into two categories:

- diffuse scleroderma, which is manifested by rapidly progressive skin and visceral involvement; and
- the CREST syndrome, a more benign disorder consisting of calcinosis, Raynaud's phenomenon (episodic vasoconstriction of the arteries and arterioles), esophageal dysmotility, sclerodactyly (hardening of the skin of the digits), and telangiectasia. (CREST is an acronym taken from the first letters of these clinical features.)

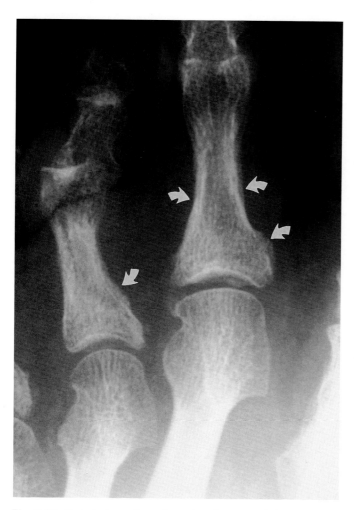
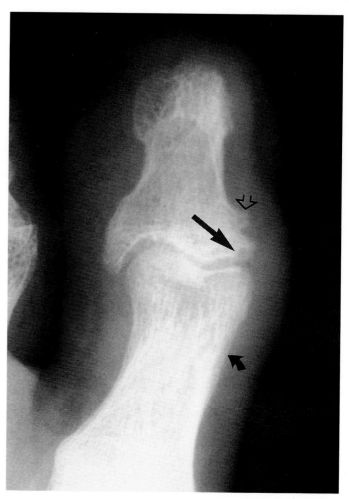

Fig. 5.33. Periosteal new bone formation due to psoriatic arthritis. **a.** AP radiograph of the second and third toes. Arrows point to multiple areas of periosteal new bone formation. **b.** Oblique radiograph of first toe. Curved arrow points to periosteal new bone, and straight solid arrow to a small 'Mickey Mouse ear' erosion. Open arrow points to a small exostosis, which is reported in psoriatic arthritis but which also can occur as a normal variant (see Chapter 1).

Soft-tissue hydroxyapatite crystal deposition is common in PSS, and is a response to tissue damage. The calcifications are usually subcutaneous, located where the skin is the tightest, such as at the fingertips, but they may be seen almost anywhere, even in joints.

Pathogenesis

Cultured fibroblasts from patients with PSS synthesize twice as much collagen as do cultured fibroblasts from normals. However, the collagen is qualitatively normal, and the cause of the increased production is unknown. The presence in affected individuals of nonspecific serologic abnormalities, such as hypergammaglobulinemia (50% of cases), antinuclear antibodies (70–90% of cases), and rheumatoid factor (25% of cases), imply an autoimmune disorder. Some patients manifest T-cell sensitization to collagen, suggesting the possibility of a delayed hypersensitivity to collagen. It is also possible that vascular damage by autoantibodies or antigen–antibody complexes may initiate injury to the endothelium, leading to perivascular edema, which is followed by periadventitial fibrosis with widespread narrowing of the microvasculature.[54]

Inflammatory synovitis is common, with infiltrates of lymphocytes and plasma cells associated with hyperplasia and hypertrophy of the synovium. Fibrosis develops, resulting in generalized joint pain and stiffness. Similarly, a myositis which progresses to fibrosis may be seen.

Distribution of PSS in the musculoskeletal system

The hands are most commonly affected, with involvement of the feet being less common and less extensive. There is often myositis, which begins with the proximal muscle groups.

Radiographic findings

Although the diagnostic changes of PSS predominate in the hands, thay may be seen to a lesser extent in the feet. Fibrous tissue replaces the subcutaneous fat and thickens the capsules of the small pedal joints. The toes develop flexion deformities, which may progress to subluxations and dislocations (Figs 5.35, 5.36). A hallux valgus deformity may occur. Atrophy and ulceration of the soft-tissue pulp may be associated with subcutaneous calcinosis circumscripta, especially of the plantar tissues (see Figs 5.35, 5.36). Resorption of the terminal tufts of the distal

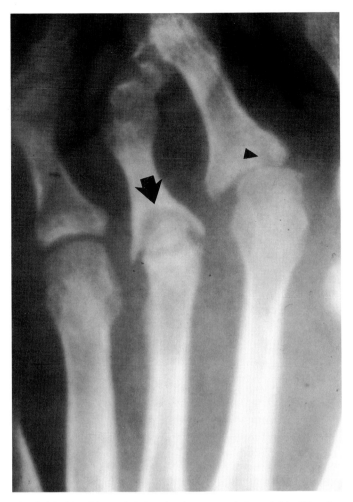

Fig. 5.34. 'Pencil in cup' deformity due to psoriatic arthritis. AP radiograph of the metatarsophalangeal joints. The third metatarsal head is eroded and fits like a pencil into the corresponding cup (arrow) formed by the base of the proximal phalanx. Less severe arthritic changes are seen in the second metatarsophalangeal joint, with joint narrowing, lateral subluxation, and small erosions (arrowhead).

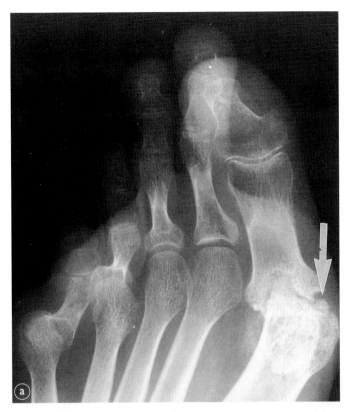

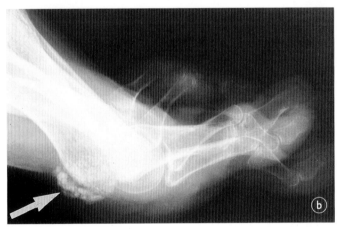

Fig. 5.35. Progressive systemic sclerosis seen on AP (a) and lateral (b) weight-bearing radiographs. Dorsiflexion of the fourth and fifth metatarsophalangeal joints has evolved into subluxation. Destruction and subchondral sclerosis of the first metatarsophalangeal joint is associated with a hallux valgus deformity. Calcinosis circumscripta (arrows) is present within the first metatarsophalangeal joint as well as in the vicinity of the medial sesamoid.

phalanges (Fig. 5.37) usually begins on their plantar surface, wheras in psoriatic arthritis and Reiter's syndrome it tends to occur on their dorsal surface in association with overlying thickened and deformed nails.[55]

Pressure and frictional forces result in thinning of the articular cartilage of the metatarsophlangeal joints, progressing to irregular destruction and sclerosis of subchondral bone (see Figs 5.35–5.37). Calcifications may occasionally occur in joints, usually in association with extensive destruction[56] (see Fig. 5.35). Diffuse osteoporosis, a variable finding, is more likely to occur in the presence of severe joint destruction and deformity (see Fig. 5.36).

In a review of 55 patients with diffuse scleroderma in which those with overlap syndromes, such as the CREST syndrome and mixed connective tissue disease, were excluded, 12 patients showed radiographic evidence of inflammatory arthritis in the hands. This radiographic evidence ranged from isolated joint erosion to generalized joint erosion similar to that shown in Figs 5.35–5.37. Four of the 12 patients with joint erosion in the hands also had erosive arthritis in the feet, but in no instance were erosions in the feet found in the abscence of erosions in the hands. Resorption of the terminal tufts of the distal phalanges of the toes was far less common and always less severe than that in the fingers.[55]

Patients with the CREST syndrome may have subcutaneous calcifications as their only musculoskeletal radiologic abnormality (see Fig. 5.38). Terminal tuft resorption of the distal phalanges is seen with far less frequency in the CREST syndrome than in scleroderma.[57]

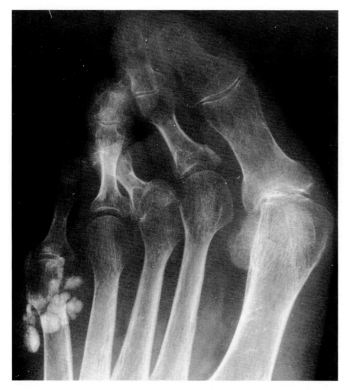

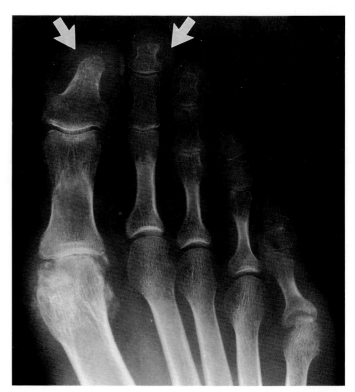

Fig. 5.36. Progressive systemic sclerosis. AP weight-bearing radiograph. Arthritis of the first metatarsophalangeal joint is associated with subchondral sclerosis and hallux valgus deformity. There is fibular deviation of the second and third toes, and hyperextension deformity of the third metatarsophalangeal joint. Calcinosis is seen along the plantar aspect of the head of the fifth metatarsal. Diffuse osteoporosis, a variable feature of progressive systemic sclerosis, is obvious in this patient.

Fig. 5.37. Progressive systemic sclerosis. AP weight-bearing radiograph. Erosions of the 1st and 5th metatarsal heads are associated with destruction of the articular cartilage. Calcinosis is present medial and plantar to the head of the 1st metatarsal The distal soft tissue and terminal tufts of the 1st and 2nd toes are partially resorbed (arrows).

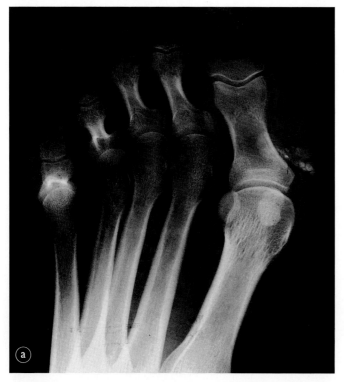

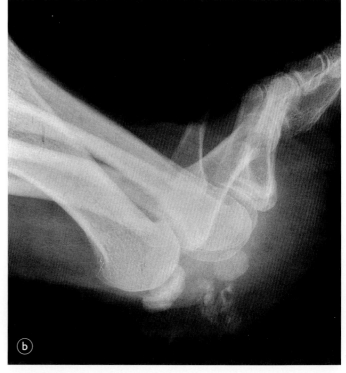

Fig. 5.38. CREST syndrome. **a** AP and **b** lateral weight-bearing radiographs. Hyperextension of the metatarsophalangeal joints with flexion deformities of the toes are seen, in association with calcinosis circumscripta in the subcutaneous fat beneath the base of the proximal phalanx of the great toe. Erosions and osteoporosis are absent.

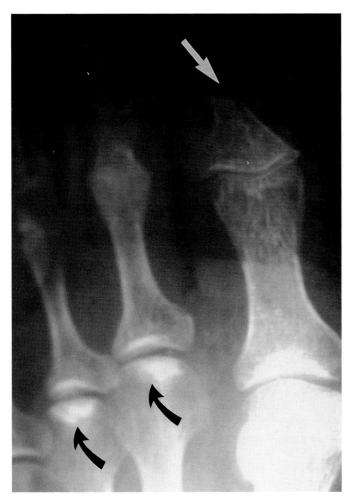

Fig. 5.39. Systemic lupus erythematosis. AP radiograph of the toes. Avascular necrosis (curved arrow) is present in the second and third metatarsal heads. The appearance is similar to Freiberg's infraction (see below), but is due to either the vasculitis of SLE or to steroid treatment, while Freiberg's is due to mechanical stresses. Acro-osteolysis (straight arrow) is seen in the first toe.

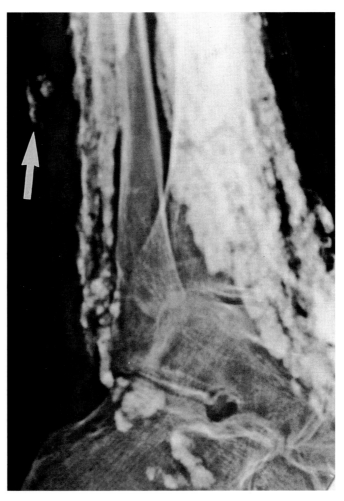

Fig. 5.40. Dermatomyositis. Mortise view of the ankle. Both subcutaneous (arrow) and muscular calcifications are present. The sheetlike configuration of the calcifications is characteristic.

Differential diagnosis

Dermatomyositis should be considered in the differential diagnosis of patients with extensive soft tissue calcifications. Another syndrome to consider is mixed connective tissue disease (MCTD). In MCTD, patients show features of systemic lupus erythematosis, scleroderma, dermatomyositis, and rheumatoid arthritis.[58]

Treatment

Steroids are the main mode of treatment, and other immunosuppressive medications are also used.

Systemic Lupus Erythematosis

Systemic lupus erythematosis (SLE) is an autoimmune disease characterized by formation of antinuclear antibodies that cause severe, multisystem tissue injury.[59] It is much more common in women than in men, and tends to affect adults under the age of 40. Patients typically present with a malar rash, malaise, and weakness. Neurologic, cardiac, renal, and pulmonary abnormalities are common. Diagnostic tests include antinuclear antigen (ANA) and LE cell prep. Rheumatoid factor may be positive.

Radiographic findings and differential diagnosis

Ninety percent of patients develop polyarthralgias, and joint effusions are common. However, although joint subluxations develop, especially in the hands, erosions are rarely seen.[59] The lack of erosions allows inflammatory arthritis to be excluded.

Avascular necrosis (Fig. 5.39) and bone infarcts are common. Erosion of the terminal tufts of the phalanges (acro-osteolysis) may be seen.

Treatment

Steroids are the main mode of treatment, though other immunosuppressive medications are also used.

Polymyositis and Dermatomyositis

Polymyositis and dermatomyositis are characterized by inflammation and degeneration of the musculature.[60] In dermatomyositis (50% of patients), a diffuse rash is present as well. Polymyositis–dermatomyositis may develop in children or adults. When it develops in older adults, it is often associated with a malignancy.

Patients present with muscle weakness and tenderness. Involvement is first seen in the proximal musculature. Eventually, muscle contractures develop. Raynaud's phenomenon is present in about one-third of patients. Arthralgias are common, but radiographic findings of arthritis are absent.

Radiographic findings
Initially, subcutaneous calcifications are seen. Sheet-like calcifications develop along muscle and fascial planes (Fig. 5.40).

Differential diagnosis
When calcifications are not extensive, hyperparathyroidism, systemic sclerosis, SLE, and MCTD should be considered. However, the presence of extensive sheets of calcification along myofascial planes is most likely due to polymyositis–dermatomyositis. Myositis ossificans (see Chapter 11) can be distinguished from polymyositis–dermatomyositis because it features ossification rather than calcification of soft tissue.

Treatment
Steroids are the main mode of treatment, though other immunosuppressive medications are also used.

Lyme Arthritis

Lyme disease is a multisystem disorder caused by the bacterium Borrelia burgdorferi and transmitted by ticks. Arthritis in Lyme disease is most frequently seen in the knee,[61] but it can involve other joints, including the ankles and the digits. Radiographs are often normal, but Lyme disease can mimic rheumatoid arthritis or Reiter's syndrome radiographically. Faller et al[62] retrospectively reviewed 10 patients with Lyme arthritis who presented primarily with complaints related to the foot and ankle. Patients presented with joint pain, plantar fasciitis, tendinitis involving the Achilles and posterior tibial tendons, or dysesthesias. Diagnosis was often delayed, owing to the nonspecific nature of the complaints.

CRYSTAL-INDUCED ARTHROPATHIES

Gout

Gout is caused by deposition of uric acid crystals within a joint, soft tissues, or bone. Hyperuricemia is a precondition for gout, but many hyperuricemic patients are asymptomatic.[63] Only 17% of hyperuricemic patients in one study developed clinical gout.[64] Men are affected far more commonly than women. The majority of cases are idiopathic, but gout may also occur as a result of abnormalities of urate metabolism (primary gout), or because of trauma, alcohol ingestion, or side effect of medication (secondary gout).

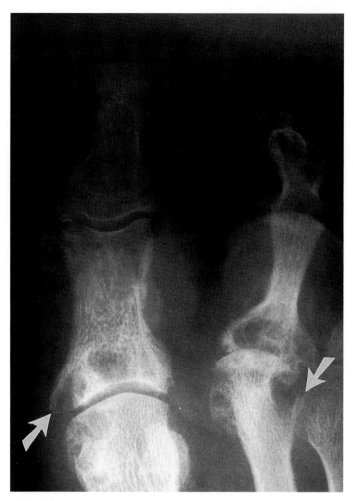

Fig. 5.41. Gout involving the first and second metatarsophalangeal joints. AP radiograph of the toes. The erosions are sharply marginated. Two erosions show a prominent 'overhanging edge' of bone (arrows), which partially encircles the tophus. The first metatarsophalangeal joint space is well-preserved. There is dislocation of the second metatarsophalangeal joint.

Gouty crystals microscopically appear needle-shaped, and are negatively birefringent under polarized light microscopy.[65] The crystals are deposited in synovium, cartilage, bone, and periarticular tissues. An acute gouty attack occurs when crystals are precipitated into the synovial fluid, causing severe pain and tenderness, and a red, swollen joint.

Distribution
Gout may involve any joint, and lacks the predictable pattern of involvement characteristic of rheumatoid arthritis. The hallux metatarsophalangeal joint is often the initial joint to be affected. The initial attack is monoarticular in 85–90% of cases.[63] In cases of polyarticular disease, findings are rarely bilaterally symmetric.

Radiographic findings
The radiographic findings of gout are attributable to tophaceous deposits of urate eroding bone. A latent period of 5–10 years is frequently seen between the clinical onset of gout and the devel-

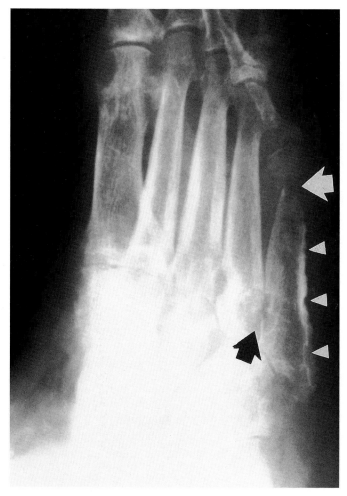

Fig. 5.42. Extensive polyarticular gout. Oblique radiograph of the foot. Erosions are seen along the fifth metatarsal shaft (arrowheads), the bases of the metatarsals (black arrow points to the largest of these), and at multiple metatarsophalangeal joints. There is pencilling of the fifth metatarsal shaft, and a pathological fracture of the metatarsal neck (white arrow). Osteomyelitis of the fifth metatarsal was suspected radiographically, but there was no clinical evidence of osteomyelitis, and radiographic findings remained stable over a period of many months.

opment of radiographic findings.[63,64] Sharply marginated bony erosions are seen, which when advanced may develop an 'overhanging edge'[66] of cortical bone (Fig. 5.41). Unlike the erosions of inflammatory arthritis, the erosions of gout may be located away from the joint. There may be diffuse tapering or 'pencilling' of bone shafts[65] (Fig. 5.42). Periosteal new bone occasionally develops (Fig. 5.43). Tophi in the soft tissue are often visible radiographically (see Fig. 5.43). They occasionally calcify,[65] usually in patients with gouty nephropathy. Osteophyte formation may be seen as a result of secondary osteoarthritis. Gout can occur in unusual locations such as the subtalar joint, and it should always be considered in an atypical erosive arthritis of the foot.

Imaging modalities other than plain radiographs are not commonly used in the diagnosis of gout. Gout is a potential cause of false-positive technetium and indium bone scans for osteomyelitis. A single case of the MRI appearance of a gout tophus has been published.[67] This case demonstrated a non-

specific appearance: heterogeneous, intermediate signal intensity of the tophus, increasing somewhat on relatively T2-weighted (SE TR/TE 2200/60) images.

Differential diagnosis

The diagnostic differentiation from rheumatoid arthritis is discussed above in the section on rheumatoid arthritis. The sharp definition of the erosions, their characteristic 'overhanging edge', and their variable location relative to the joint should allow radiologic differentiation from other arthritides.

Treatment

Treatment is primarily medical, with uricosuric drugs and allopurinol. Occasionally a large tophus may be surgically excised.

Calcium Pyrophosphate Dihydrate Deposition Disease

Calcium pyrophosphate dihydrate deposition disease (CPPD) is a crystal-induced arthropathy that is uncommon in the foot and ankle. In distinction to the needle-like, negatively birefringent urate crystals, calcium pyrophosphate crystals have a rhomboid shape and are weakly positively birefringent.[63] Calcium pyrophosphate crystals are deposited in cartilage, synovium, and joint fluid, and also periarticularly. The crystal deposition may be asymptomatic, or at the other end of the clinical spectrum, it may cause acute gout-like attacks called pseudogout, which can lead to joint destruction sometimes as extensive as neuropathic joint disease. In milder cases, the resultant arthritis resembles osteoarthritis, except for a different distribution – CPPD has a predilection for the radiocarpal joint of the wrist, the patellofemoral joint of the knee, the pubic symphysis, and the glenohumeral joint. CPPD uncommonly involves the foot but, when it does, it usually involves the talonavicular or ankle joints. It has been reported as a cause of tendon rupture.[68]

Radiographic findings

Chondrocalcinosis is characteristic (see Figs 5.44, 5.45), but it is not present in all cases. Calcification can also involve the joint capsule, periarticular soft tissues, and tendons and ligaments. Like osteoarthritis, CPPD may result in osteophyte formation, bony sclerosis and nonuniform narrowing of the joint space. When it is highly destructive, it mimics neuropathic joint disease.

Differential diagnosis

Chondrocalcinosis can be seen in osteoarthritis as well as CPPD, but it is generally more extensive in CPPD. CPPD is best differentiated from osteoarthritis by its distribution – the talonavicular joint uncommonly has severe osteoarthritis except in the setting of posterior tibial tendon rupture, but it is the predominant location of CPPD in the foot.

CPPD mimics gout clinically, but the two arthritides are easily distinguished radiographically. CPPD shows chondrocalcinosis, prominent osteophytes and joint space narrowing. Gout will either be radiographically normal or have well-marginated bony erosions. The distinction between CPPD and neuropathic joint is usually clear by clinical history, but aspiration of CPPD crystals from the joint may occasionally be needed to aid in the diagnosis.

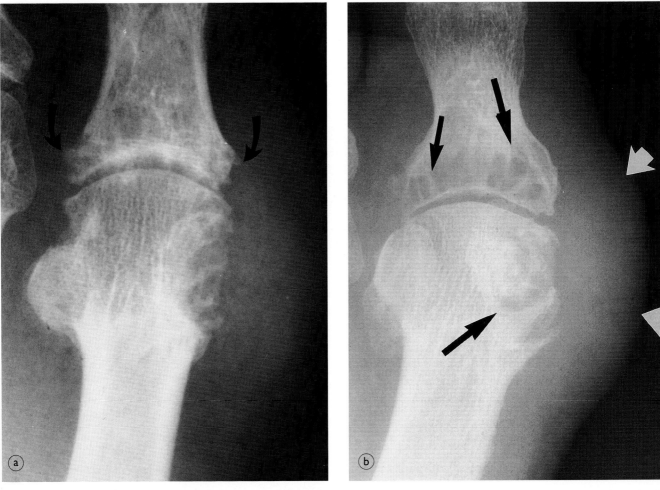

Fig. 5.43. Gout of the first metatarsophalangeal joint. **a.** AP radiograph. Small tufts of periosteal new bone are seen (arrows). There is a large erosion at the medial aspect of the first metatarsal head, a typical location for a gouty erosion. **b.** AP radiograph in another patient. A large soft-tissue tophus is present medially (white arrows). The bony erosions (black arrows) form multi-septated, lacy, sharply-marginated lucencies.

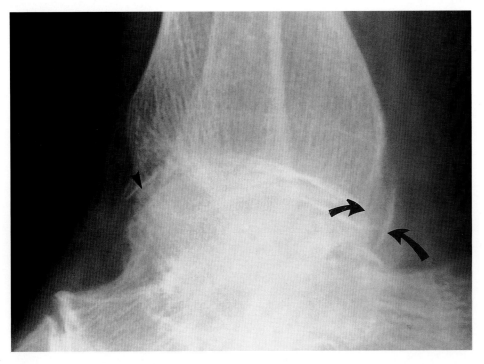

Fig. 5.44. Calcium pyrophosphate dihydrate deposition disease of the hindfoot. Lateral radiograph. Chondro-calcinosis is evident in the tibiotalar and talonavicular joints (arrowhead). Osteophytes are present at both these articulations. There is calcification of the flexor hallucis longus tendon (curved arrows).

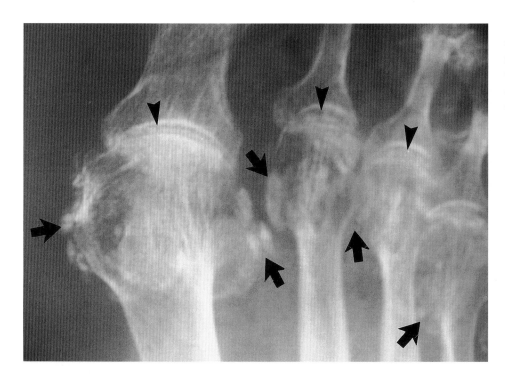

Fig. 5.45. Calcium pyrophosphate dihydrate deposition disease of the metatarsophalangeal joints. AP radiograph. Chondrocalcinosis is present (arrowheads), as well as capsular and periarticular calcifications (arrows).

Treatment

Treatment is medical, employing chiefly nonsteroidal anti-inflammatory drugs. Joint aspiration to remove crystals, and intra-articular steroid injections are used in acute attacks.

Hydroxyapatite Deposition Disease (Basic Calcium Phosphate Crystal Deposition Disease)

Basic calcium phosphate crystals include hydroxyapatite, octacalcium phosphate, and tricalcium phosphate.[69] They can deposit in and near joints, causing a painful arthropathy. Hydroxyapatite is the best known of the crystals, and the arthropathy caused by basic calcium phosphate crystals is generally termed hydroxyapatite deposition disease, or HADD. The crystals are extremely small and are visible only with electron microscopy. On light microscopy, nonbirefringent, globular aggregates of crystals are seen.[63]

Hydroxyapatite deposition disease is more common than CPPD in the foot. It tends to involve the great toe. Basic calcium phosphate crystals frequently deposit in tendons,[70] leading to tendonitis. When the crystals involve joints and bursae they produce gout-like attacks, which in most cases are monoarticular.

Radiographic findings

An amorphous calcific deposit is seen either within the joint or in a bursa (Fig. 5. 46). Unlike CPPD, chondrocalcinosis is usually absent. As a pseudogout attack caused by hydroxyapatite resolves, the calcifications may resorb.[63]

MISCELLANEOUS ARTHROPATHIES

Pigmented Villonodular Synovitis

Pigmented villonodular synovitis (PVNS) is a monoarticular, proliferative synovial process. PVNS may also arise in tendon

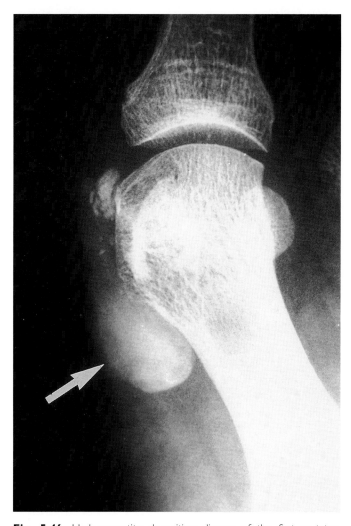

Fig. 5.46. Hydroxyapatite deposition disease of the first metatarsophalangeal joint. AP radiograph. A cloud of hazy calcification (arrow) fills the bursa medial to the head of the 1st metatarsal.

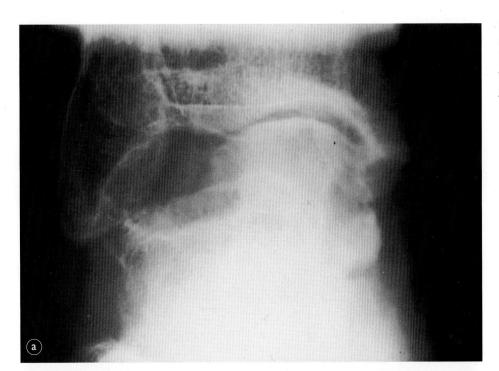

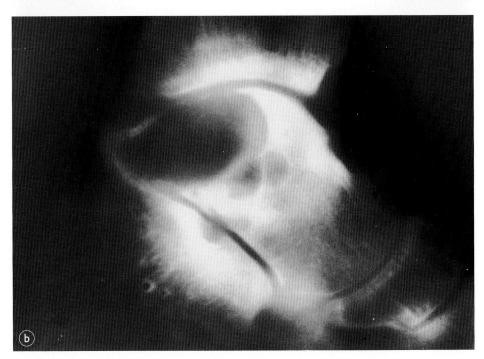

Fig. 5.47. Pigmented villonodular synovitis of the tibiotalar joint. **a.** AP radiograph. **b.** Lateral tomogram. A large cavity is seen in the talar dome laterally and posteriorly. Joint space is preserved.

sheaths, where (confusingly) it goes under the name of giant cell tumor of tendon sheath. The etiology is unknown, although it may be a post-traumatic[71] or an inflammatory process.[72] It generally occurs in patients between the ages of 20 and 50, and is more common in the ankle than in the foot. It can involve any joint. Patients complain of pain and swelling of insiduous onset.

Histologically, hemosiderin deposition is seen, as well as fibrosis and lipid-filled histiocytes. The synovium is thickened and villonodular.[73] These histologic features have distinctive correlative findings on MRI.

Radiographic findings

PLAIN RADIOGRAPHS

Plain radiographs in PVNS are often normal. Joint effusions and soft tissue masses are sometimes evident. As the disease progresses, erosions with sclerotic margins develop. Erosions arise within the joint capsule, but are often located away from the articular surface. They may be large in size (Fig. 5.47).

NUCLEAR MEDICINE STUDIES

PVNS is a highly vascular lesion, and three-phase ⁹⁹ᵐtechnetium-MDP bone scan will show increased flow and blood pool

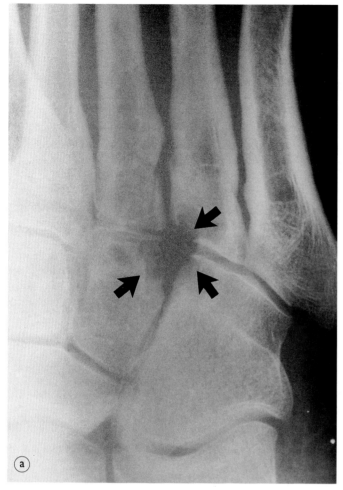

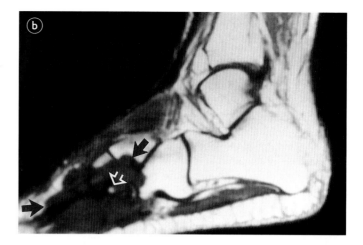

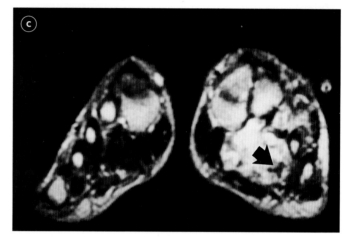

Fig. 5.48. Pigmented villonodular synovitis arising between the lateral cuneiform, cuboid and fourth metatarsal base. Patient had foot pain for eight years. Initial radiographs were normal. **a.** Oblique radiograph shows erosions (arrows) at the tarsometatarsal joints of the 3rd and 4th toes. **b.** Sagittal MRI, T1-weighted, SE 600/20. A soft-tissue mass (black arrows) is present, and is much larger than would be expected from the plain radiographic findings. Because the mass was located within the deep portion of the middle plantar soft-tissue compartment, its size was also not evident on clinical examination. The small, high-signal area within the mass (open white arrow) is an area of lipid-laden histiocytes. **c.** Coronal MRI, T2-weighted, SE 2000/80. The majority of the mass is hyperintense to muscle. A small focus of hemosiderin deposition (arrow) remains low in signal intensity.

activity. If bone erosions are present, the third phase of the scan will be abnormal as well.[72] The bone scan pattern is indistinguishable from many other processes such as infection, inflammatory arthritis, gout, and neuropathic joint.

CT AND MRI

CT will demonstrate a lobular soft-tissue mass, and bone erosions are well seen when present. The density of the soft-tissue mass may be indistinguishable from adjacent muscle, or it may be increased, owing to hemosiderin deposition.

MRI has become the imaging modality of choice, because MRI characteristics of PVNS are fairly specific.[74] PVNS appears as a heterogeneous mass. Areas of lipid-laden histiocytes show high signal on T1-weighted images, decreasing on T2-weighted images. Areas of hemosiderin deposition are of low signal intensity on all pulse sequences. They may be either large areas or punctate, relatively inconspicuous foci. The MRI diagnosis is

more difficult when only small areas of hemosiderin deposition are present.

Differential diagnosis

On plain radiographs, the findings cannot be distinguished from those of indolent infection (fungal or tubercular) or monoarticular gout. Synovial chondromatosis may have an identical appearance. A slow-growing, dense soft-tissue tumor such as desmoid should also be considered.

On MRI and histologic examination, the major differential consideration is hemosiderotic synovitis, which is caused by recurrent episodes of hemorrhage into a joint (e.g. from hemangioma or hemophilia).[73]

Treatment

Synovectomy is recommended for treatment, since if the mass is left in situ there will be continued growth. Any intraosseous extensions must be curetted and filled with bone graft. Unfortunately, the disease may recur. Radiation therapy has been used in cases where surgery is not feasible or has previously failed.

Synovial Chondromatosis

Primary synovial chondromatosis is a process in which there is metaplasia of synovium into cartilaginous nodules.[75] The nodules are usually tiny and numerous. The process is very uncommon in the ankle, and to my knowledge has not been reported in the foot. Patients present with pain and limitation of motion. They can be treated with total synovectomy.

Secondary synovial (osteo)chondromatosis refers to loose bodies within the joint, which may occur as the result of cartilaginous or osteocartilaginous fracture or osteoarthritis (see Fig. 5.5). If the loose bodies are not evident on plain radiographs, radiographic evalution is best performed with arthrotomography or CT arthrogram, as discussed in chapter 4 for the evaluation of osteochondritis dissecans. The loose bodies can be removed surgically.

Sarcoidosis

Sarcoidosis is a multisystem disease characterized by formation of noncaseating granulomata. The etiology is unknown. Between 10% and 35% of patients develop arthralgias,[76] but radiographic joint abnormalities are unusual. Joint narrowing and erosions may be seen. A review of several large series of patients found that an average of 5% showed bone abnormalities.[76] 'Lacelike' or 'punched-out' lytic lesions are the most common bone abnormality, and they typically occur in the hands and feet (Fig. 5.49).

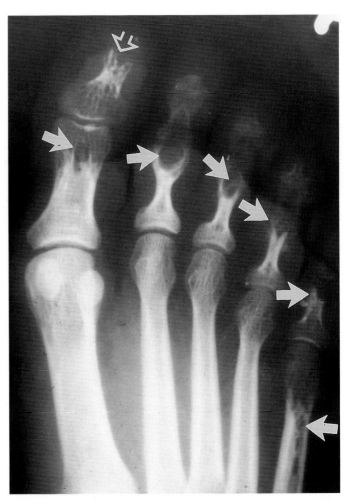

Fig. 5.49. Sarcoidosis. Acro-osteolysis is seen (open arrow). There are multiple "punched out" lesions in the proximal phalanges and the fifth metatarsal (arrows).

Diffuse Idiopathic Skeletal Hyperostosis

Diffuse idiopathic skeletal hyperostosis (DISH) is an enthesopathy associated with aging. Ossification develops at insertions of tendons and ligaments. The criteria for diagnosis are ossification of the paraspinous ligaments extending over at least four adjacent vertebral bodies[77] and absence of inflammatory changes of spondyloarthropathy. Patients who have extensive ossification of the paraspinous ligaments may complain of spinal stiffness and pain.[77] More than 70% of patients with DISH have enthesopathic changes in the foot, most commonly at the attachment of the plantar fascia. The changes in the foot may be asymptomatic, but can cause local pain.[78]

Radiographic findings
Calcification or ossification is seen at insertions of tendons and ligaments (Fig. 5.50). These enthesophytes may be large. They often have a 'whiskered' appearance, fanning out along the tendon fibers.

Differential diagnosis
Bone erosions are not present in DISH, unlike inflammatory arthritides. Although the ossification of the paraspinous ligaments may mimic the findings of psoriatic arthritis and Reiter's syndrome, DISH is distinguished by the normal appearance of the sacroiliac joints. DISH may coexist with other arthritides.

Treatment
Nonsteroidal anti-inflammatory drugs are the major form of treatment. Orthoses and local injections of steroids or anesthetic are also used. Surgical excision of spurs is rarely necessary.

Nontraumatic Synovitis of the Metatarsophalangeal Joint

Monoarticular, nontraumatic synovitis of the metatarsophalangeal joint has been reported to be a separate entity from inflammatory arthritis.[79] However, it may be a manifestation of rupture of the plantar plate (see Chapter 4).

Hemodialysis-Related Arthropathy

Patients on long-term hemodialysis develop arthropathies that are sometimes due to secondary hyperparathyroidism (see

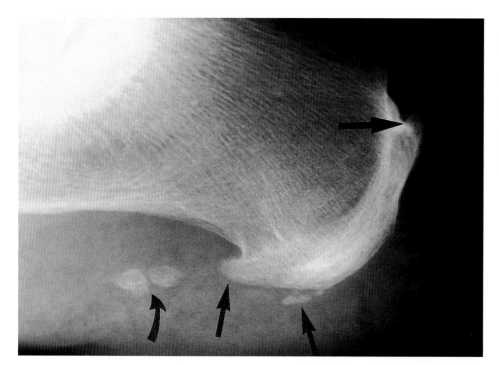

Fig. 5.50. Diffuse idiopathic skeletal hyperostosis. Lateral radiograph of the heel. There are multiple enthesophytes (straight arrows), as well as soft-tissue ossifications which may be in the plantar fascia (curved arrow). The spurs are well corticated and there is no evidence of erosions. Plantar calcaneal spurs may be asymptomatic, or may be associated with heel pain syndrome (see Chapter 8).

Chapter 12), sometimes due to deposition of an amyloid-like substance called beta-2 microglobulin in the joints,[80] and sometimes due to deposition of calcium oxalate particles.[81] Erosive changes are seen, with variable preservation of the joint space. The spine is often involved. Carpal tunnel syndrome is seen, caused by amyloid deposition, but tarsal tunnel syndrome is not reported although by analogy a similar process could be anticipated. Erosive changes may be present in the digits.

NEUROPATHIC JOINT DISEASE

Neuropathic joint disease is common in the foot. Neuropathic joints are also known as Charcot joints, after the French neurologist who originally described the abnormalities, in 1868.

Pathogenesis

Neuropathic joint disease occurs when motion of the joint is preserved but proprioception and pain sensation are diminished or lost. Charcot, as well as some more recent investigators,[82] thought that the joint destruction was due to a neurally mediated vascular reflex. Most investigators today believe that neuroarthropathy is due to repetitive trauma.[83–85] Because proprioception is lost, the patient tends to move the joint beyond its normal range. This can result in ligamentous injury and microfractures of the bone. In a normal individual, the resultant pain would induce him to rest the joint, but since pain is absent or minimal the joint continues to be used, leading to further injury. The joint may become dislocated, and fractures occur which fail to unite because the joint continues to be used. A vicious cycle develops in which instability leads to joint injury, which in turn causes worsening of the instability. This process can lead to complete destruction of a joint within weeks of the original injury.[86] Only infectious arthritis has as rapid a course.

Neuropathic changes are most commonly seen in the Lisfranc joint and the toes, but can occur in any joint. Patients typically present complaining of deformity or instability. Pain may be present, but is mild in view of the severe destructive changes. There are many causes of neuropathic joint disease. Those which affect the foot and ankle are listed in Table 5.5. By far the most common of them is diabetes mellitus. Neuropathic joints due to diabetes most commonly occur in patients with long-standing disease. A series of 96 patients who developed neuropathic joints due to diabetes found that 74% presented with foot ulcers.[100]

Radiographic findings

PLAIN RADIOGRAPHS
The earliest findings of neuropathic joints are subluxations or dislocations, fractures, joint effusions, and degenerative-appearing spurs[101] (Fig. 5.51). The joint may be either narrowed or widened. Periosteal new bone is an early finding (Figs 5.51, 5.52). As the process continues, the joint can develop either a hypertrophic or an atrophic appearance.[87–89] Hypertrophic changes are more common, especially in the hind and midfoot.

Hypertrophic neuropathic joints (Figs 5.51–5.54) are characterized by large osteophytes. Exuberant callus results from the unstable nature of the associated fractures. Osseous and carti-

Table 5.5. Causes of neuropathic joints in the foot and ankle

Diabetes mellitus[78–80]	Amyloid neuropathy[73,86]
Alcoholic neuropathy[81]	Myelomeningocele[84,87,88]
Congenital insensitivity to pain[82–84]	Leprosy[76] and other neuropathies[84]
Neurosyphilis[85]	Steroid injection[73,89,90]

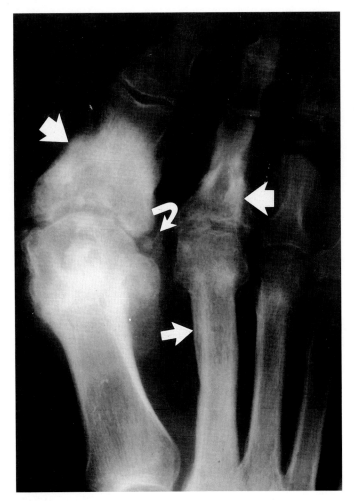

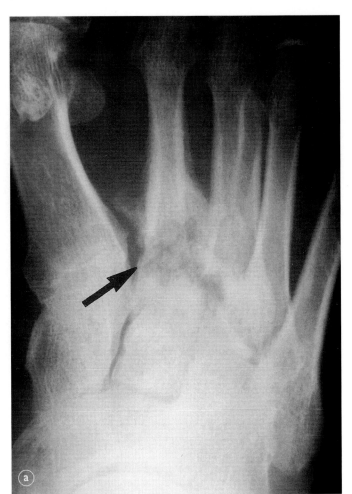

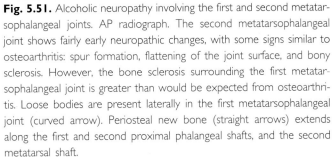

Fig. 5.51. Alcoholic neuropathy involving the first and second metatarsophalangeal joints. AP radiograph. The second metatarsophalangeal joint shows fairly early neuropathic changes, with some signs similar to osteoarthritis: spur formation, flattening of the joint surface, and bony sclerosis. However, the bone sclerosis surrounding the first metatarsophalangeal joint is greater than would be expected from osteoarthritis. Loose bodies are present laterally in the first metatarsophalangeal joint (curved arrow). Periosteal new bone (straight arrows) extends along the first and second proximal phalangeal shafts, and the second metatarsal shaft.

laginous debris from the fractures is deposited in and around the joint. The affected bone preserves its density because it continues to be used. Indeed, the bone often becomes denser than surrounding bones because of callus formation and the compression fracture of the articular surfaces. The disuse osteoporosis that is a characteristic feature of osteomyelitis is absent. Subluxation and dislocation are frequent. Severe foot deformities may develop. Neuropathic disease of the midfoot causes reversal of the normal arch of the foot, resulting in a 'rockerbottom' deformity (see Fig. 5.53).

Atrophic neuropathic joint disease usually occurs in the forefoot,[87,89] with resorption of the subarticular bone (Fig. 5.55). Resorption of the ungual tufts may also be seen.

In children, nonhealing fractures of the physis may be the major radiographic finding.[91-93,96] Periosteal new bone is prominent. Clinically, it is important to differentiate these findings from those of child abuse.

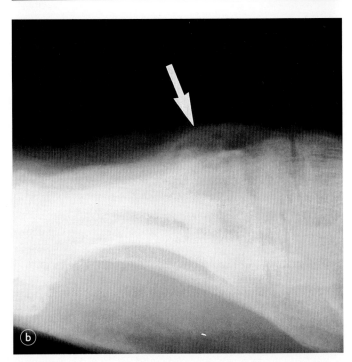

Fig. 5.52. Neuropathic Lisfranc fracture in a diabetic patient. **a.** AP radiograph. Fracture (arrow) of the base of the second metatarsal is seen. There is a large amount of callus formation. No subluxation of the joint has developed. **b.** Lateral radiograph. Periosteal reaction (arrow) is evident at the nonunited fracture, and could be mistaken for a sign of infection. Osteomyelitis is not likely because of the preservation of bone density.

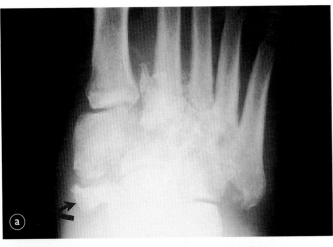

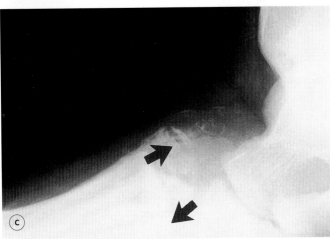

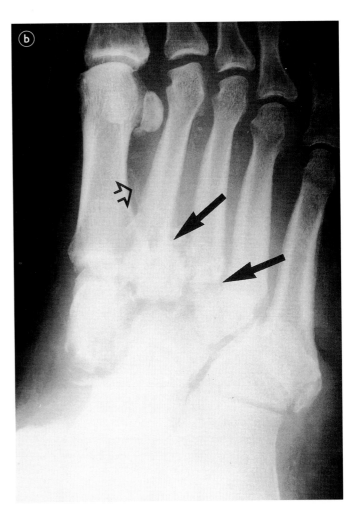

Fig. 5.53. Neuropathic changes of the midfoot in a diabetic patient. **a.** AP radiograph. The second through fifth metatarsal bases are dislocated laterally, while the first metatarsal and first cuneiform are dislocated medially, along with a fragment from the navicular (curved arrow). Increased bone density is evident; this is due to bone debris. **b.** Oblique radiograph. Fractures (arrows) through the bases of the second and third metatarsals are seen. Open arrow points to arterial calcifications, a common finding in diabetic patients. **c.** Lateral radiograph. Dorsal dislocation of the tarsometatarsal joints has led to reversal of the normal arch of the foot, the 'rocker-bottom' deformity. Arrows point to the relative positions of the second metatarsal base and the second cuneiform, which normally articulate.

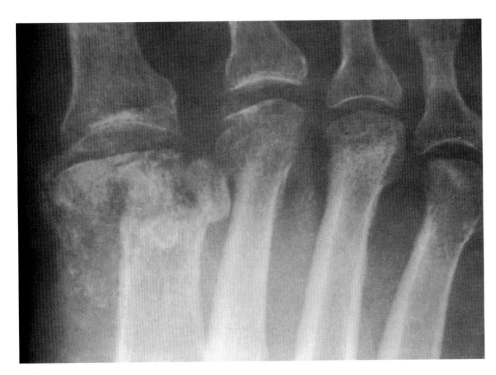

Fig. 5.54. Neuropathic disease of the first through third metatarsophalangeal joints. AP radiograph. There is a fracture of the first metatarsal head, surrounded by osseous debris. Flattening and irregularity of the second and third metatarsal heads are seen and are caused by subcortical fractures. The first and second metatarsals are in separate soft-tissue compartments, making infection unlikely. The prominent osseous debris is also unusual in infection.

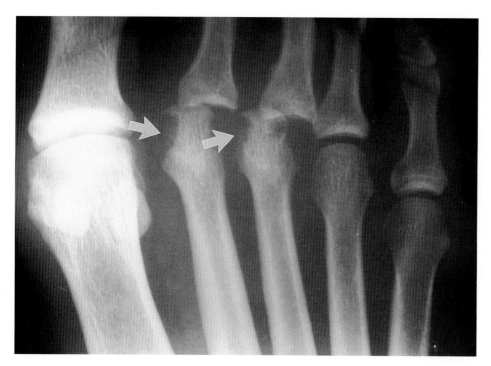

Fig. 5.55. Atrophic neuropathic changes of the second and third metatarsophalangeal joints. AP radiograph. Patient had been given steroid injections, which caused local insensitivity to pain and led to neuropathic joint disease. Erosions (arrows) at metatarsal heads could be mistaken for infection or inflammatory arthritis. Signs that suggest neuropathic diseases are the preservation of bone density, and the dislocations of the metatarsophalangeal joints. By the time that dislocations develop in rheumatoid arthritis, more severe joint erosions, involving a greater extent of the metatarsal heads, are usually present. Dislocations are unlikely in infectious arthritis. Note that although infectious arthritis is usually monoarticular, the second, third and fourth metatarsal heads occupy the same soft-tissue compartment, allowing spread of infection to the adjacent metatarsal. Therefore, the involvement of two adjacent metatarsophalangeal joints does not exclude infection.

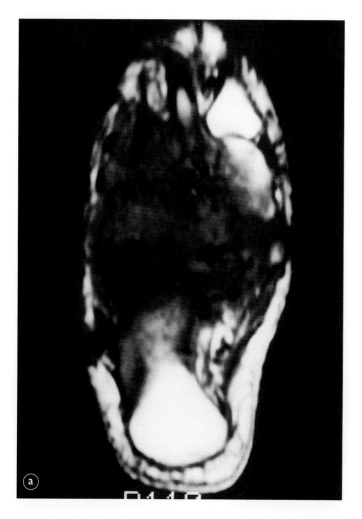

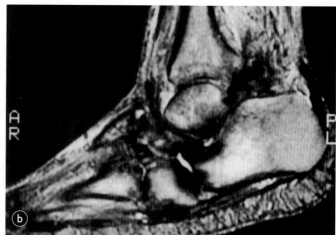

Fig. 5.56. Neuropathic disease of the midfoot on MRI. **a**. Axial T1-weighted, SE 600/20. An ill-defined mass of low-signal intensity due to callus and bone debris is seen in the midfoot, and it is difficult to distinguish the bony anatomy. **b**. Sagittal MRI T2-weighted, SE 2000/80. Rocker-bottom deformity of the foot is evident. High-signal intensity within the marrow is due to edema and trabecular trauma. Bone sclerosis at the calcaneocuboid joint remains low in signal intensity.

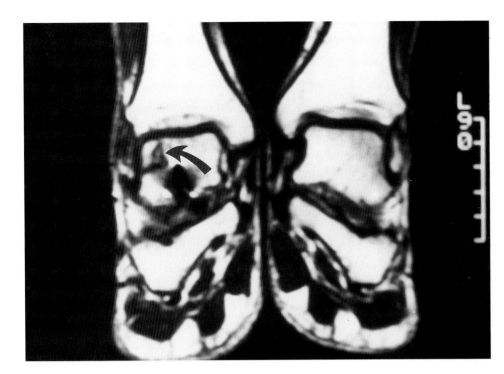

Fig. 5.57. Osteonecrosis of the talar dome. Coronal MRI T1-weighted, SE 650/20. Plain radiographs were negative. Artifact from a screw across the fracture site does not obscure the talar dome, where a focus of AVN is evident laterally (curved arrow).

RADIONUCLIDE IMAGING

Acute neuropathic joint disease is usually positive on [99m]technetium diphosphonate three-phase bone scans[102] (see Chapter 6). Chronic neuropathic joints may be positive on the delayed phase of the bone scan only. Up to 31% of neuropathic joints are positive on indium-labelled white blood cell scans.[103] A negative indium-labelled WBC scan can fairly reliably exclude infection, but a positive scan does not necessarily indicate that infection is present.

MRI

MRI demonstrates bone marrow signal abnormalities that are centered on a joint. There is decreased marrow signal on T1-weighted images, and increased signal on T2-weighted and STIR images (Fig. 5.56). Abnormalities on T2-weighted images are less prominent in long-standing cases. Joint effusion, disruption of the joint, a soft-tissue mass, and osseous debris may be evident. The findings often cannot be differentiated from those of infection. Neuropathic joint is suggested if the marrow abnormalities involve multiple adjacent bones, since in most infections no more than two adjacent bones are involved.

Differential diagnosis

The main mimic of neuropathic joint is infection. This differential diagnosis is discussed in detail in Chapter 6. Calcium pyrophosphate deposition sometimes causes severe destruction similar to neuropathic joint, but it rarely does so in the foot. Osteoarthritis is often identical in appearance to early neuropathic joint, but it does not show the same rapid course.

Avascular Necrosis

A bone becomes necrotic when its blood supply is interrupted by any of a large number of causes (Table 5.6). The most

Table 5.6. Causes of avascular necrosis. (From Steinberg and Steinberg.[104])

Trauma	Emboli
Sickle cell disease	Pancreatitis
Idiopathic	Radiation
Steroids	Caisson's disease
Vasculitis	Gaucher's disease

common causes are fracture, steroid use, sickle-cell disease, postoperative causes, and idiopathic.

A bone may undergo necrosis either in its epiphysis or its shaft. When necrosis occurs in the epiphysis, it is referred to as avascular necrosis, aseptic necrosis, or osteonecrosis. When it occurs in the shaft of a bone, it is referred to as an infarct. Although histologically the process is the same regardless of location, it is useful to maintain this distinction, because the radiographic findings and clinical course of avascular necrosis differ from the findings and clinical course of infarcts. Bone infarcts mimic bone tumors in their presentation, and are discussed in Chapter 11.

Repair of a focus of osteonecrosis occurs as new blood vessels grow into the necrotic bone. Granulation tissue is seen primarily at the periphery of the abnormal area. New bone is deposited within the osteonecrotic area. The subarticular bone is weakened by deposition of disorganized new bone and resorption of existing trabeculae. Fracture and articular collapse may occur, leading to joint incongruity and secondary osteoarthritis.

Sites of avascular necrosis in the foot

Avascular necrosis occurs at several characteristic sites in the foot: the talar dome, the metatarsal heads (most commonly the second), and the navicular.

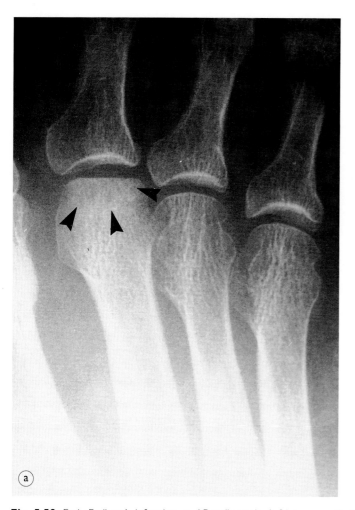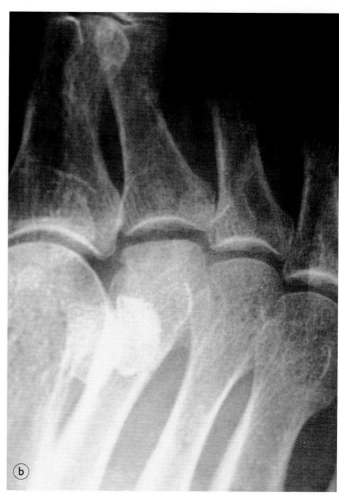

Fig. 5.58. Early Freiberg's infraction. **a**. AP radiograph. A faint crescentic line can be seen in the metatarsal head. Flattening of the metatarsal head should not be considered a sign of osteonecrosis, since it may be a normal variant. **b**. Oblique radiograph. The oblique view is useful to confirm the subtle findings.

Talar dome osteonecrosis

Osteonecrosis is a complication of displaced fractures of the neck of the talus, or a dislocation of the ankle, which disrupt the blood supply to the talar dome (Fig. 5.57; see Chapter 4, Figs 4.10, 4.11). Osteochondritis dissecans of the talar dome is an osteochondral fracture leading to bone necrosis (see Chapter 4).

Freiberg's infraction

Freiberg's infraction is avascular necrosis of a metatarsal head, most commonly the second.[105–107] It is thought to be due to repetitive trauma, and is associated with conditions that increase stress on the metatarsal head: high-heeled shoes, cowboy boots, short first toe, and surgery on the first toe (Figs 5.58, 5.59). It may also be associated with congenital absence of the second metatarsal artery.[106] It has been reported in diabetic patients, where it may be due to altered mechanics of the foot.[107]

Koehler's disease

Koehler's disease refers to osteonecrosis of the navicular in children. A normally-developing, asymptomatic navicular bone can have a sclerotic, fragmented, irregular appearance in children (see Chapter 1, Fig. 1.19). Radiographically this normal variant is indistinguishable from Koehler's disease.[108] The diagnosis is made when radiographic findings are present and the child has pain and tenderness in the area of the navicular. Koehler's disease occurs between the ages of 2 and 9 years, with an average age of 6 years.[108,109] It is a benign, self-limited process.[109]

Adult-onset osteonecrosis of the navicular

Osteonecrosis is seen in adults, probably caused by repetitive trauma.[110] It is often bilateral. The bone becomes sclerotic and has a flattened contour. It may occur following stress fractures (see Chaper 4) of the navicular.

Osteonecrosis of the hallux sesamoids

Idiopathic osteonecrosis of the sesamoids which are plantar to the first metatarsal head has been reported.[111]

Radiographic findings

PLAIN RADIOGRAPHS

The earliest stage of avascular necrosis is not detectable on plain radiographs, but can be diagnosed by MRI or bone scan

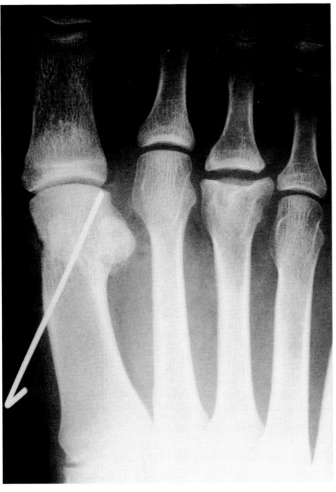

Fig. 5.59. Advanced Freiberg's infraction of the 3rd metatarsal head occuring after bunion surgery. AP radiograph. There is sclerosis of the metatarsal head, and the articular surface is concave rather than the normal convex shape. Secondary osteoarthritis has developed.

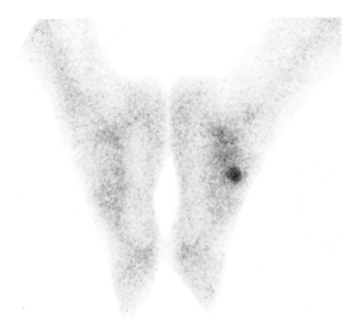

Fig. 5.60. Avascular necrosis of the navicular. ^{99m}Tc-MDP bone scan, lateral projection. A focus of increased activity is seen in the navicular. Plain radiographs were normal.

findings. As bony repair progresses, irregular areas of sclerosis can be seen (Fig. 5.58). A semicircular line of sclerosis is especially characteristic. It occurs at the interface between normal and necrotic bone. A thin lucency due to infraction of the subcortical bone is often seen in the hip, but uncommonly identified in the foot and ankle. This lucency should be distinguished from the Hawkins sign (see Chapter 4), which is a subcortical lucency that develops because of hyperemia and osteoporosis occuring after a fracture. A Hawkins sign indicates that vascularity is intact, and therefore indirectly signifies that osteonecrosis is absent. In advanced avascular necrosis, collapse of the articular surface develops, leading to secondary osteoarthritis (Fig. 5.59).

The diagnosis of avascular necrosis can often be made by assessing the patient's history and the radiographs. A bone scan is an inexpensive screening test in cases where radiographs are normal, but if the diagnosis is in doubt following bone scan, MRI can be performed.

TECHNETIUM BONE SCAN

In early avascular necrosis, radionuclide uptake on ^{99m}technetium diphosphonate bone scan is absent. Radionuclide uptake in more advanced cases is increased, owing to the deposition of reparative new bone at the periphery of the necrotic area (Fig. 5.60). An area of centrally absent uptake surrounded by increased activity can often be discerned, especially with the use of converging or pinhole collimators.

Bone marrow scans employing ^{99m}technetium sulfur colloid have been used to evaluate avascular necrosis of the hip. However, sulfur colloid is taken up by phagocytosis primarily in erythropoietic marrow, and thus it is not useful in evaluating the fatty marrow of the foot and ankle.

MRI

MRI has been shown to have superior sensitivity and specificity for osteonecrosis compared to ^{99m}technetium bone scan. A study of 85 hips found MRI sensitivity of 88.8% and specificity of 100%, compared to sensitivity of 77.5% and specificity of 75% for bone scan.[112]

The majority of the reports of MRI findings of avascular necrosis are focused on findings in the hip. However, analagous changes are seen in other areas. As in bone infarcts, the central portion may show signal characteristics of fat, fibrous tissue, or fluid. It is usually demarcated by a jagged, crescentic, low-signal intensity line (Fig. 5.57), which on T2-weighted images may be paralleled by a high-signal intensity line.[112–114]

Another reported pattern of marrow abnormality is diffuse low-signal intensity on T1-weighted images, increasing to high signal intensity on T2-weighted images.[115] Although some patients with this pattern do go on to develop radiographic findings of avascular necrosis, many do not. This pattern is nonspecific, and other entities, listed in Table 5.7, should be considered.

Table 5.7. Causes of MRI evidence of diffuse marrow abnormality in subarticular bone

Bone bruise

Transient osteoporosis

Neuropathic joint

Osteomyelitis

Tumor infiltration

Early avascular necrosis

Differential diagnosis

Advanced avascular necrosis may radiographically be indistinguishable from severe osteoarthritis. If sequential radiographs are available, they are helpful, because in avascular necrosis, collapse of the articular surface precedes the development of joint abnormalities.

On MRI, avascular necrosis may have the same appearance as osteochondritis dissecans (see Chapter 4). Often the margin of an area of osteonecrosis will be serpentine, whereas the margin of an osteochondral fracture forms a smooth arc. The patient's history is also helpful. A diffuse pattern of marrow abnormality is not specific for avascular necrosis (Table 5.7).

Treatment

Treatment of avascular necrosis is site-specific. When avascular necrosis develops in the talar dome following a fracture, patients are usually treated with limitation of weight bearing. In recalcitrant cases, treatment options include revascularization of the talar dome[116] and arthrodesis. Freiberg's infraction can be treated with debridement, joint prosthesis, or rotational osteotomy.[105]

REFERENCES

1. ARA nomenclature and classification of arthritis and rheumatism. *JAMA* (suppl) 1973; **224:**662–812.

2. Hamerman D. The biology of osteoarthritis. *N Engl J Med* 1989; **320:**1322–30.

3. O'Donoghue DH. Impingement exostoses of the talus and tibia. *J Bone Joint Surg [Am]* 1957; **39A:**835–52.

4. Kleiger B. Anterior tibiotalar impingement syndromes in dancers. *Foot Ankle* 1983; **3:**69–73.

5. Guhl JF, Stone JW, Ferkel RD. Other osteochondral pathology – fractures and fracture defects. In: Guhl JF. *Foot and Ankle Arthroscopy*, 2nd edn. (Slack: Thorofare NJ, 1993), 131–4.

6. Stoller SM, Hekmat F, Kleiger B. A comparative study of the frequency of anterior impingement exostoses of the ankle in dancers and nondancers. *Foot Ankle* 1984; **4:**201–3.

7. St Pierre RK, Velzco A, Fleming LL. Impingement exostoses of the talus and fibula secondary to an inversion sprain: a case report. *Foot Ankle* 1983; **3:**282–5.

8. Hawkins BJ, Haddad RJ. Hallux Rigidus. *Clin Sports Med* 1988; **7:**37–49.

9. Karasick D, Wapner KL. Hallux rigidus deformity: radiologic assessment. *Am J Roentgenol* 1991; **157:**1029–33.

10. Cracchiolo A, Weltmer JB, Lian G, Dalseth T, Dorey F. Arthroplasty of the first metatarsophalangeal joint with a double stem silicone implant. Results in patients who have degenerative joint disease, failure of previous operations or rheumatoid arthritis. *J Bone Joint Surg [Am]* 1992; **74A:**552-63

11. Alarcon GS. Seronegative polyarthritis. In: Kelley WN, Harris ED, Ruddy S, Sledge CB (eds). *Textbook of Rheumatology*, 3rd edn. (WB Saunders: Philadelphia, 1989), 905-11.

12. Arnett FC, Edworthy S, Bloch DA, et al. The 1987 revised criteria for rheumatoid arthritis. *Arthritis Rheum* 1987; **30:**S17.

13. Thould AK, Simon GG. Assessment of radiological changes in the hands and feet in rheumatoid arthritis. Their correlation with prognosis. *Ann Rheum Dis* 1966; **25:**220–8.

14. Brook A, Corbett M. Radiographic changes in early rheumatoid disease. *Ann Rheum Dis* 1977; **36:**71–3.

15. Minaker K, Little H. Painful feet in rheumatoid arthritis. *Can Med Assoc J* 1973; **109:**724–30.

16. Mottonen TT, Hannonen PO, Toivanen J, Rekonen A, Oka M. Value of joint scintigraphy in the prediction of erosiveness in early rheumatoid arthritis. *Ann Rheum Dis* 1988; **47:**183–9.

17. De Haas WH, De Boer W, Griffioen F, Oosten-Elst P. Rheumatoid arthritis of the robust reaction type. *Ann Rheum Dis* 1974; **33:**81–4.

18. Gubler FM, Maas M, Dijkstra PF, De Jongh HR. Cystic rheumatoid arthritis: description of a nonerosive form. *Radiology* 1990; **177:**829–34.

19. Michelson J, Easley M, Wigley FM, Hellman D. Foot and ankle problems in rheumatoid arthritis. *Foot Ankle* 1994; **15:**608–13.

20. Bienstock H. Rheumatoid plantar synovial cysts. *Ann Rheum Dis* 1975; **34:**948–99.

21. D'Amico JC. The pathomechanics of adult rheumatoid arthritis affecting the foot. *J Am Pod Assoc* 1976; **4:**227-36.

22. Rennel C, Mainzer F, Mulitz CV, Genant HK. Subchondral pseudocysts in rheumatoid arthritis. *Am J Roentgenol* 1977; **129:**1069–72.

23. Magyar E, Talerman A, Feher M, Wouters HW. The pathogenesis of the subchondral pseudocysts in rheumatoid arthritis. *Clin Orthop* 1974; **100:**341–4.

24. Rappoport AS, Sosman JL, Weissman BN. Lesions resembling gout in patients with rheumatoid arthritis. *Am J Med* 1976; **126:**41–5.

25. El-Khoury GY, Larson RK, Kathol MH, et al. Seronegative and seropositive rheumatoid arthritis: radiographic differences. *Radiology* 1988; **168:**517–20.

26. Burns TM, Calin A. The hand radiograph as a diagnostic discriminant between seropositive and seronegative 'rheumatoid arthritis': a controlled study. *Ann Rheum Dis* 1983; **42:**605–12.

27. Brower AC. Use of the radiograph to measure the course of rheumatoid arthritis. *Arthritis Rheum* 1990; **33:**316–24.

28. Scott DL, Grindulis KA, Struthers GR, et al. Progression of radiological changes in rheumatoid arthritis. *Ann Rheum Dis* 1984; **43:**8–17.

29. Cracchiolo A. Management of the arthritic forefoot. *Foot Ankle* 1982; **3:**17-23.

30. Cracchiolo A, Person S, Kitaoka HB, Grace D. Hindfoot arthrodesis in adults utilizing a dowel graft technique. *Clin Orthop* 1990; **257:**193-203.

31. Al-Janabi MA, Critchley M, Maltby P, Britton KE. Radiolabelled white blood cell imaging in arthritis. Is it a blood pool effect? *Nucl Med Commun* 1991; **12**:1013–24.

32. Uno K, Suguro T, Nohira K, et al. Comparison of Indium-labelled leukocyte scintigraphy and Technetium-99m joint scintigraphy in rheumatoid arthritis and osteoarthritis. *Ann Nuclear Med* 1992; **6**:247–51.

33. Foley-Nolan D, Stack JP, Ryan M, et al. Magnetic resonance imaging in the assessment of rheumatoid arthritis: a comparison with plain film radiographs. *Br J Rheumatol* 1991; **30**:101–6.

34. Korsunoglu-Brahme S, Riccio T, Weisman MH et al. Rheumatoid knee: role of gadopentate-enhanced MR imaging. *Radiology* 1990; **155**:176:831–5.

35. Poleksic L, Zdravkovic D, Jablanovic D, Watt I, Bacic G. Magnetic resonance imaging of bone destruction in rheumatoid arthritis: comparison with radiography. *Skeletal Radiol* 1993; **22**:557–80.

36. Cracchiolo A. Office practice footwear and orthosis. *Foot Ankle* 1982; **4**:242-8.

37. Cracchiolo A. The rheumatoid foot and ankle: Pathology and treatment. *Foot* 1993; **3**:126–34.

38. Moeckel BH, Sculco TP, Alexiades MM, et all. The double-stemmed silicone-rubber implant for rheumatoid arthritis of the first metatarsophalangeal joint: long-term results. *J Bone Joint Surg [Am]* 1992; **74A**:564–70.

39. Gold RH, Cracchiolo A III, Bassett LW. Prosthetic procedures of the joints of the ankle and foot. *Semin Roentgenol* 1986; **21**:75–83.

40. Cracchiolo A, Cimino W, Lian G. Arthrodesis of the ankle in patients who have rheumatoid arthritis. *J Bone Joint Surg [Am]* 1992; **74A**:903–9.

41. Schaller JG. Chronic arthritis in children. Juvenile rheumatoid arthritis. *Clin Orthop* 1984; **182**:79–89.

42. Resnick D, Niwayama G. Juvenile chronic arthritis. In: Resnick D, Niwayama G (eds). *Diagnosis of Bone and Joint Disorders*, 2nd edn. (WB Saunders: Philadelphia, 1988), 1068–1102.

43. Wilkinson RH, Weissman BN. Arthritis in children. *Radiol Clin N Am* 1988; **26**:1247–65.

44. Cassidy JT, Levinson JE, Brewer EJ Jr. The development of classification criteria for children with juvenile rheumatoid arthritis. *Bull Rheum Dis* 1989; **38**:1–7.

45. Martel W, Holt JF, Cassidy JT. Roentgenologic manifestations of juvenile chronic arthritis. *Am J Roentgenol* 1962; **83**:400–23.

46. Rana NA. Juvenile rheumatoid arthritis of the foot. *Foot Ankle* 1982; **3**:2–11.

47. Gold RH, Bassett LW. Radiologic evaluation of the arthritic foot. *Foot Ankle* 1982; **2**:332–41.

48. Resnick D, Niwayama G. Ankylosing spondylitis. In: Resnick D, Niwayama G (eds). *Diagnosis of Bone and Joint Disorders*, 2nd edn. (WB Saunders: Philadelphia, 1988), 1103–70.

49. Ford DK. Reiter's syndrome. *Bull Rheum Dis* 1970; **20**:588–91.

50. Resnick D. Reiter's Syndrome. In: Resnick D, Niwayama G (eds). *Diagnosis of Bone and Joint Disorders*, 2nd edn. (WB Saunders: Philadelphia, 1988), 1199–1217.

51. Resnick, D, Niwayama G. Psoriatic Arthritis. In: Resnick D, Niwayama G (eds). *Diagnosis of Bone and Joint Disorders*, 2nd edn. (WB Saunders: Philadelphia, 1988), 1171–98.

52. Resnick D, Feingold ML, Curd J, et al. Calcaneal abnormalities in articular disorders: rheumatoid arthritis, ankylosing spondylitis, psoriatic arthritis and Reiter's syndrome. *Radiology* 1977; **125**:355–66.

53. Khalkhali IJ, Stadalnik RC, Wiesner KB, Shapiro RF. Bone imaging of the heel in Reiter's syndrome. *Am J Roentgenol* 1979; **132**:110–2.

54. Haustein UF, Herrman K, Boehme H. Pathogenesis of progressive systemic sclerosis. *Int J Dermatol* 1986; **25**:286–93.

55. Bassett LW, Blocka KLN, Furst DE, Clements PJ, Gold RH. Skeletal findings in progressive systemic sclerosis (scleroderma). *Am J Roentgenol* 1981; **136**:1121–6.

56. Resnick D, Scavulli JF, Goergen TG, Genant HK, Niwayama G. Intra-articular calcification in scleroderma. *Radiology* 1977; **124**:685–8.

57. Velayos EE, Masi AT, Stevens MB, Shulman LE. The 'CREST' syndrome. comparison with systemic sclerosis (scleroderma). *Arch Intern Med* 1979; **139**:1240–4.

58. Resnick D. Mixed connective tissue disease and collagen vascular overlap syndromes. In: Resnick D, Niwayama G (eds). *Diagnosis of Bone and Joint Disorders*, 2nd edn. (WB Saunders: Philadelphia, 1988), 1343–52.

59. Resnick D. Systemic Lupus Erythematosis. In: Resnick D, Niwayama G (eds). *Diagnosis of Bone and Joint Disorders*, 2nd edn. (WB Saunders: Philadelphia, 1988), 1267–92.

60. Resnick D. Dermatomyositis and Polymyositis. In: Resnick D, Niwayama G (eds). *Diagnosis of Bone and Joint Disorders*, 2nd edn. (WB Saunders: Philadelphia, 1988), 1319–31.

61. Lawson JP, Steere AC. Lyme arthritis: radiologic findings. *Radiology* 1985; **154**:37–43.

62. Faller J, Thompson F, Hamilton W. Foot and ankle disorders resulting from Lyme disease. *Foot Ankle* 1991; **11**:236–8.

63. Rubenstein J, Pritzker KP. Crystal-associated arthropathies. *Am J Roentgenol* 1989; **152**:685–95.

64. Healey LA. Epidemiology of hyperuricemia. *Arthritis Rheum* 1975; **18**:709–12.

65. Bloch C, Hermann G, Yu TF. A radiologic reevaluation of gout: a study of 2,000 patients. *Am J Roentgenol* 1980; **134**:781–7.

66. Martel W. The overhanging margin of bone: a roentgenographic manifestation of gout. *Radiology* 1968; **91**:755–6.

67. Ruiz ME, Erickson SJ, Carrera GF, Hanel DP, Smith MD. Monoarticular gout following trauma: MR appearance. *J Comput Assist Tomog* 1993; **17**:151–3.

68. Tophaceous pyrophosphate deposition with extensor tendon rupture. *Br J Rheumatol* 1992; **31**:421–3.

69. Halverson PB, McCarty DJ. Basic calcium phosphate (apatite, octacalcium phosphate, tricalcium phosphate) crystal deposition diseases. In: McCarty DJ, Koopman WJ (eds). *Arthritis and Allied Conditions*, 12th edn. (Lea and Febiger: Philadelphia, 1993), 1857-72.

70. Hayes CW, Conway WF. Calcium hydroxyapatite deposition disease. *Radiographics* 1990; **10**:1031–48.

71. Dorwart RH, Genant HP, Johnston WH, et al. Pigmented villonodular synovitis: Clinical, pathologic and radiologic features. *Am J Roentgenol* 1984; **143**:877–85.

72. Flandry F, Hughston JC. Current concepts review: pigmented villonodular synovitis. *J Bone Joint Surg [Am]* 1987; **69A**:942–94.

73. Mirra JM, Picci P, Campanacci M. Pseudotumors of bone that simulate primary malignancies. In: Mirra JM, Picci P, Gold RH. *Bone Tumors: Clinical, Radiologic and Pathologic Correlations*. (Lea and Febiger: Philadelphia, 1989), 1766–75.

74. Jelinek S, Kransdorf MJ, Utz JA, Berrey BH, Thomson JD. Imaging of pigmented villonodular synovitis with emphasis on MR imaging. *Am J Roentgenol* 1989; **152**:337–42.

75. Jeffreys TE. Synovial chondromatosis. *J Bone Joint Surg [Br]* 1967; **49B:**530–41.

76. Resnick D, Niwayama G. Sarcoidosis. In: Resnick D, Niwayama G (eds). *Diagnosis of Bone and Joint Disorders*, 2nd edn. (WB Saunders: Philadelphia, 1988), 4013–32.

77. Resnick D, Shapiro RF, Wiener KB, Niwayama G, Utsinger PD, Shaul SR. Diffuse idiopathic skeletal hyperostosis (DISH) (ankylosing hyperostosis of Forestier and Rotes-Querol). *Semin Arthritis Rheum* 1978; **7:**153–87.

78. Garber EK, Silver S. Pedal Manifestations of DISH. *Foot Ankle* 1982; **3:**12–6.

79. Mann RA, Mizel MS. Monarticular nontraumatic synovitis of the metatarsophlangeal joint: a new diagnosis? *Foot Ankle* 1985; **6:**18–21.

80. Campistol JM, Skinner M. Beta 2-microglobulin amyloidosis: an overview. *Semin Dialysis* 1993; **6:**117–26.

81. Reginato AJ. Calcium oxalate and other crystals or particles associated with arthritis. In: McCarty DJ, Koopman WJ. *Arthritis and Allied Conditions*, 12th edn. (Lea & Febiger: Philadelphia, 1993), 1873–93.

82. Brower AC, Allman RM. Pathogenesis of the neurotrophic joint. Neurotraumatic versus neurovascular. *Radiology* 1981; **139:**349–54.

83. Kidd JG Jr. The Charcot joint: some pathologic and pathogenetic considerations. *South Med J* 1974; **67:**597–602.

84. The pathogenesis of Charcot's joint. *Am J Roentgenol* 1946; **56:**189–200.

85. Zlatkin MB, Pathria M, Sartoris DJ, et al. The diabetic foot. *Radiol Clin North Am* 1987; **25:**1095–105.

86. Norman A, Robbins H, Milgram JE. The acute neuropathic arthropathy – a rapid severely disorganizing form of arthritis. *Radiology* 1968; **90:**1159–64.

87. Kraft I, Spyropoulos E, Finby N. Neurogenic disorders of the foot in diabetes mellitus. *Am J Roentgenol* 1975; **124:**17–24.

88. Clouse ME Gramm HF, Legg M, Flood T. Diabetic osteoarthropathy. Clinical and roentgenographic observations in 90 cases. *Am J Roentgenol* 1974; **121:**22–34.

89. Schwarz GS, Berenyi MR, Siegel MW. Atrophic arthropathy and diabetic neuritis. *Am J Roentgenol* 1969; **106:**523–9.

90. Thornhill HL, Richter RW, Shelton ML, Johnson CA. Neuropathic arthropathy (Charcot forefeet) in alcoholics. *Orthop Clin North Am* 1973; **4:**7–20.

91. Murray RO. Congenital indifference to pain with special reference to skeletal changes. *Br J Radiol* 1957; **30:**2–6.

92. Silverman FN, Gilden JJ. Congenital insensitivity to pain: a neurologic syndrome with bizarre skeletal lesions. *Radiology* 1959; **72:**176–89.

93. Schneider R, Goldman AB, Bohne WH. Neuropathic injuries to the lower extremities in children. *Radiology* 1978; **128:**713–8 .

94. Steindler A. The tabetic arthropathies. *JAMA* 1931; **96:**250–6.

95. Peitzman SJ, Miller JL, Ortega L, Schumacher HR, Fernandez PX. Charcot arthropathy secondary to amyloid neuropathy. *JAMA* 1976; **235:**1345–7.

96. Gyepes MT, Newbern DH, Neuhauser EBD. Metaphyseal and physeal injuries in children with spina bifida and meningomyeloceles. *Am J Roentgenol* 1965; **95:**168–77.

97. Nellhaus G. Neurogenic arthropathies (Charcot's joints) in children. Description of a case traces to occult spinal dysraphism. *Clin Pediatr* 1975; **14:**647–53.

98. Chandler GN, Jones DT, Wright V, Hartfall SJ. Charcot's arthropathy following intra-articular hydrocortisone. *BMJ* 1959; **1:**952–3.

99. Alarcon-Segovia D, Ward LE. Charcot-like arthropathy in rheumatoid arthritis. Consequence of overuse of a joint repeatedly injected with hydrocortisone. *JAMA* 1965; **193:**1052–4.

100. Cofield RH, Morrison MJ, Beabout JW. Diabetic neuroarthropathy in the foot: Patient characteristics and patterns of radiographic change. *Foot Ankle* 1983; **4:**15–22.

101. Katz I, Radinowitz JG, Dziadiw R. Early changes in Charcot's joints. *Am J Roentgenol* 1961; **86:**965–74.

102. Schauwecker DS, Park HM, Burt RW et al. Combined bone scintigraphy and indium-111 leukocyte scans in neuropathic foot disease. *J Nucl Med* 1988; **29:**1651–5.

103. Seabold JE, Flickinger FW, Kao SCS, et al. Indium-111-leukocyte/technetium-99m-MDP bone and magnetic resonance imaging: difficulty of diagnosing osteomyelitis in patients with neuropathic osteoarthropathy. *J Nucl Med* 1990; **31:**549–56.

104. Steinberg ME, Steinberg DR. Osteonecrosis. In: Kelley WN, Harris ED Jr, Ruddy S, Sledge CB (eds). *Textbook of Rheumatology*, 3rd edn. (WB Saunders: Philadelphia, 1989), 1749–73.

105. Gauthier G, Elbaz R. Freiberg's infraction: a subchondral bone fatigue fracture. *Clin Orthop* 1978; **142:**93–5.

106. Wiley JJ, Thurston P. Freiberg's disease. *J Bone Joint Surg [Br]* 1981; **63B:**459.

107. Nguyen VD, Keh RA, Daehler RW. Freiberg's disease in diabetes mellitus. *Skeletal Radiol* 1991; **20:**425–8.

108. Williams GA, Cowell HR. Koehler's disease of the tarsal navicular. *Clin Orthop Rel Res* 1981; **158:**53–8.

109. Ippolito E, Ricciardi Pollini PT, Falez F. Koehler's disease of the tarsal navicular: long-term follow-up of 12 cases. *J Pediatr Orthop* 1984; **4:**416–7.

110. Haller J, Sartoris DJ, Resnick D et al. Spontaneous osteonecrosis of the tarsal navicular in adults: Imaging findings. *Am J Roentgenol* 1988; **151:**355-8.

111. Ogata K, Sugioka Y, Urano Y, Chikama H. Idiopathic osteonecrosis of the first metatarsal sesamoid. *Skeletal Radiol* 1986; **15:**141–5.

112. Beltran J, Herman LJ, Burk JM. Femoral head avascular necrosis: MR imaging with clinical-pathologic and radionuclide correlation. *Radiology* 1988; **166:**215–20.

113. Coleman BG, Kressell HY, Dalinka MK et al. Radiographically negative avascular necrosis: Detection with MR imaging. *Radiology* 1988; **168:**525–8.

114. Mitchell DG, Kressel HY. MR imaging of early avascular necrosis. *Radiology* 1988; **169:**281–2.

115. Turner DA, Templeton AC, Selzer PM, et al. Femoral capital osteonecrosis: MR finding of diffuse marrow abnormalities without focal lesions. *Radiology* 1989; **171:**135–40.

116. DePalma AF, Ahamad I, Flannery G, Gandhi OP. Aseptic necrosis of the talus: revascularization after bone grafting. *Clin Orthop* 1974; **234:** 232–5.

6. BONE AND SOFT-TISSUE INFECTION

There are several clinically distinct types of infection in the foot and ankle:
- acute osteomyelitis in diabetic patients;
- acute osteomyelitis in nondiabetic patients;
- Brodie's abscess;
- chronic osteomyelitis following trauma or surgery;
- septic arthritis;
- soft-tissue infections.

Because the presentation and best means of radiologic diagnosis are different in each of these groups they are discussed separately in this chapter.

OSTEOMYELITIS IN THE DIABETIC POPULATION

Osteomyelitis of the foot is a common and serious problem in diabetic patients. Owing to insensitivity to pain or to ischemia, diabetics develop foot ulcers, generally on the plantar aspect of the foot. The ulcers become infected and the infection can spread to the underlying bone. Diabetic osteomyelitis frequently is associated with septic arthritis. The infections are generally polymicrobial.

Ulcers most commonly occur at pressure points: on the plantar skin over the metatarsal heads, posterior process of the calcaneus, interphalangeal joints, and ungual tufts. In one series,[1] 63% of cases of osteomyelitis involved the metatarsal heads, 57% were in the phalanges, and 8% involved the tarsal bones, usually the calcaneus. Osteomyelitis can occur in a pre-existing neuropathic joint, because the necrotic debris in a neuropathic joint is an excellent nidus for infection. Ninety-four percent of cases of diabetic osteomyelitis in the foot are associated with ulcers,[1] so if an ulcer is absent, osteomyelitis is unlikely.

It is generally accepted that osteomyelitis develops in about one-third of deep ulcers that do not resolve with local care.[2,3] However, a recent study[4] suggests that osteomyelitis is much more common. Using bone biopsy (avoiding the ulcer site) and culture as a gold standard, this study found an underlying osteomyelitis in 68% of 41 foot ulcers. Only 32% of cases had been diagnosed clinically. The majority occured in outpatients who had no evidence of inflammation on physical examination, and were associated with ulcers that did not expose bone. If these findings are confirmed by further studies, a more aggressive diagnostic approach to rule out osteomyelitis in diabetic foot ulcers will be needed.

Clinical Findings

Osteomyelitis of the foot may be difficult to diagnose clinically, because fever and bacteremia are uncommon,[1] and erythrocyte sedimentation rate may be normal.[2] Local signs of inflammation are indistinguishable from those of cellulitis.

Percutaneous core bone biopsy can be used to diagnose osteomyelitis,[4,5] although some authors avoid it because of fear of inducing bone necrosis.[1] If performed, biopsy should avoid the ulcer site, because the organisms in the ulcer may not be the same as those in the bone.[6,7] Specimens should be sent for anaerobic as well as aerobic culture. Bone biopsy makes specific therapy possible, and a medical cure without amputation is more likely[1] when specific antibiotics against an isolated pathogen are given.

Imaging of Osteomyelitis, Emphasizing Diabetic Patients

Table 6.1 is a chronologic list of major studies of osteomyelitis in the diabetic population, summarizing the accuracy of the most commonly used imaging techniques. Note that the initial evaluations of a given technique tend to be more optimistic about its accuracy than are subsequent studies.

Plain radiographs

Plain radiographs do not generally become positive in cases of bone infection until 10–20 days after the onset of symptoms.[19–21] However, when the bone radiograph is positive at the time that the patient presents, further imaging studies may not be needed. Radiographic signs of osteomyelitis are osteopenia, small, ill-defined lucencies in the medullary bone and cortex, periosteal new bone and cortical breakthrough (Fig. 6.1–6.3). Concommitant septic arthritis is indicated by the presence of ill-defined erosions of the articular surface.

Plain radiographs should be interpreted with caution, since neuropathic joints may mimic osteomylitis. A full discussion of neuropathic joints is found in Chapter 5. In brief, there are several radiographic findings that aid in the differentiation of infection from neuropathy. Neuropathic joints in the hindfoot and midfoot are hypertrophic, with a large amount of reactive bone proliferation and debris (see Fig. 5.52–5.53), which is not seen in osteomyelitis. In the forefoot, neuropathic joints are often atrophic (see Fig. 5.55) and differentiation of the two entities is more difficult. However, the presence of osteoporosis and ill-

Table 6.1. Accuracy of imaging techniques in diabetic pedal osteomyelitis. (Within each category, studies are in chronologic order.)

Study	Patients (n)	Sensitivity%.	Specificity %
Plain Radiographs			
Park[8]	36	62	69
Seldin[9]	30	93	50
Larcos[10]	49	43	83
Newman[4]	41	28	92
Yuh[11]	29	75	75
Keenan[12]	88	69	82
Three-Phase Bone Scan			
Park[8]	36	83	75*
Seldin[9]	30	94	79
Larcos[10]	49	93	43
Maurer[14]	13	75	56
Israel[13]	38	82	92**
Yuh[11]	29	94	82
Keenan[12]	77	100	38
Newman[4]	41	69	39
Weinstein[15]	32	69	83
Indium Scan			
Larcos[10]	51	79	78
Schauwecker[16]	35	100	83***
Maurer[14]	13	75	89
Keenan[13]	46	100	78
Seabold[17]	16	80	69***
Newman[4]	41	89	89
MRI			
Yuh[11]	44	100	95
Wang[18]	46	99	81
Weinstein[15]	32	100	81

* three patients with absent flow excluded from study; two of these three had osteomyelitis

** quantitative four-phase bone scan

***all patients had neuropathic foot disease, with clinical question of superimposed osteomyelitis

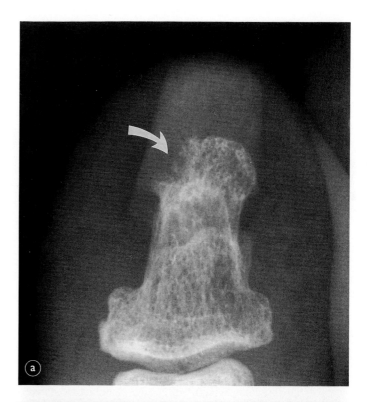

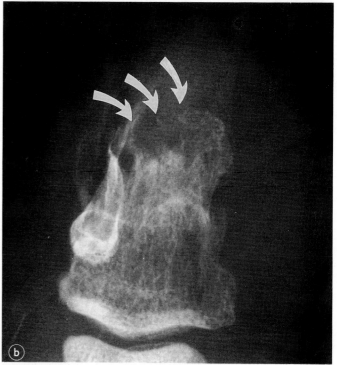

Fig. 6.1. Osteomyelitis of the first distal phalanx in a diabetic patient. **a.** Initial AP radiograph demonstrates subtle cortical erosion of the ungual tuft (arrow). Patient was treated with oral antibiotics. **b.** On radiograph 10 days later, progressive destruction is seen (arrows).

defined joint erosions point to osteomyelitis. Bone density is usually preserved in neuropathic joints.

Osteomyelitis in the diabetic population is usually epiphyseal in location, and associated with septic arthritis (Fig. 6.6). The articular erosions caused by septic arthritis can be confused with those caused by inflammatory arthritis, and this differentiation is discussed below.

In the great toe, well-defined erosions occur from pressure in patients with bunion deformity. These have been misdiagnosed as osteomyelitis (Fig. 6.4). Gout causes erosions that are well defined, unlike those of septic arthritis. Even osteoarthritis can lead to confusion: one published radiograph described as 'false positive' for osteomyelitis[9] demonstrated osteoarthritis with subchondral cysts, which should not be mistaken for osteomyelitis by the trained observer.

Technetium-labelled bone scans
After the plain radiograph, the most frequently ordered study to evaluate osteomyelitis is the three phase ^{99m}technetium-labelled diphosphonate bone scan. The first phase of the scan is a radionuclide angiogram to assess relative blood flow to the area

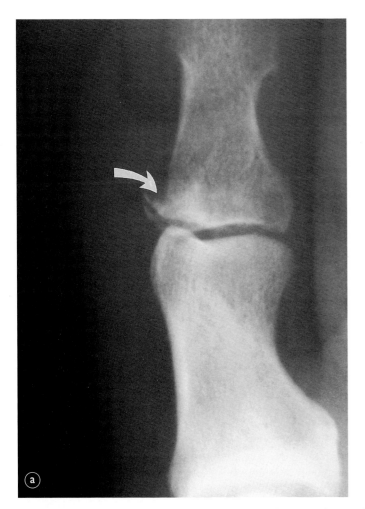
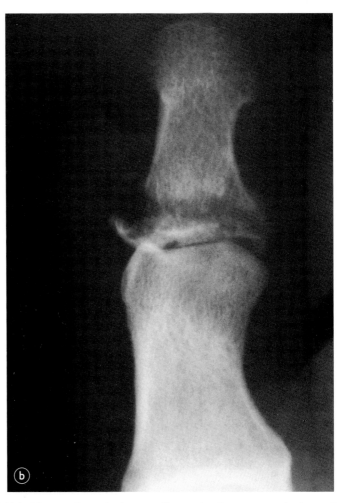

Fig. 6.2 Osteomyelitis of the first distal phalanx in a diabetic patient. **a.** Initial oblique radiograph. A saucer-like erosion is present at the base of the distal phalanx (arrow), adjacent to a soft-tissue ulcer. **b.** Oblique radiograph 14 days later. A pathologic fracture of the base of the distal phalanx has developed.

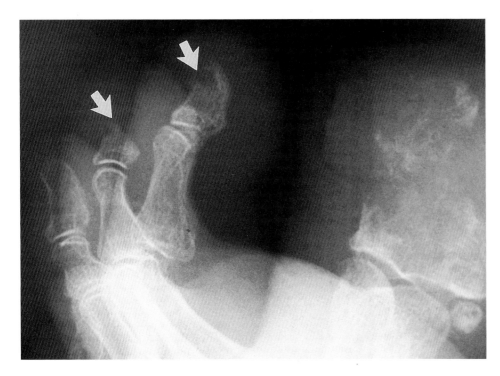

Fig. 6.3. Advanced osteomyelitis of the first toe in a diabetic patient, with less-advanced infection of the second and third toes. Oblique radiograph. The first distal phalanx is almost entirely destroyed. Resorption of the second and third ungual tufts is also seen (arrows), and was shown at amputation to be due to osteomyelitis.

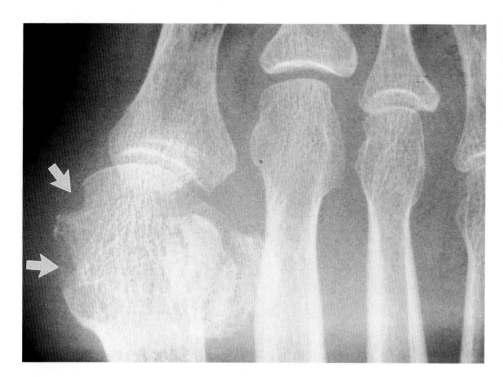

Fig. 6.4. Erosions secondary to bunion and bursitis, radiographically misdiagnosed as osteomyelitis. Attention to the well-defined nature of the erosions would have avoided this error. Review of previous radiographs showed that the findings were stable over a three year period.

in question. The second phase is a blood pool image obtained immediately following the angiogram. This shows soft-tissue activity due to hyperemia. The third phase is obtained after 3–4 hours and reflects bone uptake of radionuclide caused by osteoblastic activity (Fig. 6.5). A fourth phase at 24 hours is sometimes added in equivocal cases, since at this time the ratio of bone to soft-tissue uptake is higher.[13,24]

The bone scan diagnosis of osteomyelitis depends on the fact that, unlike most cases of cellulitis and many bone conditions, osteomyelitis results in both increased blood flow and increased osteoblastic activity.[23] A focus of osteomyelitis will almost always show increased arterial flow. Activity seen in the venous portion of the radionuclide angiogram may be due to cellulitis.[9] It should be noted that, owing to vascular compromise, diabetic patients may have absent blood flow to a region of osteomyelitis.[8]

Cellulitis is expected to demonstrate decreasing uptake between the blood pool and the delayed images, while osteomyelitis will demonstrate increasing uptake, which is visually localizable to the bone. Bone infarctions, avascular necrosis, degenerative arthritis, and many but not all bone tumors will show normal blood flow, despite abnormal uptake on delayed images.[23] There are numerous causes of positive three-phase bone scans (see Chapter 2), which must be kept in mind when interpreting a scan. Many but not all of these causes of false-positive bone scans can be differentiated from osteomyelitis on plain radiographs.

False-positive bone scans due to neuropathic joints are a difficult problem in evaluating the diabetic foot. Neuropathic joints are common in the hindfoot, and specificity of bone scan is lower there than in the forefoot. One study[12] found a specificity for osteomyelitis in the tarsometatarsal joints of only 7%. Osteomyelitis is uncommon in the tarsometatarsal joints, and a positive bone scan in this region should be viewed with suspicion.

Although the three-phase bone scan is designed to differentiate between cellulitis and osteomyelitis, cellulitis can cause false-positive bone scans. Unger[25] found that five out of 10 cases of pedal cellulitis were misdiagnosed as osteomyelitis by bone scan but were correctly diagnosed by MRI. He postulated that the false positives were due to inflammation of the periosteum from overlying cellulitis and ulcers.

Indium scans

Bone scanning with white blood cells labelled with either [67]gallium citrate or [111]indium can be used as a means of increasing the specificity of technetium bone scans. Gallium scans have not proven to be useful in the diabetic population owing to the high number of false-positive scans.[26]

Indium scanning has been reported to be positive at an earlier stage of osteomyelitis than a bone scan.[21] Antibiotic therapy does not affect the sensitivity of indium scans.[27] However, indium scans may be falsely positive in cases of fracture.[28] Another pitfall in indium scanning is its poor spatial resolution, which can make it difficult to determine if activity is in bone or soft tissue. Accuracy is increased when concomitant technetium bone scanning is performed, and the location of indium activity is compared to that of technetium[29] (see Fig. 6.5d).

Although indium-labelled white cell scans improve the specificity of three phase bone scan,[10–12,14,16,17] they may be positive in as many as 31% of noninfected neuropathic joints.[17] False-positive results are more likely to occur in rapidly progressive neuropathic joints than in ones that are long standing and radiographically stable.

CT

CT is a useful method in diagnosing osteomyelitis. One study subjectively found MRI to show infection more clearly than CT in 12 patients,[30] but no large study comparing the accuracy of

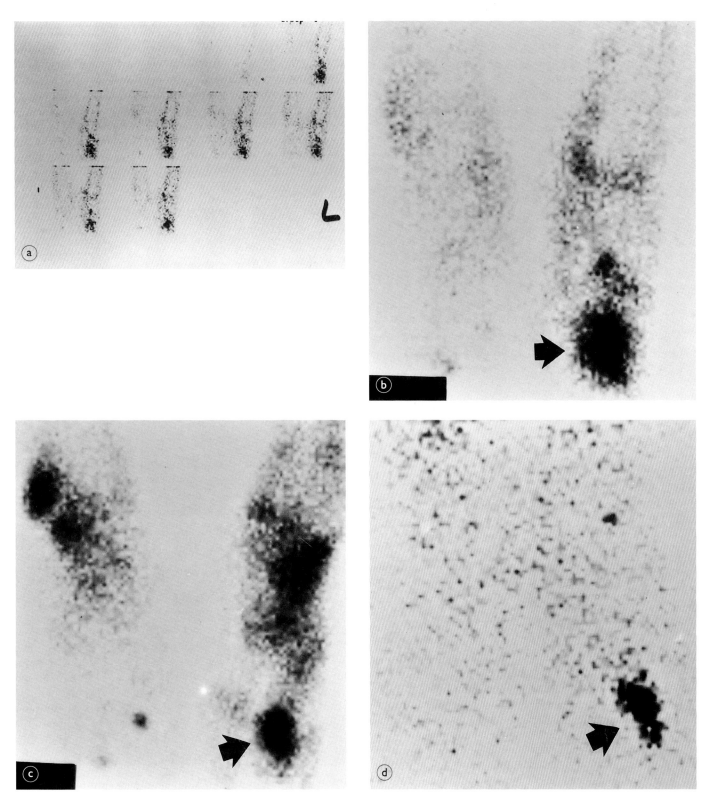

Fig. 6.5. Osteomyelitis in a diabetic patient, diagnosed by ^{99m}technetium three-phase bone scan and indium scan. Plain radiographs were normal.
a. Radionuclide angiogram, feet on detector projection. Images obtained every 4 seconds following injection of technetium methylene diphosphonate demonstrate increased arterial flow to the second or third metatarsal of the left foot. **b.** Blood pool image, anteroposterior view. There is diffusely increased activity in this region (arrow). **c.** Three-hour image, anteroposterior view. There is a relative increase in localization of activity in the second metatarsal head (arrow). Note that there is prominent activity in several other areas, owing to degenerative arthritis, seen on the delayed image only. Since these areas show normal blood flow and blood pool activity, infection there is excluded. **d.** Indium scan in the same patient shows a focus of intense activity at the second metatarsal head (arrow). Note that spatial resolution is very poor, compared to technetium bone scan.

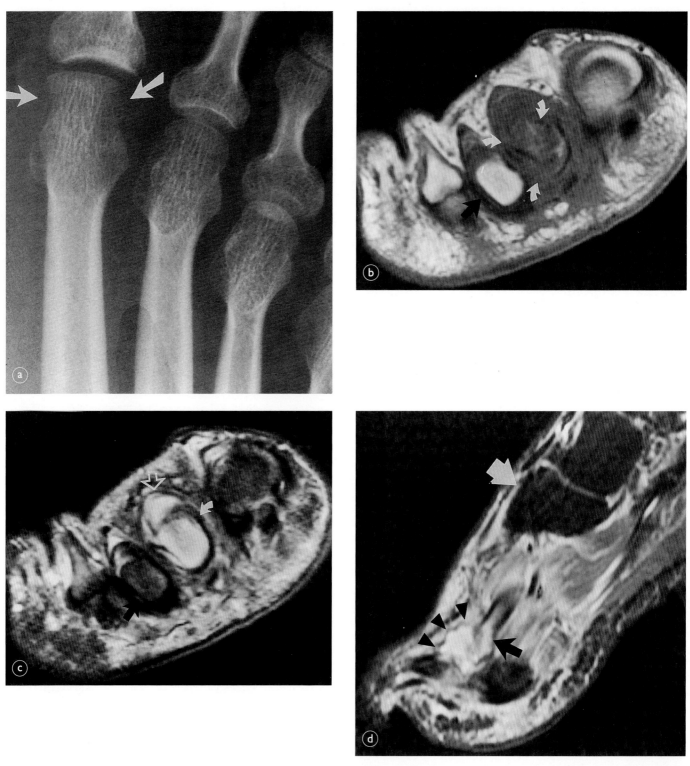

Fig. 6.6. Osteomyelitis of the second metatarsal head and septic arthritis of the metarsophalangeal joint, in a diabetic patient. **a.** Plain radiograph shows very subtle loss of cortical bone (arrows) in the second metatarsal head, compared to the third and fourth metatarsal heads. **b.** Coronal SE 500/20 MRI. On a T1-weighted sequence, the normal high-signal intensity fatty bone marrow seen in the third metatarsal head has been replaced in the second metatarsal head with low-signal intensity pus. Cortical erosions are evident, with loss of the signal-void cortical bone (white arrows). Cellulitis surrounding the metatarsal head is also low in signal intensity. **c.** Coronal FSE 4000/104. On a T2-weighted sequence, normal fatty marrow has decreased in signal intensity, while the purulent marrow in the second metatarsal (white arrow), and the surrounding cellulitis (open white arrow), have very high signal intensity. **d.** Sagittal STIR 2366.7/40/155. The difference between normal marrow (white arrow), low in signal intensity, and high-signal abnormal marrow (black arrow) is exaggerated. On this sagittal sequence, joint distension from septic arthritis (arrowheads) can be appreciated.

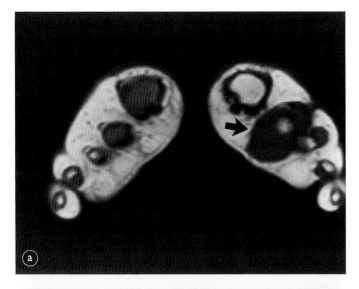

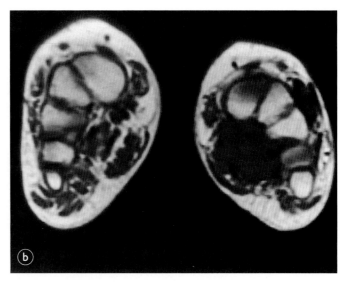

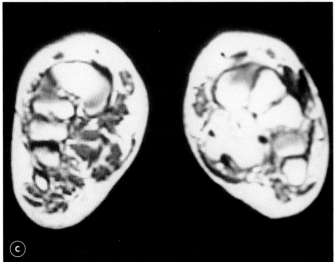

Fig. 6.7. Cellulitis surrounding the second metarsal shaft and extending into the middle plantar soft-tissue compartment of the foot. **a.** Coronal T1-weighted (SE 500/15) MR image through metatarsal shafts. Signal intensity within the marrow is normal. Low-signal intensity cellulitis (arrow) surrounds the second metatarsal shaft. Three-phase bone scan was false positive for osteomyelitis. **b.** Coronal T1-weighted (SE 500/15) MR image at level of cuneiforms. A low-signal intensity mass is seen in the plantar soft tissues. **c.** Gadolinium-enhanced coronal T1-weighted (SE 500/15) MRI at same level shows homogeneous enhancement of the cellulitis. The two, small, round low-signal foci within the mass are tendons.

CT to MRI has been published. CT will demonstrate increased density of bone marrow in cases of osteomyelitis because the fatty marrow is infiltrated with inflammatory cells and pus (see Fig. 6.14c). It will also show areas of cortical destruction, periostitis, and sequestra.[31-35] Intraosseous gas has been reported as a sign of osteomyelitis[34] visible on CT.

MRI

In multiple studies, MRI has been found to have a very high sensitivity (92–100%) for osteomyelitis.[18,30,36–40] MRI evaluation of osteomyelitis employs T1- and T2-weighted images, often supplemented by short tau inversion-recovery (STIR) sequences. A focus of osteomyelitis will demonstrate low signal intensity on T1-weighted images, and high signal intensity on T2-weighted and STIR sequences (see Fig. 6.6). Since STIR images produce high-signal intensity for tissues with long T1 or long T2 they are more sensitive than T2-weighted images, but less specific.[40] A protocol for MRI diagnosis of osteomyelitis is given in Table 6.2. I recommend obtaining T2-weighted sequences in two planes because of problems with partial-volume averaging that can result in diagnostic errors if only a single plane is used. This is especially problematic in the forefoot, where the bones are small. To demonstrate an abnormality in the toe, I generally employ an oblique sagittal plane angled to the ray, as well as the coronal plane.

The specificity of MRI for osteomyelitis is lower than its sensitivity and has been reported to be as low as 82%[40] in the general population, using criteria of abnormal signal on both T1- and T2-weighted sequences. Potential causes of false-positive scans

Table 6.2. MRI protocol for evaluation of osteomyelitis.

Coil – head or extremity
Scout – axial
Sagittal T1-weighted sequence
    angle images along affected ray for osteomyelitis of forefoot
        T1WI TR 300-600/TE 15-25
        FOV 14 cm
        slice thickness 3 mm if forefoot, 4 mm if hindfoot
        matrix 192x256, 1 excitation
Sagittal and coronal T2-weighted sequences
        T2WI TR 2000-2200/TE 20, 80
        slice thickness: 4 mm
Alternate sagittal sequence – FSE TR 3000/TE 95

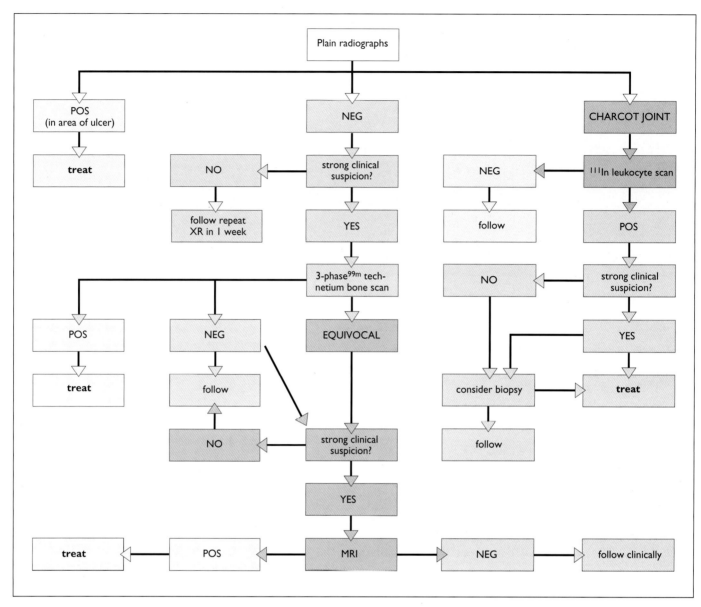

Fig. 6.8. Decision tree for imaging diagnosis of osteomyelitis in the diabetic population.

include occult fracture,[18,37,40] infarction,[40] operative changes,[35] and neuropathic joints.[18,40] Differentiation from cellulitis, sometimes difficult with bone scan, is easily made with MRI (Fig. 6.7).

Optimizing imaging diagnosis

Figure 6.8 is a decision tree based on cost and accuracy in order to optimize radiographic diagnosis in the diabetic population. It employs plain radiographs as a screening examination. If the radiograph is positive (focal osteoporosis, cortical breakthrough, joint erosions) in an area where an ulcer is present, treatment is indicated, owing to the high prevalence of osteomyelitis in this population, as well as the relatively high specificity of radiographs. If the radiograph is positive but an ulcer is absent, osteomyelitis is unlikely,[1] and radiographic changes are probably due to a resorptive neuropathic joint or to inflammatory arthritis. If the radiograph is normal, three-phase bone scan is

the next logical choice for diagnostic imaging because of its low cost. A positive scan with a normal radiograph is most likely due to osteomyelitis. If the radiograph shows a Charcot joint, [111]indium leukocyte scan can be useful to exclude infection. Since indium scans can be falsely positive in Charcot joints, a positive scan should be confirmed with biopsy if clinical suspicion is not high.

If three-phase bone scan is negative, osteomyelitis is not excluded early in the course of disease.[21] The patient can either be followed with plain radiographs, or, if clinical suspicion is high, an MRI, which has virtually 100% sensitivity, can be performed. MRI is also the procedure of choice when three-phase bone scan is equivocal, because it is able to localize abnormalities to bone, periosteum, or soft tissue more accurately than indium is. If a Charcot joint is present on radiographs, MRI is generally not useful, and indium WBC scans are preferable.

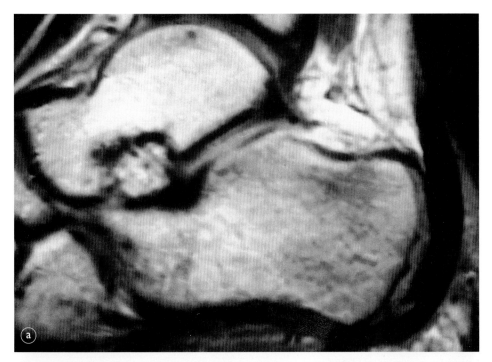

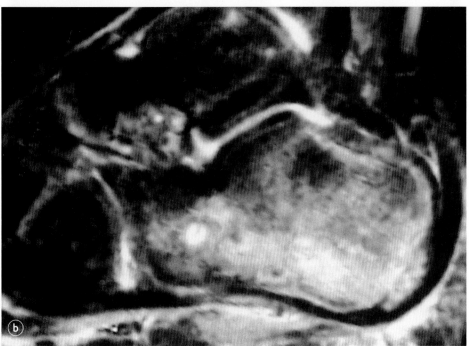

Fig. 6.9. Osteomyelitis of the calcaneus in a seven-year-old child. Patient presented with pain, fever and elevated white blood cell count. Plain radiographs were normal. **a.** Sagittal balanced (SE 2000/20) MRI. Heterogeneous areas of low signal intensity are seen within the marrow of the calcaneus. **b.** Sagittal STIR (2366.7/40/150) MRI. There is a dramatic increase in signal intensity in the marrow of the calcaneus.

Differential Diagnosis

The plain radiographic signs of infection must always be interpreted with caution, since other conditions may have similar findings. There are many causes of periosteal new bone (see Table 8.1). Localized osteopenia and a permeative appearance of the bone may be due to disuse osteoporosis or reflex sympathetic dystrophy (see Chapter 8), or rarely to tumor, as well as to osteomyelitis. Inflammatory arthritis sometimes presents with a similar radiographic picture to osteomyelitis, but can be differentiated by a combination of clinical and radiographic findings (see Chapter 5).

In diabetics, osteomyelitis must be differentiated from cellulitis and from neuropathic joint. This can be a difficult diagnostic problem, not perfectly solved by any imaging technique.

The site of the abnormality can be helpful in distinguishing osteomyelitis from neuropathic joints. Osteomyelitis occurs most frequently at the first, fifth, and second rays and in the calcaneus. Charcot joints are most common at the tarsometatarsal or intertarsal joints.

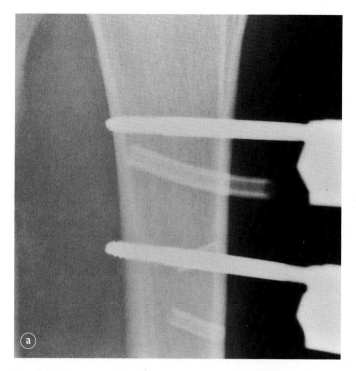
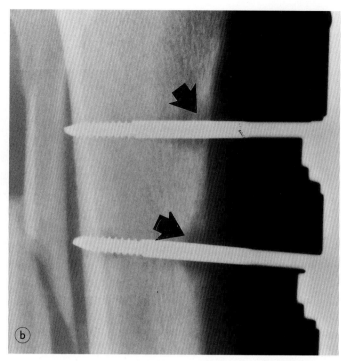

Fig. 6.10. Osteomyelitis of the tibia, occuring at the site of external fixator pins. **a.** Baseline AP radiograph shows normal bone density surrounding the pins. **b.** AP radiograph 1 month later shows lucent zones (arrows) surrounding the pins.

Treatment

Medical treatment is initially carried out with 4–6 weeks of intravenous antibiotics, which may be followed by oral antibiotics. Specific treatment against isolated pathogens is associated with a good response to antibiotic treatment; necrosis or gangrene or both are predictors of a poor clinical outcome (i.e. amputation).[1]

However, surgical treatment must be considered, as removal of a bony abnormality may be essential in order to allow a cure. Removal of a bony abnormality may also protect the patient from a recurrence. Treatment with cast immobilization, or excision of a bony prominence, may resolve the soft-tissue ulcer, and treat a neuropathic joint.

It is important to avoid overtreating patients who have soft-tissue infection or neuropathic joint with weeks of antibiotics. A careful clinical and radiologic evaluation is needed to avoid this too-common error.

ACUTE OSTEOMYELITIS IN THE NONDIABETIC POPULATION

Acute osteomyelitis of the foot and ankle is not common in the nondiabetic population. It is most most frequently seen in children, owing to hematogenous seeding (Fig. 6.9). Children present acutely, with pain, limping, and usually a fever. White blood cell count and erythrocyte sedimentation rate are elevated.

Acute osteomyelitis can also occur because of spread from cellulitis, especially if a foreign body is present. It can occur adjacent to orthopedic hardware, especially if the hardware extends from the bone to the skin (Fig. 6.10). Aseptic loosening of hardware can usually be differentiated from infection by the configuration of the lucency surrounding the hardware.

Aseptic loosening will generally have a funnel-like configuration, widest where the most motion occurs. Infection usually causes a round area of bony destruction.

Imaging diagnosis uses the same criteria as outlined above for diabetic patients. However, false-negative ^{99m}technetium bone scans are reported to be more common in children, especially neonates, than in adults.[41] In addition, care must be taken to distinguish physeal activity, which is normal in the immature skeleton, from abnormal metaphyseal activity. MRI is especially useful in children, owing to its high sensitivity and specificity early in the course of the disease (see Fig. 6.9). False-positive bone scan studies are not as common a problem in adult nondiabetic patients as in the diabetic population. However, occasionally on bone scan one can mistake a stress fracture for osteomyelitis, especially if the clinical history is confusing. MRI is useful to rule out occult fracture if the bone scan diagnosis is in doubt.

BRODIE'S ABSCESS

A Brodie's abscess is a contained focus of infection within bone. It is most common in children, but can also occur in adults. Brodie's abscess is usually metaphyseal in location, and it may cross the growth plate into the epiphysis.[42] They are usually caused by pyogenic bacteria, especially staphylococcus, but a similar picture may occur with fungal infection.

Clinical Findings

The patient may present with chronic pain and limp as well as local tenderness. Erythrocyte sedimentation rate and white blood cell count may be normal or elevated.[42]

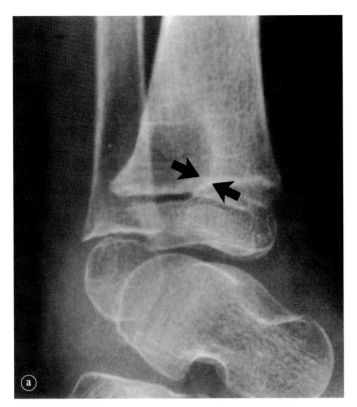 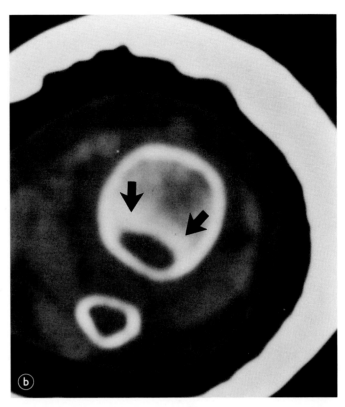

Fig. 6.11. Five-year-old girl with Brodie's abscess, presenting with pain and a limp. **a.** Lateral plain radiograph shows a lytic metaphyseal lesion with a thick, sclerotic border (between arrows). The outer margin of the sclerotic border is ill-defined, while the inner margin is sharp. **b.** Axial CT better demonstrates the thick sclerotic rind (arrows) surrounding the lesion. Other images showed that the abscess crossed the physeal plate into the epiphysis, a finding that could not be discerned on plain radiographs.

Imaging

Plain radiographs are usually the only imaging study required, although they can be supplemented by CT scanning. The abscess appears as a well-defined lytic lesion surrounded by a thick rind of sclerotic reactive bone (Figs 6.11, 6.12). The inner margin of this rind is sharply defined, while the outer margin fades gradually into normal bone. In contrast to the Brodie's abscess, similar lytic lesions of bone such as fibrous dysplasia, enchondroma, chondroblastoma, and nonossifying fibroma generally have a thin margin of sclerosis that is well-defined on both the inner and outer aspects. An osteoid osteoma, like the Brodie's abscess, has a thick rind of reactive sclerotic bone, but the lucent portion of the lesion is much smaller and is usually limited to cortical bone.

Treatment

Brodie's abscess can be treated with antibiotics, though sometimes surgical drainage is needed.

CHRONIC OSTEOMYELITIS

An untreated or inadequately treated episode of acute osteomyelitis can progress to chronic osteomyelitis, but this is rare today.

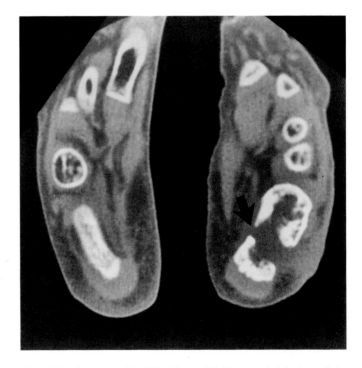

Fig. 6.12. One-year-old child with coccidioidomycosis infection of the calcaneus, caused by hematogenous spread following pulmonary infection. Axial CT. The normal fatty marrow has been replaced with soft-tissue density of purulent exudate. Sinus tract has developed medially (arrow); lateral wall defect is post-surgical.

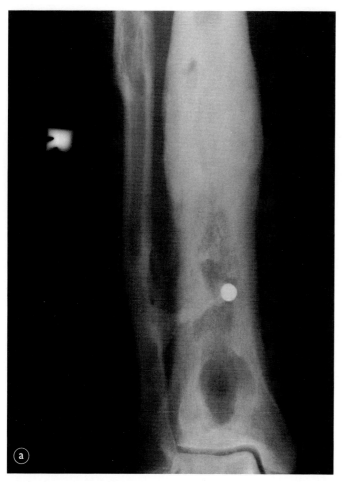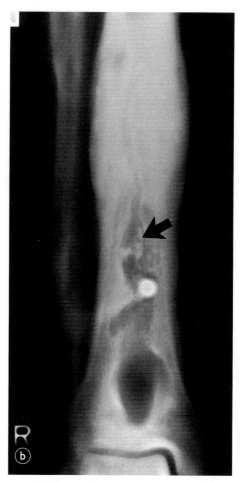

Fig. 6.13. Chronic osteomyelitis in patient who had recurrent episodes of pain, swelling and erythema following gunshot wound. **a.** AP plain radiograph shows sclerosis proximally, a retained shot pellet, and a lucent cavity distally. **b.** AP complex motion tomography shows bony sequestrum (arrow), which was surgically excised.

More commonly, a chronic, indolent infection develops in an area of bone that is ischemic because of prior fracture. It is not uncommon following open fractures of the distal tibia, where vascular supply is poor. Chronic osteomyelitis may develop at sites where metallic fixators form an avascular nidus for bacteria.

In the past, chronic osteomyelitis was caused most frequently by Staphylococcus aureus, but there has been increasing incidence of gram-negative, anaerobic, and mixed infections.[43,44]

Clinical Findings

Patients present with chronic pain and usually have an elevated erythrocyte sedimentation rate. White blood cell count may be normal.

Imaging

Because of the underlying bony abnormalities, it is difficult to assess radiographically whether active osteomyelitis is present.

Plain radiographs
Tumeh and colleagues[45] found that only one radiographic sign, the presence of a sequestrum, was specific for active infection.

However, a sequestrum was visible in only 9% of cases on plain radiographs. Conventional tomography (Fig. 6.13) can be used to increase visualization of sequestra.

Bony erosions, periosteal reaction, and soft-tissue swelling are not accurate indicators of active disease. Progressive changes on serial radiographs have a sensitivity of 14% and a specificity of 70% for active disease.[45]

Nuclear medicine
Technetium bone scan is not generally useful in chronic osteomyelitis where there are underlying bone abnormalities.[26,46] Occasionally, it may be helpful if it shows involvement of bone that was previously normal on bone scan (Fig. 6.14). Gallium scanning has been used, but its accuracy is low,[26,46] and gallium scanning may be totally normal in patients with osteomyelitis.[47] The only pattern of uptake that is accurate is when gallium uptake is more intense than that of technetium.[47]

The diagnostic procedure of choice for chronic osteomyelitis of the leg and ankle is the indium scan. In the peripheral skeleton, indium has a sensitivity of 94% and a specificity of 80%.[29]

CT and MRI
For the surgical treatment of chronic osteomyelitis to be successful, sequestra of necrotic bone must be resected. CT scanning is

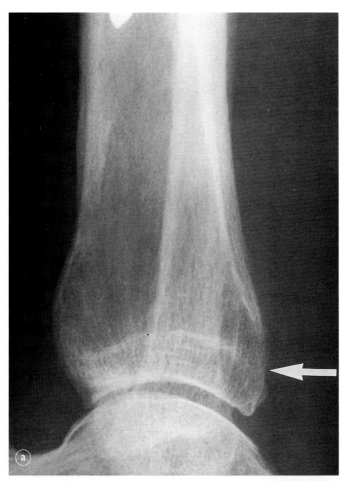

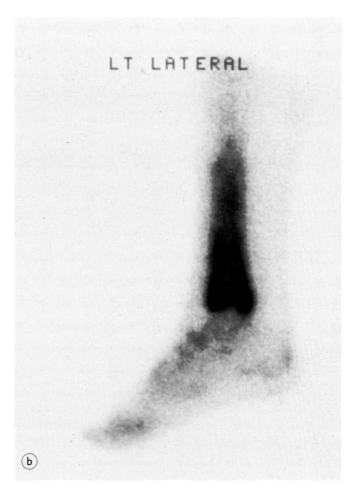

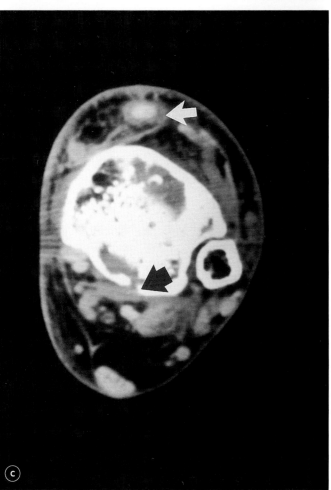

Fig. 6.14. Chronic osteomyelitis and superimposed acute osteomyelitis following intramedullary nail fixation for tibial fracture. Patient had a several-year history of osteomyelitis, treated with multiple courses of oral and intravenous antibiotics. He presented with increasing pain. **a.** Lateral radiograph shows focal osteoporosis of the distal tibia. An area of thinning of the posterior cortex is seen (arrow). **b.** ^{99m}Technetium bone scan, 3 hour image, lateral view. Previous scans had shown activity at the site of the tibial nail, but now activity is present more distally in the tibia, abutting the articular surface but without evidence of involvement of the talar dome. **c.** Axial CT, soft-tissue window. Cortical breakthrough is evident posteriorly (black arrow). The tibial marrow cavity is filled with purulent material (compare its density to the fatty marrow in the fibula). Fluid is seen in the anterior tibial tendon sheath (white arrow). Needle aspiration of the tibia showed grossly purulent fluid, as did debridement of the region of the anterior tibial tendon. Cultures grew *Staphylococcus aureus*.

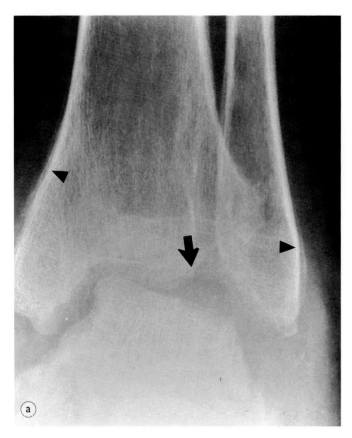
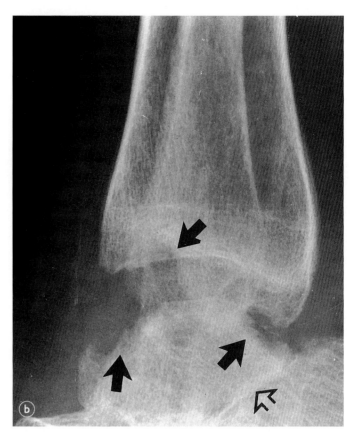

Fig. 6.15. Infectious arthritis of the ankle in a young woman. **a.** AP radiograph. **b.** Lateral radiograph. Despite aggressive treatment, the joint was rapidly destroyed by this staphylococcal infection. Bones are osteoporotic. Erosions (arrows) and joint distension are seen. In this patient there is communication between the subtalar joint and the ankle joint, and the subtalar joint (open arrow) is markedly narrowed, owing to destruction of the articular cartilage from the infection. Periosteal new bone is seen along the shafts of the tibia and fibula (arrowheads).

more sensitive than plain radiography in the detection of sequestra,[35] and therefore it can be useful in planning treatment. MRI can also be used to detect sequestra. A noncontrolled study of eight patients with chronic osteomyelitis found that MRI accurately depicted sequestra and sinus tracts and identified the extent of the infection.[48] CT or MRI can also be used to show areas of cortical breakthrough, and soft-tissue involvement (Fig. 6.14).

Treatment

Chronic osteomyelitis is generally treated with debridement followed by soft-tissue flaps to cover the wound. Some cases require amputation.[43,44] In debilitated patients, chronic supression with oral antibiotics may be used.

INFECTIOUS ARTHRITIS

Infectious arthritis can occur as a result of a puncture wound, from hematogenous seeding, or spread from cellulitis. It frequently coexists with osteomyelitis. It is almost always monoarticular. The second, third, and fourth metatarsophalangeal joints lie in a common soft-tissue compartment, and

severe cases of septic arthritis may involve these three adjacent metatarsal heads.

Septic arthritis may be caused by a variety of bacteria, including *Staphylococcus aureus* and gram-negative bacteria, as well as by mycobacteria and fungi.

Clinical Presentation

Infectious arthritis caused by pyogenic bacteria presents with fever, arthralgia, and local signs of inflammation. Joint cultures and frequently blood cultures are positive.

Imaging of Septic Arthritis

In bacterial infections, radiographs show a rapidly progressive arthritis. A joint effusion may be the earliest sign, followed by joint space narrowing and bony erosions (Fig. 6.15). The periarticular bone becomes osteoporotic. Fungal or mycobacterial organisms have a more indolent course. When the diagnosis of septic arthritis is suspected clinically or radiographically, joint aspiration is performed for gram stain and culture. Plain radiographs are usually the only imaging studies needed. MRI or CT can be performed to determine the extent of any associated osteomyelitis or deep soft-tissue abscesses.

Differential Diagnosis

Differential diagnosis of infectious arthritis is with Charcot joint and noninfectious inflammatory arthritides.

It can be difficult to differentiate neuropathic joints from infectious arthritis, since both can be rapidly progressive and both are common occurences in diabetic patients. Local osteoporosis is characteristic of infectious arthritis and is not seen in neuropathic joints. Conversely, the presence of bony debris around the joint is a sign that points to neuroarthropathy rather than infection.

Noninfectious inflammatory arthritis can be mistaken radiographically for infection, and at initial presentation the possibility of inflammatory arthritis may not have been considered. If multiple joints in different soft-tissue compartments are involved, infection is less likely than inflammatory arthritis. Radiographic examination of the opposite foot is useful, since rheumatoid arthritis is generally bilaterally symmetric. Inflammatory arthritis is slowly progressive, while a pyogenic infectious arthritis rapidly destroys a joint.

Treatment

Early treatment with irrigation and antibiotics is essential to preserve joint function.

SOFT TISSUE INFECTIONS

Soft-tissue infections can be divided into cellulitis, treated medically, and abscess, generally treated with drainage as well as antibiotics. In the forefoot, cellulitis is usually contained within one of the three plantar muscular compartments[49] (see Chapter 1).

Clinical Presentation

Soft-tissue infections generally present with the classic signs of inflammation – redness, heat, pain, and swelling. An abscess, especially in the deep compartment of the foot, may be occult clinically. Many infections are associated with some injury to the skin, especially on the plantar surface.

Imaging of Soft-Tissue Infections

On plain radiographs of cellulitis, soft-tissue swelling is seen, and blurring of the soft-tissue planes is sometimes evident. One should always look for foreign bodies such as needles, other pieces of metal, or spines of aquatic animals, even if the patient does not recall an injury. However, some foreign bodies, like wood, glass, or thorns, may not be visible on plain radiographs especially if the technique is suboptimal or the view obstructs the foreign body. Three-phase bone scan usually demonstrates increased flow to the affected area and increased activity on blood pool images, but decreasing activity on delayed images.[8,9] As discussed above, bone scans in cellulitis may be falsely positive for osteomyelitis, perhaps because of reactive periostitis.

CT scans in patients with cellulitis will show a decrease in attenuation of the involved muscles. Fat has increased attenuation due to edema. Cellulitis will be more easily seen on MRI, where it has high signal on T2-weighted images and enhances homogeneously with gadolinium administration (see figure 6.7). In diabetic patients, MRI will frequently show diffusely abnormal signal because of edema in the plantar soft-tissues of the foot,[50] and this finding does not necessarily indicate cellulitis.

MRI or CT can be used in diagnosis of occult abscess. The abscess will be low-attenuation on CT, low-signal intensity on T1-weighted MRI images, and high-signal intensity on T2-weighted images. The periphery will enhance with contrast on both CT and MRI. However, it should be remembered that other soft-tissue masses, including sarcomas, show identical findings.[51]

Differential Diagnosis

Cellulitis must be differentiated from osteomyelitis, and abscesses need to be distinguished from other soft-tissue masses such as hematoma or tumor.

REFERENCES

1. Bamberger DM, Daus GP, Gerding DN. Osteomyelitis in the feet of diabetic patients: long-term results, prognostic factors, and the role of antimicrobial and surgical therapy. *Am J Med* 1987; **83**:653–60.

2. Sugarman B, Hawes S, Muscher DM, et al. Osteomyelitis beneath pressure sores. *Arch Intern Med* 1983; **143**:683–8.

3. Wheat J. Diagnostic strategies in osteomyelitis. *Am J Med* 1985; **78(suppl 6B)**:218–24).

4. Newman LG, Waller J, Palestro CJ, et al. Unsuspected osteomyelitis in diabetic foot ulcers: diagnosis and monitoring by leukocyte scanning with indium In 111 oxyquinolone. *JAMA* 1991; **266**:1246–51.

5. Caprioli R, Testa J, Cournoyer RW Jr, Esposito FJ. Prompt diagnosis of suspected osteomyelitis by utilizing percutaneous bone culture. *J Foot Surg* 1986; **25**:263–9.

6. Sapico FL, Witte JL, Canawati HN, Montgomerie JZ, Bessman AN. The infected foot of the diabetic patient: quantitative microbiology and analysis of clinical features. *Rev Infect Dis* 1984; **6(suppl 1)**:S171–6.

7. Perry CR, Pearson RL, Miller GA. Accuracy of cultures of material from swabbing of the superficial aspect of the wound and needle biopsy in the preoperative assessment of osteomyelitis. *J Bone Joint Surg [Am]* 1991; **73A**:745–9.

8. Park HM, Wheat J, Siddiqui AR, et al. Scintigraphic evaluation of diabetic osteomyelitis: concise communicaton. *J Nucl Med* 1982; **23**:569–83.

9. Seldin DW, Heiken JP, Feldman F, Alderson PO. Effect of soft-tissue pathology on detection of pedal osteomyelitis in diabetics. *J Nucl Med* 1985; **26**:988–93.

10. Larcos G, Brown ML, Sutton RT. Diagnosis of osteomyelitis of

the foot in diabetic patients: value of ^{111}In-leukocyte scintigraphy. *Am J Roentgenol* 1991; **157:**527–31.

11. Yuh WTC, Corson JD, Baraniewski HM. Osteomyelitis of the foot in diabetic patients: evaluation with plain film, 99m-MDP Bone Scintigraphy, and MR Imaging. *Am J Roentgenol* 1989; **152:** 795–800.

12. Keenan AM. Diagnosis of pedal osteomyelitis in diabetic patients using current scintigraphic techniques. *Arch Intern Med* 1989; **149:**2262–6.

13. Israel O, Gips S, Jerushalmi J, Frenkel A, Front D. Osteomyelitis and soft-tissue infection: differential diagnosis with 24 hour/4 hour ratio of Tc-99m MDP uptake. *Radiology* 1987; **163:**725–6.

14. Maurer AH, Millmond SH, Knight LC, et al. Infection in diabetic osteoarthropathy: use of indium-labeled leukocytes for diagnosis. *Radiology* 1986; **161:**221–5.

15. Weinstein D, Wang A, Chambers R, et al. Evaluation of MRI in the diagnosis of osteomyelitis in diabetic foot infection. *Foot Ankle* 1993; **14:**18–22.

16. Schauwecker DS, Park HM, Burt RW, et al. Combined bone scintigraphy and indium-111 leukocyte scans in neuropathic foot disease. *J Nucl Med* 1988; **29:**1651–5.

17. Seabold JE, Flickinger FW, Kao SCS, et al. Indium-111-leuko-cyte/technetium-99m-MDP bone and magnetic resonance imaging: difficulty of diagnosing osteomyelitis in patients with neuropathic osteoarthropathy. *J Nucl Med* 1990; **31:**549–56.

18. Wang A, Weisntein D, Greenfield L, et al. MRI and diabetic foot infections. *Magn Reson Imaging* 1990; **8:**805–9.

19. Capitanio MA, Kirkpatrick JA. Early roentgen observations in acute osteomyelitis. *Am J Roentgenol* 1970; **130:**488–96 .

20. Waldvogel FA, Medoff G, Swartz MN. Osteomyelitis: a review of clinical features, therapeutic considerations and unusual aspects (first of three parts). *N Engl J Med* 1970; **282:**198–206.

21. Raptopoulos V, Doherty PW, Goss TP, King MA, Johnson K, Gantz NM. Acute osteomyelitis: advantage of white cell scans in early detection. *Am J Roentgenol* 1982; **139:**1077–82.

22. Mettler FA, Guiberteau MJ. Skeletal system. In: *Essentials of Nuclear Medicine Imaging.* (WB Saunders: Philadelphia, 1991), Chapter 11.

23. Maurer AH, Chen DCP, Camargo EE, Wong DF, Wagner HN, Alderson PO. Utility of three-phase skeletal scintigraphy in suspected osteomyelitis: concise communication. *J Nucl Med* 1981; **22:**941–9.

24. Alazraki N, Dries D, Datz F, Lawrence P, Greenberg E, Taylor A Jr. Value of a 24-hour image (four phase bone scan) in assessing osteomyelitis in patients with peripheral vascular disease. *J Nucl Med* 1985; **26:**711–7.

25. Unger E, Moldofsky P, Gatenby R, Hartz W, Broder G. Diagnosis of osteomyelitis by MR Imaging. *Am J Roentgenol* 1988; **150:**605–10.

26. Schauwecker DS, Park HM, Mock BH, et al. Evaluation of complicating osteomyelitis with Tc-99m MDP, In-111 granulocytes and Ga-67 citrate. *J Nucl Med* 1984; **25:**849–53.

27. Datz FL, Thorne DA. Effect of antibiotic therapy on the sensitivity of indium-11-labelled leukocyte scans. *J Nucl Med* 1986; **27:**1849–53.

28. Kim EE, Pjura GA, Lowry PA, Gobuty AH, Traina JF. Osteomyelitis complicating fracture: pitfalls of 111-In leukocyte scintigraphy. *Am J Roentgenol* 1987; **148:**927–30.

29. Schauwecker DS. Osteomyelitis: diagnosis with In-111-labeled leukocytes. *Radiology* 1989; **171:**141–6.

30. Berquist TH, Brown ML, Fitzgerald RH, May GR. Magnetic

resonance imaging: application in musculoskeletal infection. *Magn Reson Imaging* 1985; **3:**219–30.

31. Kuhn JP, Berger PE. Computed tomographic diagnosis of osteomyelitis. *Radiology* 1979; **130:**503–6.

32. Hermann G, Rose JS. Computed tomography in bone and soft tissue pathology of the extremities. *J Comput Assist Tomogr 1979;* *3:*58–66.

33. Wing VW, Jeffrey RB, Federle MP, et al. Chronic osteomyelitis examined by CT. *Radiology* 1985; **54:**171–4.

34. Ram PC, Martinez S, Korobkin M, Beriman RS, et al. CT detection of intraosseous gas: a new sign of osteomyelitis. *Am J Roentgenol* 1981; **137:**721–3.

35. Seltzer SE. Value of computed tomography in planning medical and surgical treatment of chronic osteomyelitis. *J Comput Assist Tomogr* 1984; **8:**482–7.

36. Modic MT, Feiglin DH, Piraino DW, et al. Vertebral osteomyelitis: assessment using MR. *Radiology* 1985; **157:**157–66.

37. Unger E, Moldofsky P, Gatenby R, Hartz W, Broder G. Diagnosis of osteomyelitis by MR imaging. *Am J Roentgenol* 1988; **150:**605–10.

38. Tang JSH, Gold RH, Bassett LW, Seeger LL. Musculoskeletal infection of the extremities: evaluation with MR imaging. *Radiology* 1988; **166:**205–9.

39. Mason MD, Zlatkin MB, Esterhai JL, et al. Chronic complicated osteomyelitis of the lower extremity: evaluation with MR imaging. *Radiology* 1989; **173:**355–9.

40. Erdman WA, Tamburro F, Jayson HT, et al. Osteomyelitis: characteristics and pitfalls of diagnosis with MR imaging. *Radiology* 1991; **180:**533–9.

41. Ash JA, Gilday DL. The futility of bone scanning in neonatal osteomyelitis: concise communication. *J Nucl Med* 1980; **21:**417–20.

42. Resnick D, Niwayama G. Osteomyelitis, septic arthritis, and soft tissue infection: the mechanisms and situations. In: Resnick D, Niwayama G (eds). *Diagnosis of Bone and Joint Disorders,* 2nd edn. (WB Saunders: Philadelphia, 1988), 2540–2.

43. Anthony JP, Mathes SJ. Update on chronic osteomyelitis. *Clin Plastic Surg* 1991; **18:**515–23.

44. Meadows SE, Zuckerman JD, Koval KJ. Posttraumatic tibial osteomyelitis: diagnosis, classification, and treatment. *Hosp Joint Dis Bull* 1993; **52:**11–6.

45. Tumeh SS, Aliabadi P, Weissman BN, McNeil BJ. Disease activity in osteomyelitis: role of radiography. *Radiology* 1987; **165:**781–4.

46. Merkel KD, Brown ML, Dewanjee MK, Fitzgerald RH Jr. Comparison of indium-labelled-leukocyte imaging with sequential technetium-gallium scanning in the diagnosis of low-grade musculoskeletal sepsis. *J Bone Joint Surg [Am]* 1985; **67A:**465–76.

47. Tumeh SS, Aliabadi P, Weissman BN, McNeil BJ. Chronic osteomyelitis: bone and gallium scan patterns associated with active disease. *Radiology* 1986; **158:**685–8.

48. Quinn SF, Murray W, Clark RA, Cochran C. MR imaging of chronic osteomyelitis. *J Comput Assist Tomogr* 1988; **12:**113–7.

49. Sartoris DJ, Devine S, Resnick D, et al. Plantar compartmental infection in the diabetic foot. *Invest Radiol* 1985; **20:**772–84.

50. Moore TE, Yuh WT, Kathol MH, et al. Abnormalities of the foot in patients with diabetes mellitus: findings on MR imaging. *Am J Roentgenol* 1991; **157:**813–6.

51. Crim JR, Seeger LL, Yao L, et al. Diagnosis of soft-tissue masses with MR imaging: can benign masses be differentiated from malignant ones? *Radiology* 1992; **185:**581–6.

7. TENDON ABNORMALITIES

There are many causes of tendon abnormalities in the foot:
- chronic overuse by athletes;
- acute trauma with or without associated fractures;
- abnormal mechanical stresses due to underlying foot deformity or obesity;
- iatrogenic (steroid injections); and
- systemic conditions such as rheumatoid arthritis.

The incidence of tendon injuries appears to have increased in recent decades, probably because of increased athletic activity by 'weekend athletes.'

In this chapter the most common tendon abnormalities in the ankle and foot will be discussed. For each tendon, anatomy is briefly reviewed. Further discussion of normal anatomy, and a cross-sectional atlas, is found in Chapter 1.

The importance of consistent terminology and grading of abnormalities cannot be overemphasized. Treatment of tendon abnormalities is in flux, and radiology is most useful in furthering advances in treatment if radiologic description is as precise as possible.

TERMINOLOGY

Several different terms are used to describe abnormal changes in tendons: tenosynovitis, peritendinitis, tendinitis, tendinosis, tear, and rupture. Unfortunately, there is considerable inconsistency in terminology found in the literature. The following terms will be used in this chapter:
- tenosynovitis – inflammation involving the tendon sheath, with or without changes in the underlying tendon. Tenovaginitis is a synonymous term;
- peritendonitis – inflammation involving the peritendinous structures; this term is used for tendons such as the Achilles tendon that do not have a synovial sheath.[1] Paratenonitis is a synonym;
- tendonitis – a reversible inflammatory process within the tendon;[1] and
- tendinosis – fibrinoid and mucoid degeneration within a tendon.[2]

ACHILLES TENDON

Anatomy

The Achilles tendon, or calcaneal tendon, is the conjoint tendon of the gastrocnemius and soleus muscles, which act to plantar

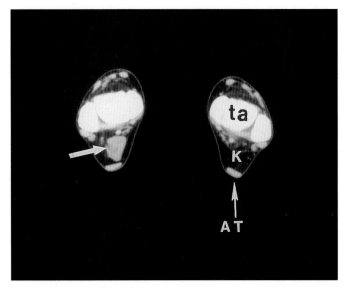

Fig. 7.1. Accessory soleus muscle. Axial CT demonstrates a mass of muscle density (arrow) deep to the Achilles tendon. Typical fatty septations of muscle are visible within the accessory soleus, helping to distinguish it from other soft-tissue masses. Sequential images will show its elongated, elliptical appearance, blending with the fibers of the soleus muscle superiorly. On contralateral side, ta – talus, AT – Achilles tendon, K – Kager's (pre-Achilles) fat.

flex the foot. The gastrocnemius muscle arises from two heads: the medial head from the posterior aspect of the medial femoral condyle and the lateral head from the lateral femoral condyle. The soleus muscle arises from the proximal tibia and fibula. The conjoint tendon inserts on the posterior tuberosity of the calcaneus. The Achilles tendon does not have a true tendon sheath, but is surrounded instead by a connective tissue paratenon.

The accessory soleus is an anomalous muscle that is located deep to the soleus. Since its muscular portion extends to near its insertion on the calcaneus, it may present as a pre-Achilles mass[3–5] visible on plain radiographs and easily diagnosable on CT or MRI (Fig. 7.1). It has been reported to be a cause of pain in athletes, perhaps because of its poor vascularity.[5]

The pre-Achilles bursa lies between the tendon and the calcaneus, and the retro-Achilles bursa lies subcutaneously behind the tendon. A triangle of fat known as Kager's triangle separates the Achilles tendon from the deep flexors of the foot.

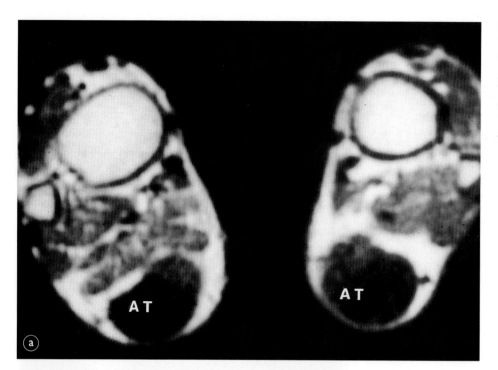

Fig. 7.2. MRI of bilateral xanthomas of the Achilles tendon. The tendons show marked, lobular enlargement, and heterogeneous signal intensity which increased on T2-weighted sequences. **a.** axial T1-weighted image, 500/20. **b.** Sagittal balanced image, SE 1000/30. AT= Achilles tendon.

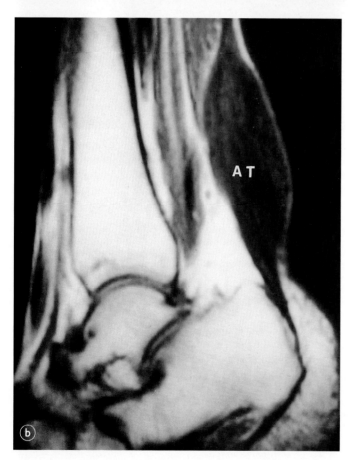

Partial or complete Achilles tendon rupture usually occurs as a result of acute injury superimposed on tendinosis. The mean age of rupture is 35 years,[12] and the injury is more common in men.

Rupture is most common 2–6 cm above the tendon insertion, where vascularity is poor.[13] Rheumatoid and seronegative arthritis, gout, hyperlipidemia, and corticosteroid injection predispose to tendon rupture.[6]

Clinical Findings

Peritendonitis is the earliest stage of injury to the Achilles tendon. Patients complain of local tenderness and burning pain that occurs after sports activities. Physical findings are scant, although crepitus may be felt. Continued stress on the tendon leads to tendinosis. Pain is related to physical activity, and morning stiffness may be present. On physical examination, the tendon is tender, and ankle dorsiflexion may be decreased. In chronic cases of tendinosis, diffuse or nodular thickening of the tendon is palpable. Partial rupture is difficult to differentiate clincally from peritendonitis and tendinosis.[14]

Patients with tendon rupture complain of posterior calf pain, and often give a history of feeling a sudden 'snap' in the calf. Physical examination discloses weakness (but usually not total loss) of plantar flexion, and a palpable defect in the tendon may be present in complete rupture. Manual compression of the midcalf will cause plantar flexion of the foot if the Achilles tendon is intact (Thompson test).[15] Physical diagnosis of rupture has been estimated to be inaccurate 25% of the time.[16]

Etiology of Achilles Tendon Injury

True tendonitis, with inflammatory cell infiltration, does not occur in the Achilles tendon. Rather, peritendinitis (inflammatory changes in the peritenon) and tendonosis (mucoid degeneration) are seen. They usually occur as a result of overuse in athletes.[2,6–11]

Classification

In a system proposed by Kuwada et al,[17] four stages of rupture are recognized. Type I is a partial rupture involving less than 50% of the tendon. Type II is a complete rupture with no more

Table 7.1. Differential diagnosis of Achilles tendon rupture.

Injury – peritendonitis, tendinosis, tear of medial head of
   gastrocnemius
Bursitis – pre-Achilles and retro-Achilles bursae
Stress fracture – calcaneus, tibia, or fibula

Table 7.2. Differential diagnosis of Achilles tendon mass.

Xanthoma (usually bilateral)
Partial or healed Achilles tendon rupture
Accessory soleus muscle
Myositis ossificans
Soft-tissue tumor

Table 7.3. Ultrasound protocol for Achilles tendon.

Patient position – prone, feet off end of table
Transducer – 7.5 or 10 mHz linear array, using gel-standoff pad
Views – sagittal and axial in neutral and dorsiflexion

than a 3 cm gap between the tendon ends. Type III has a defect of 3–6 cm, and type IV more than 6 cm.

Differential Diagnosis

Other causes of similar pain that should be considered are listed in Table 7.1. Bursitis may be palpable on clinical examination, and is visible on ultrasound, CT or MRI. A stress fracture is often occult on intial plain radiographs, but is usually visible on subsequent radiographs obtained in 1–2 weeks. In avid athletes, documentation of stress fracture by nuclear medicine scan is sometimes needed to induce the patient to rest the leg. A tear of the medial head of the gastrocnemius will be identified on MRI if the sagittal images include the distal portion of the belly of the gastrocnemius.

Table 7.2 summarizes masses that may be found in the region of the Achilles tendon. Xanthomas can be distinguished by history of hypercholesterolemia, by their bilaterality, and by imaging appearance. On CT or MRI the mass is lobular and confined to the substance of the tendon (see Fig. 7.2). Other soft-tissue tumors arising in the region of the Achilles tendon can be seen to be separate from the tendon on CT or MRI. An accessory soleus muscle (see Fig. 7.1) may present with a tender mass, and can be identified on CT or MRI. Myositis ossificans (see Chapter 11) is post-traumatic ossification of muscle, which produces a round to oval mass. A history of trauma can usually but not always be elicited. Sequential plain radiographs demonstrate maturing ossification, which is densest at the periphery. MRI is potentially confusing, since the mass will appear identical to many soft-tissue tumors.

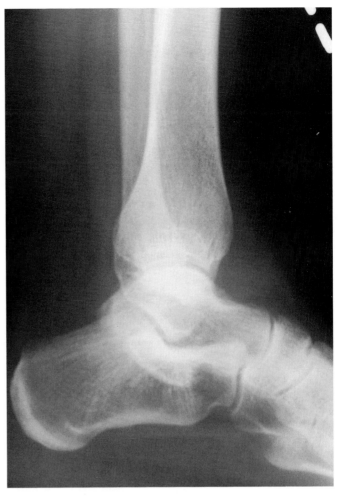

Fig. 7.3. Lateral radiograph in acute Achilles tendon rupture. Achilles tendon is not distinctly seen, and there is soft-tissue density in the pre-Achilles fat space.

Imaging the Achilles Tendon

Plain radiographs
In cases of tendon injury or bursitis, lateral plain radiographs often demonstrate blurring of the pre-Achilles fat (Fig. 7.3). Calcific tendinosis is uncommon (Fig. 7.4) and should be distinguished from the common finding of calcification at the enthesis (insertion of the tendon), which is associated with DISH (see Chapter 5). In diabetic patients, there may be an avulsion of the calcaneal insertion, rather than a tear of the tendon (see Chapter 4, Fig. 4.28).

Ultrasonography
Ultrasonography evaluates the size and echogenicity of the Achilles tendon. The ultrasound examination should be performed with the patient in a prone position with his feet extending beyond the end of the ultrasound table (Table 7.3). A 7.5 or 10 mHz linear array transducer may be used. Because of the subcutaneus location of the tendon, the use of a gel stand-off pad greatly improves the images. The tendon should be examined in both the transverse and longitudinal planes, and it should be compared to the contralateral tendon. If the tendon

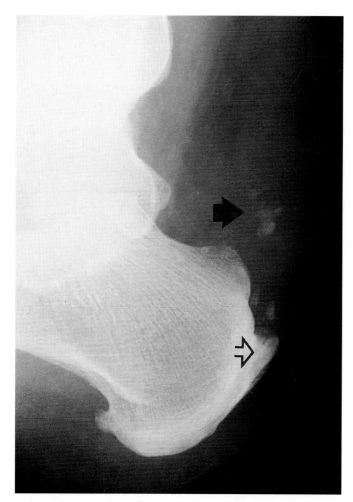

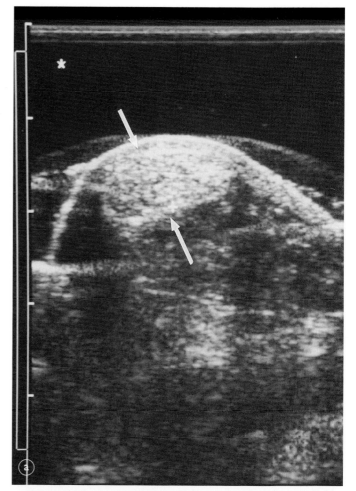

Fig. 7.4. Calcific tendinosis as well as calcification at enthesis. Patient had long-standing pain, thought clinically to be due to bursitis, but unresponsive to steroid injections into the bursa. Tendon is thickened. Small ossifications (arrow) were demonstrated by ultrasound (see Fig. 7.8) to be within the substance of the tendon. Enthesal calcifications (open arrow) are attached to the calcaneal tuberosity, and are not related to tendinosis.

is abnormal in appearance, dorsiflexion of the ankle will aid in visualization of any tear.

The normal tendon (Fig. 7.5) measures 4.5–6 mm in its shorter diameter[18] (maximum 6.7 cm in intensive athletes[19]) and has an elliptical shape on transverse images. The anterior margin of the tendon is flat or concave. Because of the oblique orientation of the tendon, measurements of thickness should be performed on transverse rather than sagittal images. The tendon shows uniform echogenicity, with what has been described as a 'honeycomb' appearance.[19]

Peritendonitis will show fluid surrounding the tendon,[19–21] and thickening of the anterior margin of the tendon[22] (Fig. 7.6). In patients with tendinosis, inhomogeneity and thickening of the tendon are seen (Figs 7.6–7.8). Most authors have reported focal or diffuse thickening ranging from 7 mm up to 17 mm at the point of maximum tendon thickness.[18–20] One report by Mathieson et al[21] found that patients with a clinical diagnosis of tendinosis had normal tendon thickness and echogenicity. These

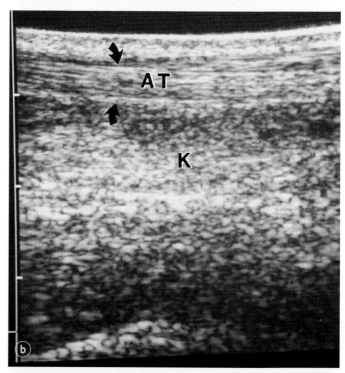

Fig. 7.5. Normal Achilles tendon ultrasound, 7.5 mHz. **a.** Axial measurement of thickness should be made along the short axis of the tendon (arrows) rather than the AP diameter, which is oblique to the tendon axis. **b.** Longitudinal scan demonstrates uniform echogenicity of the tendon. AT – Achilles tendon. Arrows show tendon margins. K – Kager's fat.

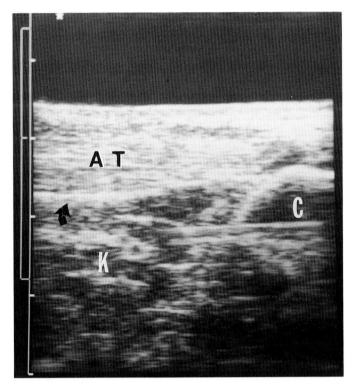

Fig. 7.6. Ultrasound of tendinosis and peritendonitis, 10 mHz. Sagittal ultrasound demonstrates a thick and inhomogeneous tendon, indicating tendinosis. Thickening of the anterior margin of the tendon (arrow) and heterogeneity of pre-Achilles fat (K) is consistent with peritendonitis. C – calcaneal tuberosity.

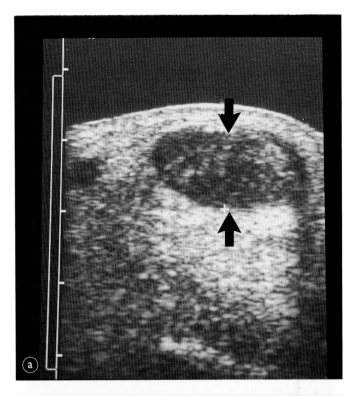

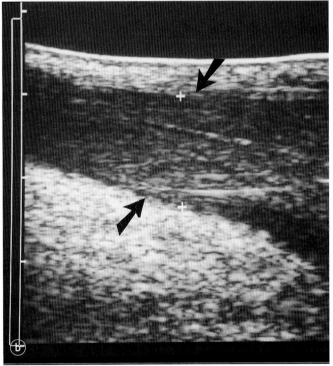

Fig. 7.7. Ultrasound of another patient with chronic tendinosis, 10 mHz. Tendon (arrows) is thickened with a maximum dimension of 14 mm, and decreased in echogenicity compared to normal. **a.** Axial image. **b.** Sagittal image.

results, at variance with those of other investigators,[23–25] are probably explained by the fact that he measured the thickness of the tendon 1 cm above the superior calcaneal surface instead of at its thickest point. Examination of the entire tendon and measurement at its thickest point rather than an arbitrary distance from the calcaneus is recommended.

Ultrasound has been reported to have a high accuracy for partial rupture,[19,23,25] although there is some overlap with findings of tendinosis.[24–26] For partial tendon rupture, Kainberger[19] used the criteria of focal decrease in tendon size, contour defect, irregular acoustic shadowing, intratendinous fluid, or thickening of the severed ends of the tendon, and he found both a false negative and a false positive rate of 12%. Kalebo[23] used the criteria of discontinuity of tendon fibers, focal sonolucencies, and localized tendon swelling, and found an overall accuracy of 95%. Weinstabl[24] found one false-negative ultrasound out of two patients with partial tears; both were diagnosed correctly on MRI. Neuhold[26] found that six out of eight patients with tendinosis had focal sonolucencies in the tendon, indicating that this finding is not specific for partial tear.

Complete tears show a gap in the tendon (Fig. 7.9); this increases in size when the foot is dorsiflexed. The gap in the tendon may be either hyperechoic, owing to hemorrhage, or hypoechoic, owing to fluid in the gap.[27] Patients who have been treated with casting show a diffusely thickened tendon, except that the tendon is of relatively normal thickness in the area of prior rupture (Fig. 7.10). Postoperative patients show marked

thickening of the Achilles tendon.[18–21] Pre-Achilles bursitis is readily visualized (Fig. 7.11).

CT scanning

CT is less useful than ultrasound or MRI in the evaluation of the Achilles tendon, because of its insensitivity to partial tears.[24–26]

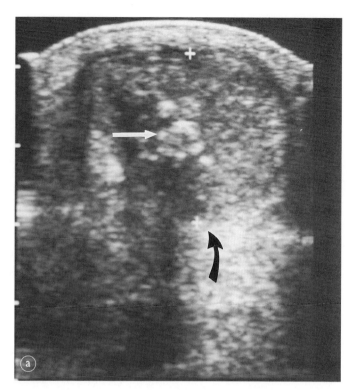
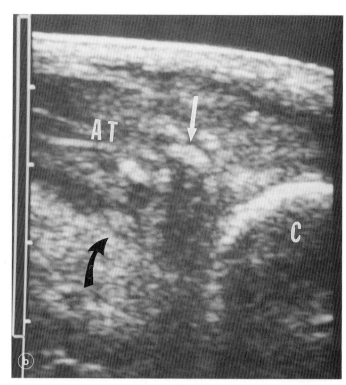

Fig. 7.8. Ultrasound of calcific tendinosis, 10 mHz (same patient as Fig.7.5). **a.** Axial image. **b.** Sagittal image. Tendon is markedly thickened (21 mm) and inhomogeneous. Curved arrow shows anterior margin of tendon. Straight arrow shows bright calcific deposits, with shadowing deep to the calcium. C – calcaneal tuberosity.

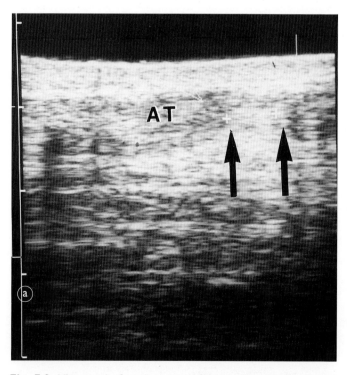
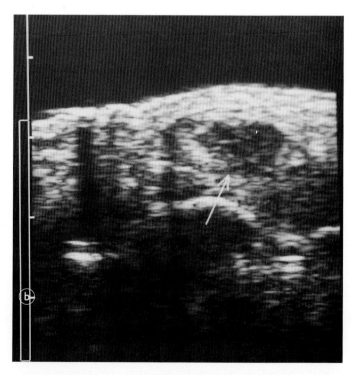

Fig. 7.9. Ultrasound of small rupture of the Achilles tendon, 1 week after the causative injury, 10 mHz. **a.** Sagittal scan. Small (6 mm) hyperechoic gap filled with echogenic debris is seen in the tendon (AT). **b.** Axial scan. Above and below the gap, tendon (arrow) appears thickened and heterogeneous. At surgery performed the same day as the ultrasound, a less than 1 cm complete rupture was confirmed.

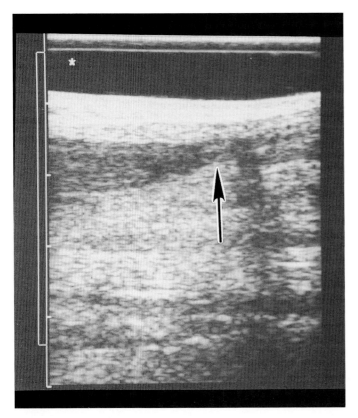

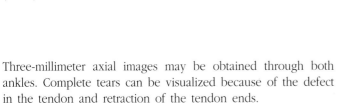

Fig. 7.10. Sagittal ultrasound of Achilles tendon following treatment of complete rupture with casting, 7.5 mHz. The majority of the tendon appears thickened. A focal area of normal thickness (5 mm) is seen (arrow) at the site of previous rupture.

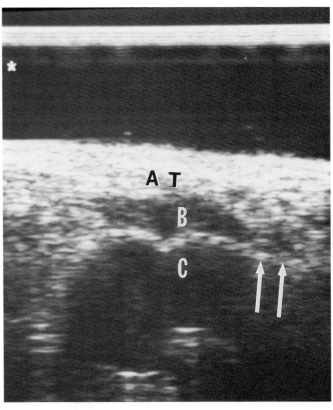

Fig. 7.11. Sagittal ultrasound of pre-Achilles bursitis in a patient who had recently increased athletic activity, 7.5 mHz. The hypoechoic bursa (B), filled with fluid, is seen separating the tendon (AT) from the tuberosity of the calcaneus (C). Arrows show site of tendon insertion.

Three-millimeter axial images may be obtained through both ankles. Complete tears can be visualized because of the defect in the tendon and retraction of the tendon ends.

MRI

MRI should be performed with images in both the sagittal and axial planes (Table 7.4). Sagittal T1-weighted images and T2-weighted images should have a 3–4 mm slice thickness. Field of view should be not smaller than 18 cm, so that the entire tendon and the distal belly of the gastrocnemius (where injuries may also occur) are visualized. Axial T2-weighted images may be performed with a 14–16 cm field of view and 5 mm slice thickness.

The normal Achilles tendon is signal-void on MRI. It is oval in shape, and the anterior contour is flat or concave[28,29] (Fig. 7.12). Tendinosis will demonstrate thickening of the tendon. The tendon may remain signal void, or may show a moderate increase in signal intensity presumably because of mucoid degeneration (signal less than that of fluid on T2-weighted image – Figs 7.13, 7.14). Peritendonitis is evident as strands of fluid in the pre-Achilles space. A partial tear will show a focal region of high signal, equal to that of fluid on T2-weighted image, within the substance of the tendon (Figs 7.15, 7.16). With complete tears, the length of the gap should be recorded, and the position of the foot noted (Fig. 7.17).

As on ultrasound and CT, the postoperative tendon will appear thickened on MRI. Areas of increased signal intensity are

Table 7.4. MRI protocol for Achilles tendon.

Coil – extremity or head
Scout – sagittal
Axial images – T2W (SE TR 2200 to 2400/TE 20–80
      FOV 14–16 cm
      slice thickness – 5 mm
      matrix: 128×256, 2 excitations
sagittal images – T1W (SE TR 300 to 500/TE 15–25)
      FOV 18–20 cm
      slice thickness: 3–4 mm
      matrix: 256×256, 1 excitation
    T2W (SE TR 2000/TE 20–80)
      same FOV, slice thickness as for T1W sagittal
      matrix – 128×256, 2 excitations
alternate coronal sequence – FSE TR 3000/TE 95

sometimes seen in asymptomatic patients, and are probably not significant as long as no fluid signal is seen in the tendon. A prosthetic tendon implant will be void of signal.[30]

Most reports of the accuracy of MRI in evaluating the Achilles tendon are anecdotal. Weinstabl[25] found MRI to give an accurate assessment of the degree of injury in thirteen cases confirmed operatively. Marcus[31] found that MRI accurately diagnosed partial

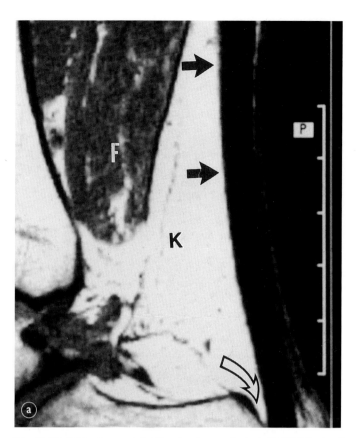

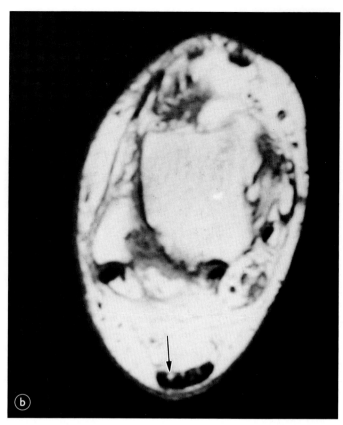

Fig. 7.12. MRI of normal Achilles tendon. **a.** Sagittal SE 500/20. Achilles tendon is a well-defined subcutaneous structure void of signal (arrows). Kager's fat triangle is located anteriorly (K), separating the Achilles tendon from the deep flexors of the foot (F). Curved arrow shows potential space of preAchilles bursa. **b.** Axial SE 2000/20. Anterior margin of tendon may be either flat or concave. Irregularity of the anterior margin of the tendon near its insertion is a normal finding due to interdigitation of fat between tendon fibers.

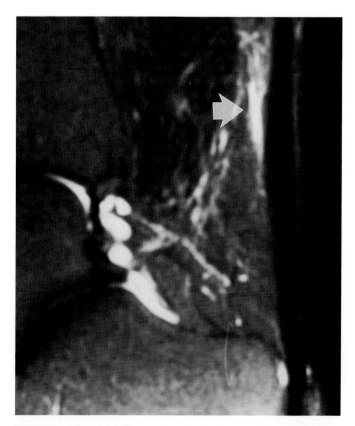

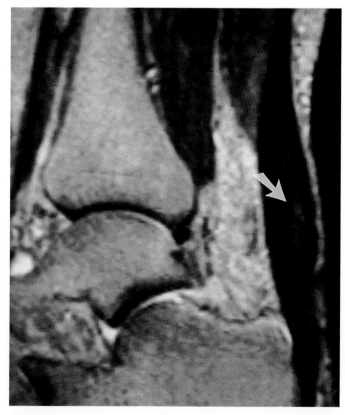

Fig. 7.13. MRI of Achilles peritendonitis. Sagittal FSE 4100/95. High signal intensity (arrow) anterior to the Achilles tendon is consistent with peritendonitis.

Fig. 7.14. MRI of Achilles tendinosis. Sagittal SE 2200/80. AT is thickened, and a small amount of slightly increased signal intensity (arrow), which remains less than the signal intensity of fluid, is present within it.

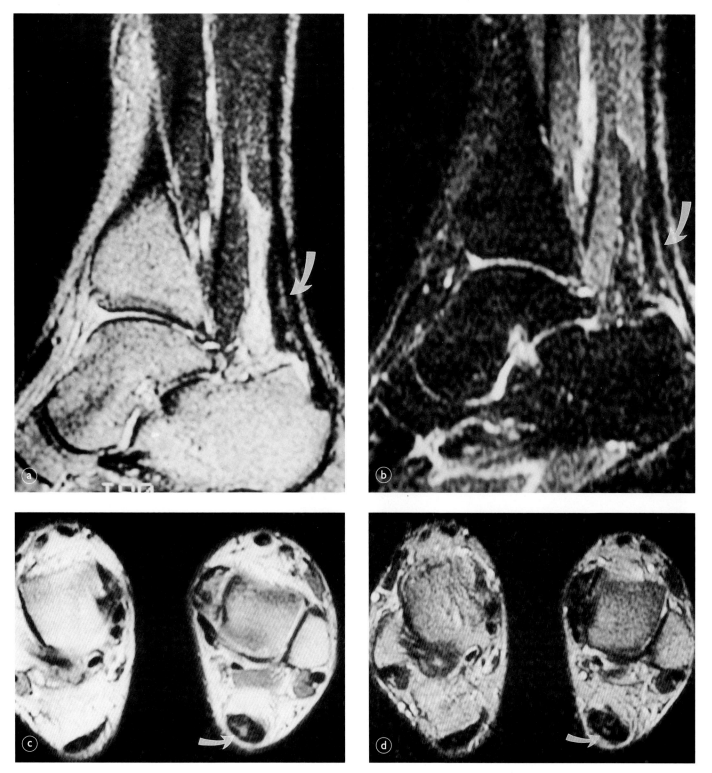

Fig. 7.15. MRI of partial tear of the Achilles tendon. **a.** Sagittal T2-weighted image, SE 2000/80. The tendon is attenuated near its insertion. A line of high signal intensity (arrow) is seen extending vertically between the tendon fibers. **b.** Sagittal STIR 2000/40/140. The vertical split in the tendon (arrow) is more easily seen. **c.** Axial balanced image, SE 2000/40. The tendon (arrow) is convex anteriorly, and contains several foci of high signal intensity. **d.** Axial T2-weighted image, SE 2000/80. Foci of abnormal signal intensity (arrow) have increased in signal compared to the balanced image.

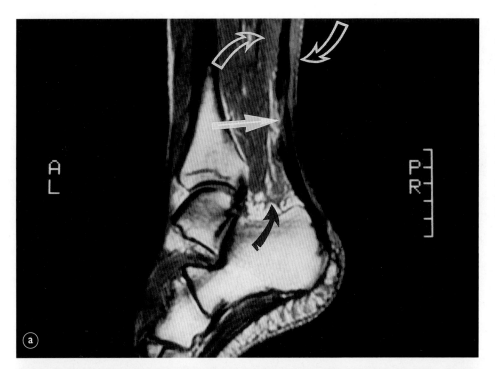

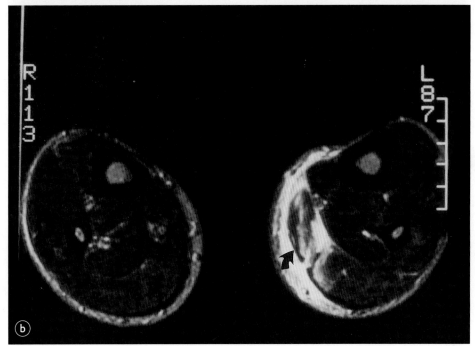

Fig. 7.16. MRI of partial rupture of Achilles tendon extending vertically into the medial head of the gastrocnemius muscle. **a.** Sagittal SE T1-weighted image, 600/20. Disruption of tendon fibers is seen anteriorly (straight solid arrow). There is hemorrhage in the pre-Achilles fat (curved solid arrow). Fluid is also seen around the proximal Achilles tendon (open arrows) **b.** Axial T2-weighted image, SE 2000/70. Partial rupture of the medial head of the gastrocnemius (arrow) is evident, with extensive high-signal fluid surrounding it.

or complete tears in five patients, of whom one had a palpable defect, three had a positive Thompson test, and four had plantar flexion weakness.

Treatment

Peritendonitis and tendinosis are usually treated conservatively with rest, nonsteroidal medications or casting,[6,10,32] but recalcitrant cases may require release of the peritenon[10,33] Partial ruptures of the tendon may be treated conservatively, or with surgical excision of the abnormal region of tendon.[14]

The debate over treatment of complete ruptures is ongoing,[16,17,30,32-34] and a full review is beyond the scope of this book. Support for nonoperative treatment was given by Nistor et al,[34] who in a prospective, randomized study of 105 patients found that results of operative and nonoperative treatment resulted in similar levels of strength and in the ability to return to athletic activity. There were two reruptures in the surgically treated group and five in the nonsurgically treated group. The preponderance of the literature has been in favor of operative treatment. Wills et al[35] reviewed 20 studies of treatment of Achilles tendon rupture that had been published between 1959 and 1981. They found that, overall, surgical therapy reduced the

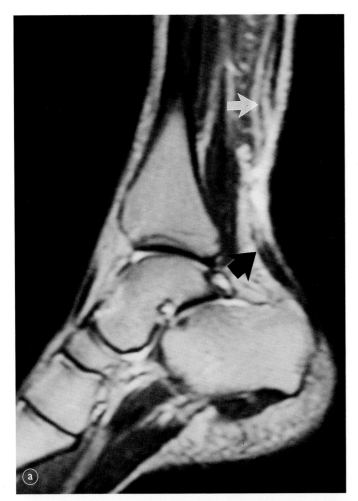

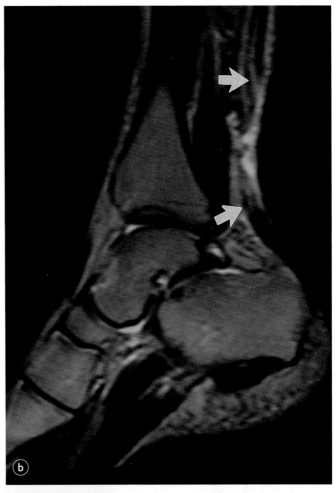

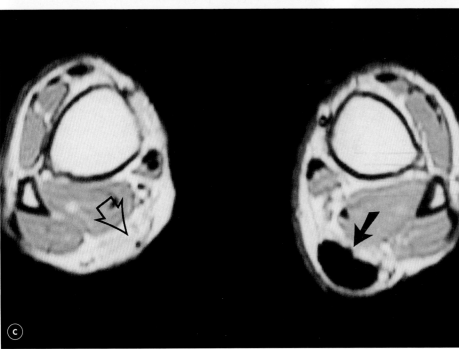

Fig. 7.17. Complete rupture of Achilles tendon. **a.** Balanced sagittal image, SE 2000/20 **b.** T2-weighted sagittal image, SE 2000/80. There is a gap in the tendon, and irregularity of the retracted tendon ends (arrows). **c.** Axial balanced image, SE 2000/20. The right Achilles tendon is completely absent at this level. Open arrow points to expected site of Achilles tendon. The patient also had tendinosis of the left Achilles tendon, with thickening of the anteroposterior dimension of the tendon (closed arrow).

risk of rerupture (1.7% risk of rerupture for surgically treated, and 17.7% for nonsurgically treated patients). However, they also found a significant morbidity associated with surgical treatment, including skin sloughs and infection.

In current orthopedic practice, older and less athletic patients are more likely to be treated conservatively. Young or athletic patients are usually treated with surgical repair of the tendon.[9,17,36] The size of the defect in the tendon should also be considered in determining treatment. A tendon rupture in which there is only a small gap between the tendon ends may be treated by casting the foot in plantar flexion[17] or functional bracing with dorsiflexion blocked. In long gaps, surgery may be needed to provide adequate apposition of the torn tendon ends. Neglected ruptures are more likely to have separation of the tendon ends, and they generally require surgery. Autogenous tissue is used in the majority of cases, although silastic implants have been used occasionally in large ruptures.[19]

POSTERIOR TIBIAL TENDON

Anatomy

The tibialis posterior muscle arises from the posterior surfaces of the tibia, the interosseous membrane, and the fibula. It becomes tendinous immediately above the ankle joint, and the tendon curves behind the medial malleolus, inserting predominantly on the tuberosity of the navicular bone. Smaller tendon slips insert on the plantar aspects of the cuneiforms, the cuboid, the bases of the second through fourth metatarsals, and the sustentaculum tali. The tibialis posterior acts to supinate the foot and adduct the forefoot, and it is crucial to maintaining the medial aspect of the longitudinal arch.

Etiology of Posterior Tibial Tendon Rupture

Rupture of the posterior tibial tendon is a fairly common occurrence, seen primarily in middle-aged and elderly women. The rupture is usually spontaneous, caused by abnormal stresses such as obesity, pre-existing flatfoot deformity, or prior trauma to the medial aspect of the foot or steroid use.[37] A 1.5 cm hypovascular zone in the tendon, extending distally from a point approximately 1 cm distal to the medial malleolus, has been postulated as a predisposing factor to tendon rupture.[38] Inflammatory arthritis, either seronegative[39] or rheumatoid,[40] may cause tenosynovitis and rupture.

In a small percentage of patients, tenosynovitis and rupture occur as a result of athletic activity, in which case the pain may be misattributed to joint pain in the midtarsal joints.[41] Rupture has also been reported as a result of ankle fracture.[42,43]

Clinical Presentation

Posterior tibial tendon rupture leads to a painful flatfoot deformity. The site of rupture is characteristically between the medial malleolus and the insertion of the tendon on the navicular, and physical examination demonstrates tenderness in this region. There is weakness when attempting a one-legged toe stand and

Table 7.5. Differential diagnosis of posterior tibial tendon rupture

Tenosynovitis
Arthritis: degenerative or inflammatory
Spring ligament injury
Foot fracture
Type 2 accessory navicular
tarsal coalition

also with inversion of the plantarflexed foot. Flatfoot deformity, abduction of the forefoot and valgus heel are usually present. The accuracy of physical diagnosis is unknown. A case has been reported[44] in which navicular tubercle tenderness was present, but without pes planus or weakness of inversion. In this case, MRI demonstrated a complete posterior tibial tendon rupture verified at surgery.

Classification

Rupture of the posterior tibial tendon progresses gradually over a period of months to years. Detection of the early stages of rupture is important because early surgical repair can prevent the development of deformity, which may require hindfoot arthrodesis.[45–48] Rupture has been divided into three main stages or grades.[49] In stage I, longitudinal splits develop in the tendon, which appears enlarged. In stage II, there is thinning of the tendon. In Stage III, a complete rupture with discontinuity of the tendon is seen.

Differential Diagnosis

The differential diagnosis is summarized in Table 7.5. Tenosynovitis of the posterior tibial or flexor digitorum longus tendons may mimic rupture. Acquired flatfoot deformity can also be due to degenerative or rheumatoid arthritis, abnormalities of the spring ligament, or fracture of the foot.[50,51] An accessory navicular can cause pain in a patient with flatfoot deformity, and may be associated with tenosynovitis of the posterior tibial tendon. Tarsal coalition will cause a painful, rigid flatfoot.

Imaging of Posterior Tibial Tendon Rupture

Plain radiographs
Standing radiographs of the foot show characteristic findings, although the various stages of injury cannot be differentiated. Pes planus is present (Fig. 7.18) with a sagging of the longitudinal arch at the talonavicular joint. The head of the talus subluxes inferior and medial to the navicular (see Fig. 7.18), and there is abduction of the forefoot. Radiographically evident osteoarthritis is a very late finding.

Ultrasonography
Ultrasound has been used to document posterior tibial tendon rupture[52] and tenosynovitis,[53] although no series has been

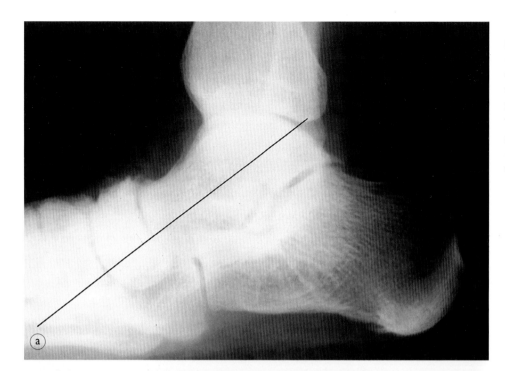

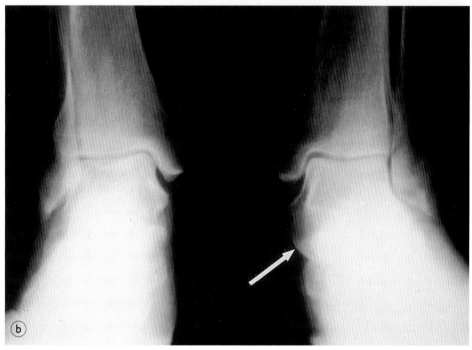

Fig. 7.18. Plain radiographic findings in posterior tibial tendon rupture. **a.** Lateral radiograph. Pes planus is present: a line drawn along the long axis of the talus extends below the axis of the first metatarsal. There is plantar flexion of the talus. **b.** AP radiograph. There is medial subluxation of the head of the talus (arrow) relative to navicular. The heel is in valgus.

published evaluating its accuracy. Given the superficial location of the tendon, ultrasound is a promising technique (Fig. 7.19).

CT

CT is performed with direct axial and coronal scans (see Chapter 2). Slice thickness can be 3–4 mm. Both feet are usually imaged.

The tendon is evaluated for thickening or thinning; normally the posterior tibial tendon should be approximately twice the diameter of the flexor digitorum longus tendon, which is located directly posterolateral to the posterior tibial tendon. Heterogeneity and thickening of the tendon are seen in grade I tears, and thinning is seen in grade II. In grade III tears an area of fluid density replaces the soft-tissue density of the tendon.

CT is relatively insensitive to longitudinal splits within the tendon,[54,55] which are difficult to distinguish from tendinosis, and it is difficult to distinguish fluid surrounding the tendon from thickening of the tendon.[55] A reported secondary sign of rupture is a posterior spur of the medial malleolus.[52]

In an initial report, Rosenberg et al[54] found that CT detected 96% of 28 suspected ruptures that underwent surgery. In 14%, the degree of injury was underestimated, for an overall accuracy of 82%. Her subsequent study[55] of 22 tendon ruptures assessed with both CT and MRI found a 90% accuracy in detecting rupture for CT, and a 95% accuracy for MRI. Accuracy of classification of type of rupture was 59% for CT and 73% for MRI compared to surgical inspection.

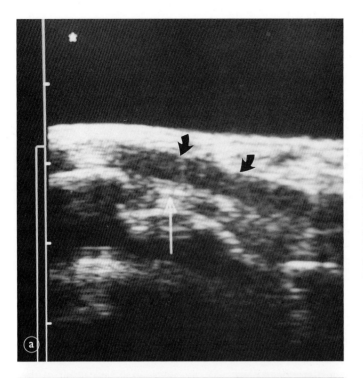

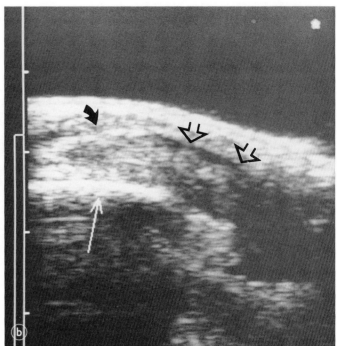

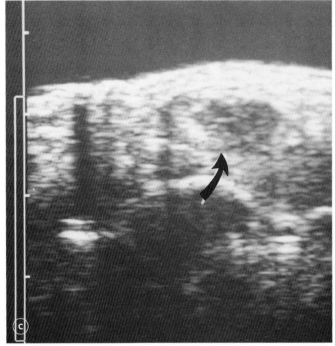

Fig. 7.19. Ultrasound of the posterior tibial tendon at 10 mHz. **a.** Longitudinal scan of normal posterior tibial tendon. Tendon (closed arrows) is of uniform thickness and echogenicity, and well-demarcated from adjacent fat. **b.** Longitudinal scan of Stage II posterior tibial tendon rupture. Proximally (closed arrow) the tendon is thickened and heterogeneous. Distally the tendon sheath is filled with fluid (open arrows). A few intact fibers are seen within the fluid. **c.** Transverse scan, same patient, demonstrates the irregular-appearing tendon (closed arrow). (Case courtesy of Dr Hector Hidalgo, Durham, North Carolina.)

MRI

In order to evaluate subtle abnormalities of the tendon, it is useful for the inexperienced radiologist to image both feet. In the axial planes through the hindfoot, 3–4 mm T2-weighted sequences are obtained (Table 7.6). Fast spin echo (FSE) sequence may be substituted for one of the T2-weighted sequences. Additional T1-weighted images are obtained in either the coronal or the axial plane, primarily for evaluation of bony abnormalities.

The normal tendon is signal-void and about twice the size of the adjacent flexor digitorum longus tendon (Figs 7.20–7.21). The tendon may increase slightly in signal intensity on T1-weighted

or balanced images at its navicular insertion (see Fig. 7.20), and this should not be mistaken for a rupture.

Care should be taken to avoid overdiagnosis of apparent tendon abnormalities, which are due to the 'magic angle' phenomenon described by Erickson et al[56] This term refers to increased signal intensity seen in tendons on T1-weighted images when the tendon is oriented obliquely to the static magnetic field. The increased signal is maximal at an angle of 55°. Curved tendons such as the posterior tibial and peroneal tendons will frequently demonstrate this spurious signal intensity. Unlike increased signal that is due to a true abnormality of the tendon, signal that is due to the 'magic angle' phenomenon

Table 7.6. MRI protocols for posterior tibial tendon.

Protocol A: best used by inexperienced examiners
coil – head or extremity, containing both hindfeet
scout – sagittal
axial and coronal T2WI TR 2000–2200/TE 20, 80
      FOV 20 cm
      slice thickness: 3–4 mm
      matrix: 192×256, 1 excitation
    alternate coronal sequence: FSE TR 3000/TE 95
coronal T1WI TR 300-500/TE 15–25
      FOV 20 cm
      slice thickness – 3–4 mm
      matrix –192×256, 1 acquisition
Protocol B: superior resolution
coil – head or extremity, containing only affected hindfoot
decrease FOV to 14 cm, other parameters and sequences remain the same

will not be present on the second echo of a T2-weighted sequence.

On MRI, tenosynovitis will demonstrate thickening of the tendon and fluid in the tendon sheath (Fig. 7.21). A grade I rupture will show thickening of the tendon and foci of high signal within the tendon on T2-weighted images (Fig. 7.22). Grade II rupture will show attenuation of the tendon (Figs 7.23, 7.24), and grade III will show a gap in the tendon (Fig. 7.25).

Rosenberg[55] found a 73% accuracy for MRI compared to surgery in determining the stage of posterior tibial tendon rupture. The question has recently been raised as to whether

MRI is more accurate than surgery. Conti et al[57] studied 20 cases of posterior tibial tendon rupture which were followed for an average of two years after surgery. He found a significant disparity between the grade of rupture as determined by MRI and that determined by surgical inspection: of 17 surgical stage I ruptures, seven were type I by MRI, and 10 were stage II by MRI. In 11 of the 20 cases, the injury was shown to be more extensive by MRI than could be detected by inspection at surgery. Only one patient had more extensive injury seen at time of surgery than MRI predicted. MRI stage I ruptures had a significantly better outcome from tendon reconstruction.

The MRI grading of the tendon injury more accurately predicted the failure of tendon repair, defined as recurrent pain or deformity. Further studies are needed to confirm if MRI rather than surgical inspection should serve as the 'gold standard' to guide choice of treatment between tendon repair and triple arthrodesis.

Treatment

Treatment of posterior tibial tendon rupture is in a state of evolution. Stages I and II can be treated with surgical repair of the tendon and possibly tendon transfer. Stage III may be treated with tendon transfer or with hindfoot arthrodesis, depending on the severity of deformity and rigidity of the foot.[49]

Dislocation of the Posterior Tibial Tendon

Dislocation of the posterior tibial tendon has rarely been reported. Recently Ouzounian and Myerson[58] reviewed the English literature and presented a series of seven additional patients. Dislocation occurs most commonly in young patients and is caused trauma. Patients are often misdiagnosed as having

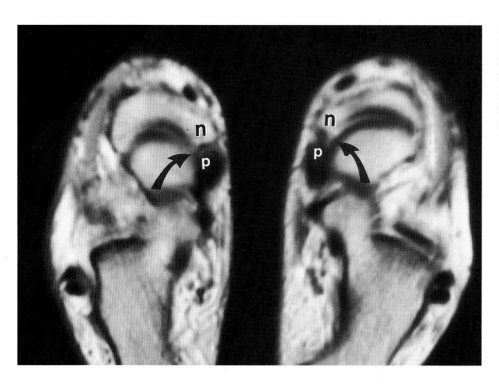

Fig. 7.20. Normal MRI appearance of the posterior tibial tendon at level of navicular insertion. Axial balanced image SE 2000/20. Slight increase in tendon signal (arrow) is seen at the navicular insertion. Signal was normal on T2-weighted images. n=navicular. p= posterior tibial tendon.

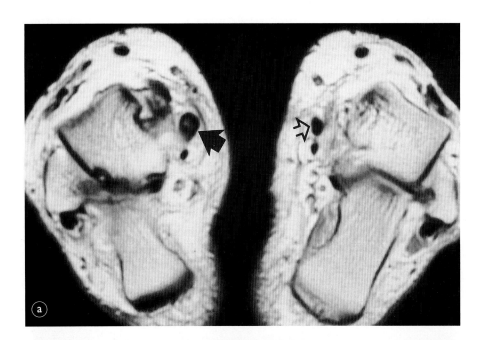

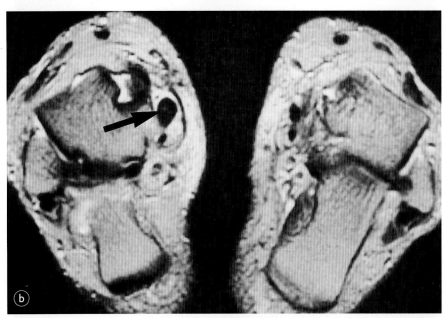

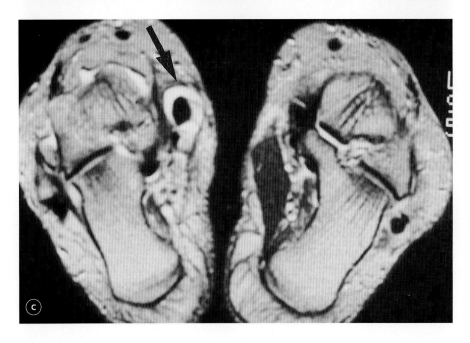

Fig. 7.21. MRI of tenosynovitis and stage I tear of posterior tibial tendon. **a.** Axial balanced image, SE 3000/20. The right posterior tibial tendon (solid arrow) is enlarged and contains a small focus of abnormal signal. Compare to the normal left posterior tibial tendon (open arrow). **b.** Axial T2-weighted image, SE 3000/70. High signal (arrow) is seen centrally within the tendon. **c.** Axial T2-weighted image, SE 3000/70. More distally, fluid (arrow) is seen within the tendon sheath, surrounding the thickened right posterior tibial tendon.

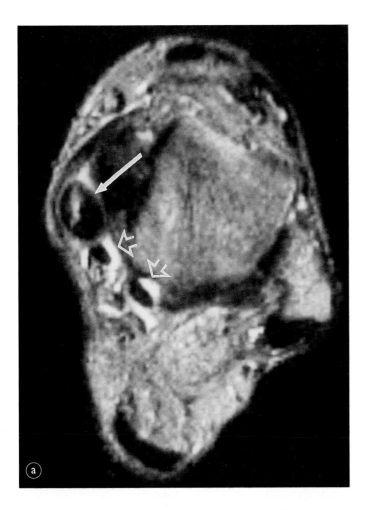

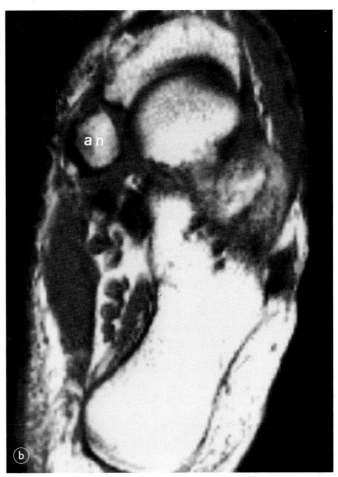

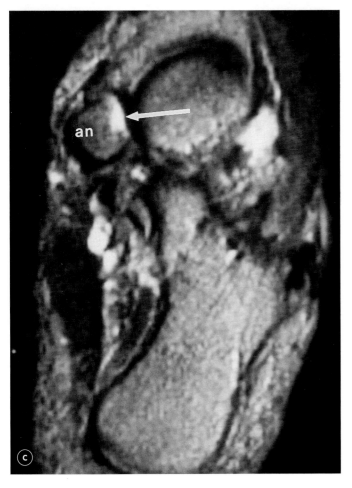

Fig. 7.22. MRI of stage I posterior tibial tendon rupture and avulsion of an accessory navicular. **a.** Axial T2-weighted image, SE 2200/70 demonstrates enlarged tendon (arrow) with disrupted fibers centrally. Note that fluid is also present around the flexor digitorum longus and flexor hallucis longus tendons (open arrow), a common and nonspecific finding. **b.** Axial balanced image, SE2200/20. **c.** Axial T2-weighted image, SE 2200/70. This patient also had avulsion of a type 2 accessory navicular bone (see Chapter 1). Posterior tibial tendon tears are associated with the presence of an accessory navicular. Arrow shows fluid related to the avulsion.

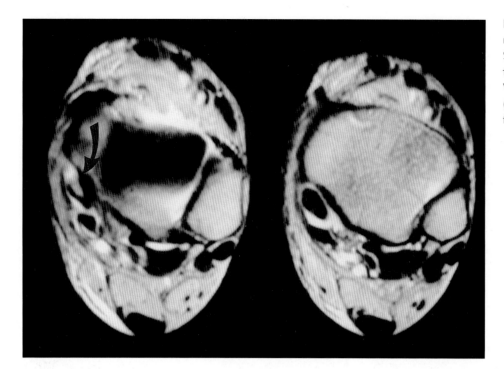

Fig. 7.23. MRI of stage II rupture of posterior tibial tendon. Axial T2-weighted image, SE 2000/80. Two sequential axial images through the left ankle demonstrate a large, V-shaped cleft in the posterior tibial tendon (arrow). At a higher level (image on right), fluid is seen surrounding the tendon.

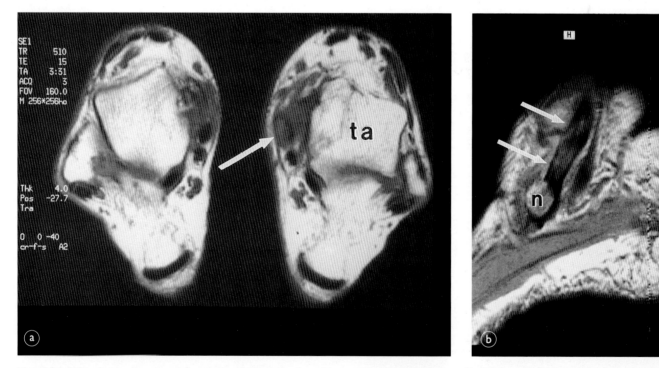

Fig. 7.24. MRI of stage II rupture of posterior tibial tendon in another patient (same patient as Fig. 7.19). **a.** Axial T1-weighted image, SE 510/15. Tendon (arrow) is nearly completely ruptured, with a few intact fibers still seen. Fluid in tendon sheath is of intermediate signal intensity. ta – talus. **b.** Sagittal T1-weighted image, SE 510/15. In general, sagittal images are not helpful in diagnosis of posterior tibial tendon rupture, but in this case one image serendipitously shows the tendon (arrows) from the level of the medial malleolus to its navicular insertion (n). The tendon fibers and sheath are signal void, and the fluid is of intermediate signal intensity.

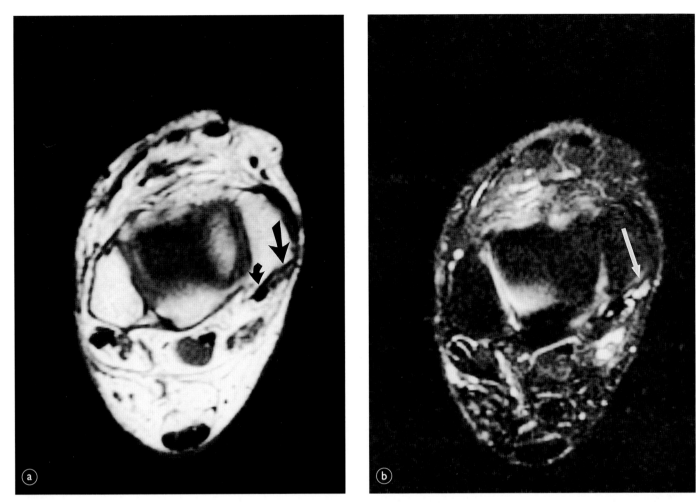

Fig. 7.25. Axial MRI of stage III rupture of posterior tibial tendon. **a.** SE 500/15. The posterior tibial tendon is absent at the level of the medial malleolus. Straight arrow points to expected location of tendon. Curved arrow points to flexor digitorum longus tendon. **b.** FSE 3000/95. High signal intensity due to fluid (arrow) is seen in the expected location of the posterior tibial tendon.

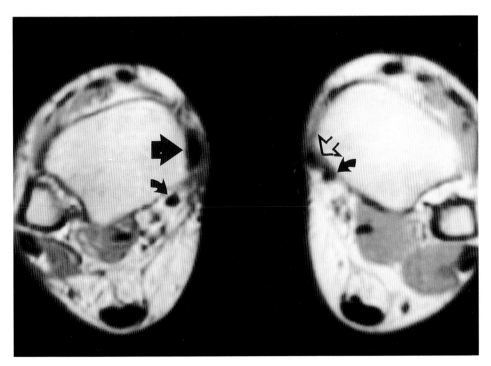

Fig. 7.26. MRI of dislocation of posterior tibial tendon. Axial SE 2000/20 immediately above the level of the mortise joint. The right posterior tibial tendon (closed arrow) is dislocated anteromedially. Compare the normal position of the left posterior tibial tendon (open arrow). Curved arrows show normal flexor digitorum longus tendon bilaterally.

an ankle sprain. Physical examination is nonspecific, revealing pain and tenderness in the region of the medial malleolus. Patients sometimes complain of a popping sensation. Conservative treatment is unsatisfactory, and repair of the flexor retinaculum is needed. Given the difficulty of diagnosis and the need for surgical repair, MRI is recommended[58,59] (Fig. 7.26).

FLEXOR HALLUCIS LONGUS TENDON

Anatomy

The flexor hallucis longus arises from the posterior surface of the midfibula and lower fibula. It becomes tendinous just below the level of the mortise joint, where it courses behind the medial malleolus to take a horizontal course in the foot. It runs below the sustentaculum tali of the calcaneus and inserts on the distal phalanx of the first toe.

Etiology of Injury

Injury to the flexor hallucis longus tendon can be divided into two main categories by the location in which it occurs: either proximally, around the ankle, or distally, close to the tendon insertion.

Ballet dancers may develop tenosynovitis and rupture of the flexor hallucis longus tendon around the region of the medial malleolus.[60–62] The injury is thought to be due to the stress of the en pointe and demi pointe positions. Ballet dancers also may have impingement of the soft tissue structures of the ankle by the os trigonum or a prominent lateral posterior process of the talus, and this can lead secondarily to flexor hallucis longus tenosynovitis.[63,64]

Injury at the level of the midcalcaneus may occur because of calcaneal fracture. Rupture near the head of the talus has been reported in a long distance runner.[65]

Runners develop a stenosing tenosynovitis near the sesamoids of the great toe.[66] Rupture of the tendon close to its insertion has been reported following a twisting injury[67] and forced dorsiflexion against a contracted muscle.[68]

Clinical Presentation

Dancers experience pain and tenderness behind the medial malleolus. Runners usually have pain at the first metatarsophalangeal joint.

Differential Diagnosis

Pain and tenderness behind the medial malleolus may be due to posterior tibial tendon rupture or dislocation, or rarely to tenosynovitis of the flexor digitorum longus. Os trigonum syndrome, subtalar arthropathy, Achilles tendonitis, and osteochondritis dissecans of the talus should be considered.

Pain at the level of the first metatarsophalangeal joint may be due to problems of the sesamoids: synovitis, stress fracture,

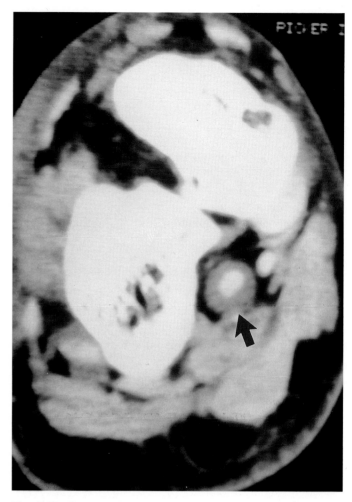

Fig. 7.27. Coronal CT at level of anterior facet of subtalar joint in patient with flexor hallucis longus injury. Patient with calcaneal fracture had weakness of flexion of first toe. CT demonstrates fluid surrounding the tendon (arrow).

subluxation, or dislocation. Arthritis of the first metatarsophalangeal joint is common.

Imaging of the Flexor Hallucis Longus

Plain radiographs are not contributory. CT using the calcaneal fracture protocol (see Chapter 4) is preferable to MRI in cases of calcaneal fracture, since it will optimally demonstrate the salient features of the fracture as well as tendon injury. MRI should employ the same protocol as for posterior tibial tendon rupture.

Fluid surrounding the tendon within the tendon sheath has been reported as a sign of tenosynovitis[69] (Fig. 7.27). However, fluid may be seen within the tendon sheath owing to communication of the synovial sheath with the ankle joint. Therefore, patients may have fluid in the tendon sheaths either unilaterally or bilaterally, without signs or symptoms referable to the flexor hallucis longus (Fig. 7.28).

A tear of the tendon will show high-signal intensity on T2-weighted images (Fig. 7.29). Fluid usually extends along the tendon sheath.

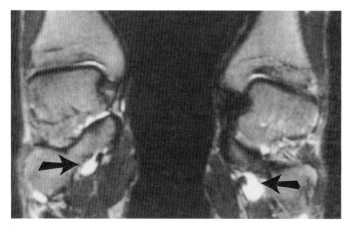

Fig. 7.28. Coronal MRI demonstrating incidental fluid (arrows) within the flexor hallucis longus tendon sheath bilaterally. SE 2200/80. Patient had pain in the left ankle only, and no symptoms or signs referable to the flexor hallucis longus tendon.

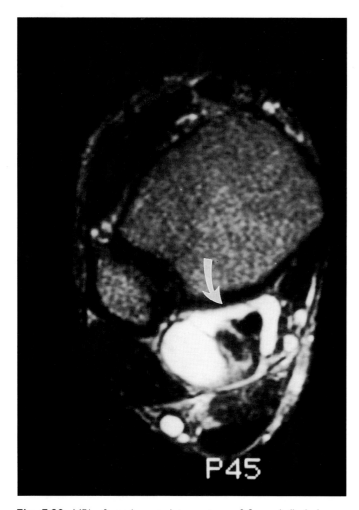

P45

Fig. 7.29. MRI of nearly complete rupture of flexor hallucis longus musculotendinous junction in college football player. Patient experienced a sudden 'snap' during practice, and was unable to either plantarflex or dorsiflex foot because of pain. Axial FSE 3000/90 immediately above mortise joint. High signal intensity fluid (arrow) is seen occupying the majority of the flexor hallucis longus muscle.

Treatment

Tenosynovitis in dancers is usually treated conservatively, since scar tissue from surgical release can be problematic,[60] although if the problem is secondary to os trigonum syndrome the ossicle can be excised.[63,64] Lidocaine injection may be used for the stenosing tenosynovitis seen in runners.[66] Ruptures are generally treated surgically.

PERONEAL TENDONS

Anatomy

The peroneus longus muscle originates from the proximal fibula and interosseous membrane. It is superficial to the peroneus brevis throughout the calf but it comes to lie posterior to the peroneus brevis slightly above the level of the lateral malleolus. It courses behind the lateral malleolus, and then changes to a horizontal orientation in the hindfoot. It runs behind and below the peroneal tubercle of the calcaneus, extends beneath the cuboid deep to the long plantar ligament, and inserts on the medial cuneiform and the base of the first metatarsal. A sesamoid bone, the os peroneum, may be present in the peroneus longus tendon at the level of the calcaneocuboid joint.

The peroneus brevis arises from the distal third of the fibula and interosseous membrane. It runs with the peroneus longus muscle behind the fibula and horizontally in the hindfoot in front of and above the peroneal tubercle of the calcaneus and the peroneus longus. It inserts on the lateral tubercle of the fifth metatarsal.

As the peroneal tendons change orientation from a vertical course in the calf to a horizontal course in the hindfoot, they are held in place by the superior and inferior peroneal retinacula. The superior peroneal retinaculum holds the tendons in the peroneal groove of the fibula, and the inferior retinaculum holds them against the lateral aspect of the calcaneus. The peroneus longus and brevis have a common tendon sheath, which originates slightly above the lateral malleolus and extends below the inferior retinaculum.

Accessory tendon slips may occur[70–72] and may cause lateral ankle pain. Absence of the peroneus longus is a rare anomaly. It has been reported in a ballet dancer who developed a peroneus brevis rupture.[73]

Subluxation of the Peroneal Tendons

The superior peroneal retinaculum may be ruptured during skiing[33] or other severe inversion injuries of the ankle, and this will result in anterior subluxation or dislocation of the tendons. A small cortical avulsion fracture of the lateral margin of the fibula, at or above the lateral malleolus, may be present.[74–75]

Subluxation of the tendons may also occur because of congenital absence of the peroneal groove of the fibula. The subluxed tendons can be palpated on physical examination, more prominently with dorsiflexion of the foot. Treatment is generally surgical.[33] Because of the ease of physical diagnosis, imaging does not have a significant role to play, although CT has been used.[76–77]

Table 7.7. Differential diagnosis of chronic lateral ankle pain.

Instability from chronic laxity of the lateral collateral ligaments

Arthritis: ankle or subtalar joint

Fracture: osteochondritis dissecans, fracture of lateral process of talus, stress fracture of cuboid or fifth metatarsal

Sinus tarsi syndrome

Anterolateral ankle impingement syndrome

Anomalous peroneal tendon or os peroneum syndrome

Table 7.8. MRI protocol for lateral ankle pain

Use same sequences as for posterior tibial tendon, except substitute:

T1WI in sagittal rather than coronal plane

add:

3DFT FISP sagittal plane TR40/TE10/FA40

  FOV 18 cm, slab 7 cm

  32 partitions for 2.18 mm effective slice thickness

  64 partitions for 1.09 mm effective slice thickness

  matrix 192×256, 1 acquisition

Tenosynovitis

Tenosynovitis is usually secondary to an intra-articular fracture of the calcaneus, with impingement or entrapment of the peroneal tendons by bony fragments.[78] Uncommonly, it may be due to inflammatory arthritis or abnormal foot mechanics.[77,79–81]

Peroneal Tendon Rupture

Longitudinal splits in the peroneal brevis tendon are generally due to inversion injury to the ankle.[82–84] Patients may present with pain, instability, and less commonly weakness of eversion. Complete rupture is rare. Treatment is usually surgical.

Sobel et al[85] found attrition of the peroneus brevis tendon in 11.3% of cadaveric ankles, and significant longitudinal splits in 7%. These changes were thought to be due to impingement in the peroneal groove. This study raises the question of how often longitudinal splits of the peroneus brevis tendon are clinically significant. Positive MRI scans may occur in asymptomatic patients, and MRI findings of splits in the peroneus brevis tendon should be interpreted with caution.

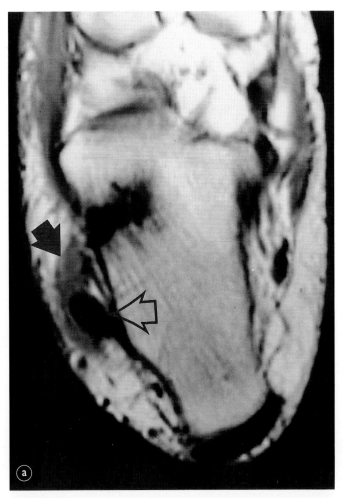 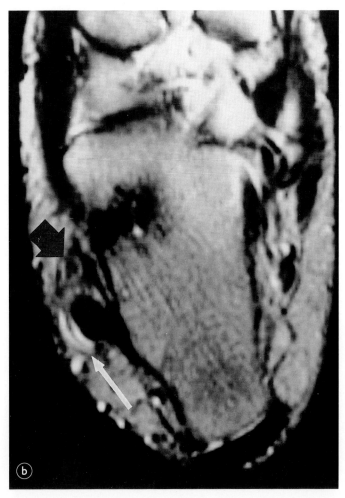

Fig. 7.30. MRI showing partial rupture of the peroneus brevis tendon in a patient with rheumatoid arthritis. **a.** Balanced axial image, SE 2000/30. Approximately two-thirds of the tendon is torn (black arrow), with intact fibers seen medially. Open arrow points to peroneus longus tendon. **b.** T2-weighted axial image, SE 2000/70. The intact fibers of the peroneus brevis tendon are better seen, outlined by fluid (black arrow). Fluid is also seen in the common peroneal tendon sheath (white arrow).

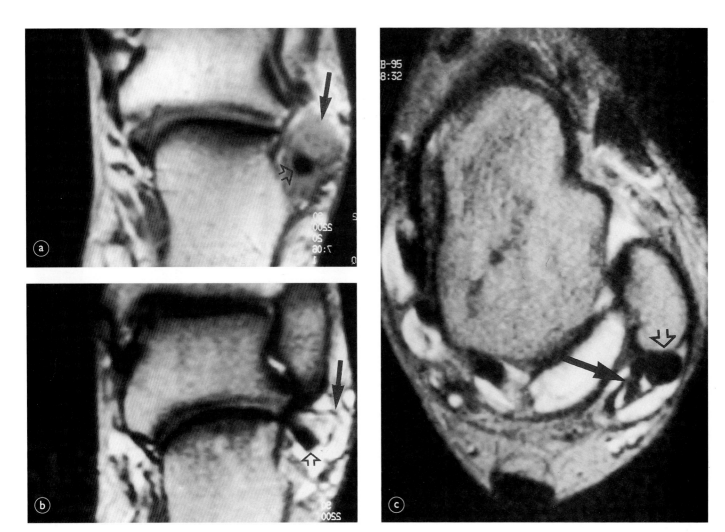

Fig. 7.31. MRI of complete tear of the peroneus brevis tendon due to inversion injury. **a.** Coronal balanced image SE 2200/20. Amorphous material of intermediate signal intensity (closed arrow) is seen in the expected location of the peroneus brevis tendon, superior to the peroneus longus tendon (open arrow). **b.** Coronal T2-weighted image SE 2200/80. Fluid fills the common tendon sheaths of the peroneus brevis and longus. A few strands of wavy, low-signal-intensity peroneus brevis tendon fibers are seen (arrow). Tendon was completely ruptured at surgical exploration. Open arrow points to peroneus longus tendon. **c.** Axial T2-weighted image, at the level of the lateral malleolus. The peroneus brevis tendon, located deep to the peroneus longus tendon, is attenuated but visible at this level. There is fluid surrounding the flexor tendons secondary to the patient's ankle effusion.

Rupture of the peroneus longus tendon is very rare.[86,87] It has been reported as causing peroneal compartment syndrome.[88]

Differential Diagnosis of Peroneal Tendon Injury

Peroneal tendon injury must be differentiated from other causes of lateral ankle pain (Table 7.7). The entities listed can usually be diagnosed by a combination of physical examination, plain radiographs, and MRI.

Imaging of the Peroneal Tendons

Plain radiographs

Findings are usually nonspecific, with lateral soft-tissue swelling evident. Calcific tendinosis can occur. Posterior displacement of the os peronei, a sesamoid in the peroneus longus, has been reported as a sign of peroneus longus rupture.[86] Chip fracture of the lateral malleolus may be seen in cases of tendon subluxation.[74,75]

Tenosynography

Tenosynography has been used to diagnose tynosynovitis and rupture.[81] It is seldom used today, since unlike MRI it cannot examine for the other, more common injuries (Table 7.7) which may cause chronic lateral ankle pain.

CT

CT scanning is the optimal method to evaluate the peroneal tendon in cases of calcaneal fracture (see Chapter 4, Fig. 4.24) because of its excellent spatial resolution and its ability to show small bone fragments. In cases of chronic pain, MRI is preferable because it can more completely evaluate other causes of lateral ankle pain as well as possible peroneal tendon abnormalities.

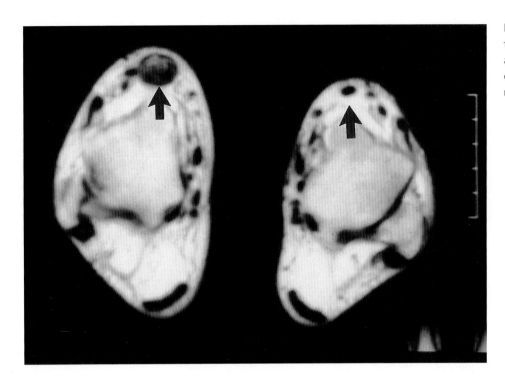

Fig. 7.32. MRI of laceration of the anterior tibial tendon. SE 2000/20. The injured right anterior tibial tendon (arrow) is markedly enlarged and irregular compared to the normal left side (arrow).

MRI

The protocol for MRI examination (Table 7.8) is designed to evaluate other causes of ankle pain as well as peroneal tendon injury. Sagittal T1-weighted images and thin-slice three-dimensional full-thickness sequences are used for optimal visualization of the sinus tarsi.

MRI has been advocated as the method of choice for evaluating the peroneal tendons,[72,10] although, because of the rarity of injuries, there are no series examining its accuracy. As with the posterior tibial tendon (see above), care must be taken to avoid misdiagnosis due to artefact from the 'magic angle' phenomenon when the tendons change direction. Abnormalities should be diagnosed only when signal is abnormal on T2-weighted as well as T1-weighted or balanced images (Figs 7.30, 7.31).

ANTERIOR TIBIAL TENDON

Anatomy

The tibialis anterior muscle arises from the tibia, from the interosseous membrane, and from an intermuscular septum that separates it from the extensor digitorum longus. It becomes tendinous in the distal third of the tibia, and inserts on the plantar and medial aspects of the medial cuneiform and the base of the first metatarsal. As it changes course at the ankle, it is held in place by the superior and inferior extensor retinacula. The tibialis anterior acts to dorsiflex and invert the foot.

Etiology of Injury

Tenosynovitis may occur in runners or hikers because of overuse going down hills.[11] Spontaneous rupture, which occurs near the tendon insertion, is rare.[11,89–93]

Clinical Presentation

Patients usually have mild symptoms and present with foot drop late following injury.[91] On physical examination, dorsiflexion of the foot is weak.

Differential Diagnosis

Peroneal nerve injury or L4–L5 disk herniation should also be considered.

Imaging of the Anterior Tibial Tendon

Plain radiographs are generally not contributory, although a case with ossification of the tendon secondary to injury has been reported.[59] CT or MRI may be performed as for posterior tibial tendon (Fig. 7.32).

Treatment

Acute injuries are treated surgically. Repair is generally not performed if diagnosis is delayed, especially in older patients.[11]

REFERENCES

1. Williams JGP. Achilles tendon lesions in sport. *Sports Med* 1986; **3**:114–35.

2. Puddu G, Ippolito E, Postacchini F. A classification of Achilles tendon disease. *Am J Sports Med* 1976; **4**:145–50.

3. Nidecker A, von Hochstetter A, Fredenhagen H. Accessory muscles of the lower calf. *Radiology* 1984; **151**:47–8.

4. Dunn A. Anomalous muscles simulating soft-tissue tumors in the lower extremities. Report of three cases. *J Bone Joint Surg [Am]* 1965; **47A**:1397–400.

5. Nichols GW, Kalenak A. The accessory soleus muscle. *Clin Orthop* 1984; **190**:279–80.

6. Reinherz RP, Granoff SR, Westerfield M, Pathologic afflictions of the Achilles tendon. *J Foot Surg* 1991; **30**:117–21.

7. Fox JM, Blazina ME, Jobe EW, et al. Degeneration and rupture of the Achilles tendon. *Clin Orthop* 1975; **107**:221–4.

8. Hattrup SJ, Johnson KA. A review of ruptures of the Achilles tendon. *Foot Ankle* 1985; **6**:34–8.

9. Clement P, Taunton J, Smart G. Achilles tendinitis and peritendinitis: etiology and treatment. *Am J Sports Med* 1984; **12**:179–84.

10. Galloway, MT, Jokl P, Dayton OW. Achilles tendon overuse injuries. *Clin Sports Med* 1992; **11**:771–82.

11. Frey CC, Shereff MJ. Tendon injuries about the ankle in athletes. *Clin Sports Med* 1988; **7**:103–18.

12. Jozsa L, Kvist M, Balint BJ et al. The role of recreational sport activity in Achilles tendon rupture. *Am J Sports Med* 1989; **17**:338–43.

13. Lagergren C, Lindholm A. Vascular distribution in the Achilles tendon: an angiographic and microangiographic study. *Acta Chir Scand* 1958; **116**:491–5.

14. Allenmark C. Partial Achilles tendon tears. *Clin Sports Med* 1992; **11**:759–69.

15. Thompson, TC, Doherty JH. Spontaneous rupture of tendon of Achilles: a new diagnostic clinical test. *J Trauma* 1962; **2**:126–9.

16. Inglis AE, Scott WN, Sculco TP, Patterson AH. Ruptures of the tendo achillis. An objective assessment of surgical and non-surgical treatment. *J Bone Joint Surg [Am]* 1976; **58A**:990–3.

17. Kuwada GT. Classification of tendon Achillis rupture with consideration of surgical repair techniques. *J Foot Surg* 1990; **29**:212–7.

18. Fornago BD. Achilles tendon: US examination. *Radiology* 1986; **159**:759–64.

19. Kainberger FM, Engel A, Barton P, et al. Injury of the Achilles tendon: Diagnosis with sonography. *Am J Roentgenol* 1990; **155**:1031–6.

20. Blei CL, Nirschl RP, Grant EG. Achilles tendon: US diagnosis of pathologic conditions. *Radiology* 1986; **159**:765–7.

21. Mathieson JR, Connell DG, Cooperber PL, Lloyd-Smith DR. Sonography of the Achilles tendon and adjacent bursae. *Am J Roentgenol* 1988; **151**:127–31.

22. Maffulli N, Regine R, Angelillo M, Capasso G, Filice S. Ultrasound diagnosis of achilles tendon pathology in runners. *Br J Sports Med* 1987; **21**:158–62.

23. Kalebo P, Allenmark C, Peterson L, Sward L. Diagnostic value of ultrasonography in partial ruptures of the Achilles tendon. *Am J Sports Med* 1992; **20**:378–81.

24. Kalebo P, Goksor LA, Sward L, Peterson L. Soft-tissue radiography, computed tomography, and ultrasonography of partial Achilles tendon ruptures. *Acta Radiol* 1990; **31**:565–70.

25. Weinstabl R, Stiskal M, Neuhold A, Aamlid B, Hertz H. Classifying calcaneal tendon injury according to MRI findings. *J Bone Joint Surg [Br]* 1991; **73B**:683–4.

26. Neuhold A, Stiskal M, Kainberger F, Schwaighofer B. Degenerative Achilles tendon disease: assessment by magnetic resonance and ultrasonography. *Eur J Radiol* 1992; **14**:213–20.

27. Fornage BD, Rifkin MD. Ultrasound examination of tendons. *Radiol Clin North Am* 1988; **26**:87–107.

28. Keene JS, Lash EG, Fisher DR, et al. Magnetic resonance imaging of achilles tendon ruptures. *Am J Sports Med* 1989; **17**:333–7.

29. Quinn SF, Murray WT, Clark RA, Cochran CF. Achilles tendon: MR imaging at 1.5 T. *Radiology* 1987; **164**:767–70.

30. Liem MD, Zegel HG, Balduini FC, et al. Repair of Achilles tendon ruptures with a polylactic acid implant: Assessment with MR imaging. *Am J Radiol* 1991; **156**:769–73.

31. Marcus DS, Reicher MA, Kellerhouse LE. Achilles tendon injuries: the role of MR imaging. *J Comput Assist Tomogr* 1989; **13**:480–6.

32. Inglis AE, Sculco TP. Surgical repair of ruptures of the tendon Achilles. *Clin Orthop* 1981; **156**:160–9.

33. Oden, R. Tendon injuries about the ankle resulting from skiing. *Clin Orthop* 1987; **216**:63–9.

34. Nistor L. Nonsurgical treatment of Achilles tendon ruptures. *J Bone Joint Surg [Am]* 1981; **63A**;394–9.

35. Wills CA, Washburn S, Caiozzo V, Prietto CA. Achilles tendon rupture: a review of the literature comparing surgical versus nonsurgical treatment. *Clin Orthop* 1986; **207**:156–63.

36. Landvater SJ, Renstrom PA. Complete Achilles tendon ruptures. *Clin Sports Med* 1992; **11**:741–58.

37. Holmes GB Jr., Mann RA. Possible epidemiological factors associated with rupture of the posterior tibial tendon. *Foot Ankle* 1992; **13**:70–9.

38. Frey C, Shereff M, Greenidge N. Vascularity of the posterior tibial tendon. *J Bone Joint Surg [Am]* 1992; **72A**:884–8.

39. Myerson M, Solomon G, Shereff M. Posterior tibial tendon dysfunction: its association with seronegative inflammatory disease. *Foot Ankle* 1989; **9**:219–25.

40. Downey DJ, Simkin PA, Mack LA, Richardson ML, Kilcoyne RF, Hansen ST. Tibialis posterior tendon rupture: a cause of rheumatoid flat foot. *Arthritis Rheum* 1988; **31**:441–6.

41. Woods L, Leach RE. Posterior tibial tendon rupture in athletic people. *Am J Sports Med* 1991; **19**:495–8.

42. Dezwart DF, Davidson JSA. Rupture of the posterior tibial tendon associated with ankle fractures. *J Bone Joint Surg [Am]* 1983; **65A**:260–1.

43. Monto RR, Moorman CT, Mallon WJ, Nunley JA. Rupture of the posterior tibial tendon associated with closed ankle fracture. *Foot Ankle* 1991; **11**:400–3.

44. Alexander IJ, Johnson KA, Berquist TH. Magnetic resonance imaging in the diagnosis of disruption of the posterior tibial tendon. *Foot Ankle* 1987; **8**:144–7.

45. Jahss MH. Spontaneous rupture of the tibialis posterior tendon: Clinical findings, tenographic studies, and a new technique of repair. *Foot Ankle* 1982; **3**:158–66.

46. Johnson KA. Tibialis posterior tendon rupture. *Clin Orthop* 1983; **177**:140–7.

47. Mann RA, Thompson FM. Rupture of the posterior tibial tendon causing flat foot. *J Bone Joint Surg [Am]* 1985; **67A**:556–61.

48. Funk DA, Cass JR, Johnson KA. Acquired adult flat foot secondary to posterior tibial tendon pathology. *J Bone Joint Surg [Am]* 1986; **68A:**95–102.

49. Jahss MH. *Disorders of the Foot and Ankle*, 2nd edn. (WB Saunders: Philadelphia, 1991), Chapter 50.

50. Leach RE, Dilorio E, Harney RA. Pathologic hindfoot conditions in the athlete. *Clin Orthop* 1983; **177:**116–21.

51. Henceroth WD II, Deyerle WM. The acquired unilateral flatfoot in the adult: some causative factors. *Foot Ankle* 1982; **2:**304–8.

52. van Holsbeeck M, Introcaso JH. Musculoskeletal ultrasonography. *Radiol Clin North Am* 1992; **30:**907–25.

53. Stephenson CA, Seibert JJ, McAndrew MP, et al. Sonographic diagnosis of tenosynovitis of the posterior tibial tendon. *J Clin Ultrasound* 1990; **18:**114–6.

54. Rosenberg ZS, Jahss MH, Noto AM, Shereff MJ, Cheung Y, Frey CC, Norman A. Rupture of the posterior tibial tendon: CT and surgical findings. *Radiology* 1988; **176:**489–93.

55. Rosenberg ZS, Cheung Y, Jahss MH, Noto AM, Norman A, Leeds NE. Rupture of the posterior tibial tendon: CT and MR imaging with surgical correlation. *Radiology* 1988; **169:**229–35.

56. Erickson SJ, Cox IH, Hyde JS, et al. Effect of tendon orientation on MR imaging signal intensity: a manifestation of the 'magic angle' phenomenon. *Radiology* 1990; **181:**389–92.

57. Conti S, Michelson J, Jahss M. Clinical significance of magnetic resonance imaging in preoperative planning for reconstruction of posterior tibial tendon ruptures. *Foot Ankle* 1990; **13:**208–14.

58. Ouzonian TY, Myerson MS. Dislocation of the posterior tibial tendon. *Foot Ankle* 1992; **13:**215–9.

59. Cheung Y, Rosenberg ZS, Magee T, Chinitz L. Normal anatomy and pathologic conditions of ankle tendons: current imaging techniques. *Radiographics* 1992; **12:**429–44.

60. Hamilton, WG. Tendonitis about the ankle joint in classical ballet dancers. *Am J Sports Med* 1977; **5:**84–7.

61. Hamilton WG. Foot and ankle injuries in dancers. *Clin Sports Med* 1988; **7:**143–7.

62. Sammarco GJ, Miller EH. Partial rupture of the flexor hallucis longus tendon in classical ballet dancers. *J Bone Joint Surg [Am]* 1979; **61A:**149–50.

63. Hamilton W. Stenosing tenosynovitis of the flexor hallucis longus tendon and posterior impingement upon the os trigonum in ballet dancers. *Foot Ankle* 1982; **3:**74–80.

64. Wredmark T, Carlstedt CA, Bauer H, Saartok T. Os trigonum syndrome: a clinical entity in ballet dancers. *Foot Ankle* 1991; **11:**404–6.

65. Holt KW, Cross MJ. Isolated rupture of the flexor hallucis longus tendon: a case report. *Am J Sports Med* 1990; **18:**645–6.

66. Gould N. Stenosing tenosynovitis of the flexor hallucis longus tendon at the great toe. *Foot Ankle* 1981; **2:**46–8.

67. Krackow, KA. Acute traumatic rupture of the flexor hallucis longus tendon. *Clin Orthop* 1980; **150:**261-2.

68. Rasmussen RB, Thyssen EP. Rupture of the flexor hallucis longus tendon: case report. *Foot Ankle* 1990; **10:**288–9.

69. Ferkel RD, Flannigan BD, Elkins BS. Magnetic resonance imaging of the foot and ankle: correlation of normal anatomy with pathologic conditions. *Foot Ankle* 1991; **11:**289-305.

70. Regan TP, Hughston JL. Chronic ankle 'sprain' secondary to anomalous peroneal tendon: a case report. *Clin Orthop* 1977; **123:**52–4.

71. White AA, Johnson D, Griswald DM. Chronic ankle pain associated with peroneus accessorium. *Clin Orthop* 1974; **103:**53–5.

72. Sobel M, Bohne WHO, Markisz JA. Cadaver correlation of peroneal tendon changes with magnetic resonance imaging. *Foot Ankle* 1990; **11:**384–8.

73. Cross MJ, Crichton KJ, Gordon H, Mackie IG. Peroneus brevis rupture in the absence of the peroneus longus muscle and tendon in a classical ballet dancer: A case report. *Am J Sports Med* 1988; **16:**677–8.

74. Murr S. Dislocation of the peroneal tendons with marginal fracture of the lateral malleolus. *J Bone Joint Surg [Br]* 1961; **43B:**563–5.

75. Church CC. Radiographic diagnosis of acute peroneal tendon dislocation. *Am J Roentgenol* 1977; **129:**1065–8.

76. Szczukowski M, Pierre RK, Fleming LL, Somogyi J. Computerized tomography in the evaluation of peroneal tendon dislocation: a report of two cases. *Am J Sports Med* 1983; **11:**444–7.

77. Rosenberg ZS, Feldman F, Singson RD. Peroneal tendon injuries: CT analysis. *Radiology* 1986; **161:**743–8.

78. Rosenberg ZS, Feldman F, Singson RD. Peroneal tendon injury associated with calcaneal fractures: CT findings. *Am J Roentgen* 1987; **149:**125–9.

79. Palmer DG. Tendon sheaths and bursae involved by rheumatoid disease at the foot and ankle. *Australas Radiol* 1970; **14:**419–28.

80. Schweitzer GJ. Stenosing peroneal tenovaginitis. *S Afr Med J* 1982; **61:**521–3.

81. Gilula LA, Oloff L, Caputi R, Destouet JM, Jacobs A, Solomon MA. Ankle tenography: a key to unexplained symptomatology. II. Diagnosis of chronic tendon disabilities. *Radiology* 1984; **151:**581–7.

82. Munk RL, Davis PH. Longitudinal ruptures of the peroneus brevis tendon. *J Trauma* 1976; **16:**803–6.

83. Larsen, E. Longitudinal rupture of the peroneus brevis tendon. *J Bone Joint Surg [Br]* 1987; **69B:**340–1.

84. Sammarco GJ, DiRaimondo CV. Chronic peroneus brevis tendon lesions. *Foot Ankle* 1989; **9:**163–70.

85. Sobel M, Bohne WHO, Levy ME. Longitudinal attrition of the peroneus brevis tendon in the fibular groove: an anatomic study. *Foot Ankle* 1990; **11:**124–8.

86. Thompson F, Patterson A. Rupture of the peroneus longus tendon. Report of three cases. *J Bone Joint Surg [Am]* 1989; **71A:**293–5.

87. Tehranzadeh J, Stoll DA, Gabriele OM. Case report 271: Posterior migration of the os peroneum of the left foot, indicating a tear of the peroneal tendon. *Skeletal Radiol* 1984; **12:**44–7.

88. Davies JA. Peroneal compartment syndrome secondary to rupture of the peroneus longus tendon. *J Bone Joint Surg [Am]* 1979; **61A:**783–4.

89. Burman MS. Subcutaneous rupture of the tendon of the tibialis anticus. *Ann Surg* 1934; **100:**368–72.

90. Dooley BJ, Kudelka P, Menelaus MB. Subcutaneous rupture of the tendon of tibialis anterior. *J Bone Joint Surg [Br]* 1965; **62B:**686–9.

91. Mensor MC, Ordway GL. Traumatic subcutaneous rupture of the tibialis anterior tendon. *J Bone Joint Surg [Am]* 1953; **35A:**675–80.

92. Moskowitz E. Rupture of the tibialis anterior tendon simulating peroneal nerve palsy. *Arch Phys Med Rehabil* 1971; **52:**431–3.

93. Rimoldi RL, Oberlander MA, Waldrop JI, Hunter SC. Acute rupture of the tibialis anterior tendon: a case report. *Foot Ankle* 1991; **12:**176–7.

8. MISCELLANEOUS DISORDERS

REFLEX SYMPATHETIC DYSTROPHY, TRANSIENT OSTEOPOROSIS, AND TRANSIENT MARROW EDEMA

Reflex sympathetic dystrophy syndrome (RSD or RSDS), which is also known by many terms including Sudeck's atrophy and causalgia, is a painful condition of unknown etiology that affects the extremities and commonly involves the foot. It usually follows an injury, which may be minor, to the affected extremity. It may also occur following one or more surgical procedures to the foot. RSD is probably due to local overactivity of sympathetic nerves, a theory supported by the fact that it often improves after sympathetic nerve block.[1] It usually occurs in adults, but it has been reported in children and adolescents.[2-3]

RSD is divided into three phases. In the first phase, patients develop soft-tissue swelling, and local hypothermia or hyperthermia. Pain can be severe, often disproportionate to the initial injury, and usually involves most if not all of the foot. There is hyperemia of the affected extremity, which leads to osteoporosis. The first phase lasts from 1–7 weeks.

In the second phase, patients complain of hypersensitivity of the skin to touch and changes in temperature. Atrophy of the skin and muscles begins to develop. The second phase lasts from 3–24 months.

In the final, irreversible stage, pain persists and skin and muscle atrophy is prominent.[1,4-6] RSD may spontaneously regress rather than continuing to the third and final stage.

Transient Osteoporosis

Transient osteoporosis is often considered to be a separate syndrome, but it is probably a variant of RSD. Patients present with pain and swelling, and osteoporosis is present radiographically or by bone densitometry. Transient osteoporosis may affect several joints in succession, and it is then called transient migratory osteoporosis. The syndrome is more common in men than in women. In women it is often associated with pregnancy and usually involves the hip. MRI shows bone marrow edema, and the designation transient bone marrow edema has been suggested to include cases where osteoporosis is not radiographically detectable.[7-9]

Distribution of RSD

Although the pain in RSD may be limited to one extremity, the contralateral extremity may show abnormal blood flow and soft tissue and bone changes as well, although often to a much lesser extent. RSD may involve an entire extremity, or it may be limited to the foot or hand. Occasionally, RSD may involve only a portion of the hand or foot,[10] either extending along one ray (radial type), or involving a limited zone (zonal type) with normal bone beyond. Radiographically, RSD is most severe in the periarticular bone, but transient bone marrow edema has been reported to involve the tibial diaphysis exclusively.[9]

Radiographic findings

Plain radiographs are normal early in the course of the syndrome. Later, patchy osteoporosis, which is greatest in the para-articular regions, develops (Fig. 8.1). Intracortical tunneling is seen, and there is endosteal and subperiosteal bone resorption. The bone has a 'moth-eaten' appearance. Small subchondral erosions may be seen.[4] However, Johnson[11] reports that radiographic findings may be absent in up to one third of patients. He also found that the osteoporosis seen in RSD, in contrast to that seen in disuse osteoporosis, may not completely resolve radiographically, even though the signs and symptoms of RSD disappear.

Three-phase ^{99m}technetium-MDP bone scans demonstrate increased activity in the radionuclide angiogram, owing to hyperemia, increased activity on the blood pool image, and increased activity (centered on the joints) on the delayed images[12] (see Fig. 8.1). This pattern is also seen in inflammatory arthritis. Decreased activity in the affected limb has also been reported.[13]

The MRI findings in RSD are variable. One study found that only one of 17 patients with RSD showed bone marrow abnormalities on MRI, and six showed soft-tissue edema or bone marrow sclerosis.[6] Transient bone marrow edema is evident on MRI as diffuse decreased signal on T1-weighted images, and increased signal on T2-weighted images (Fig. 8.2).

Differential diagnosis

Although RSD is associated with trauma or surgery, if the injury is slight no history of trauma may be elicited; this should not prevent making the diagnosis. Extremity pain and local osteoporosis could be due to an inflammatory arthritis as well as to RSD. However, in RSD the joint spaces are preserved, and erosions are usually minimal compared to the degree of pain present. Radiographically, RSD is indistinguishable from disuse osteoporosis. Hyperparathyroidism has a similar appearance, but involves the entire skeleton whereas RSD is limited to one or two extremities. The osteoporosis seen in osteomyelitis has a more limited distribution than that seen in RSD, involving one bone or two adjacent bones. Lytic bone tumors also have a more

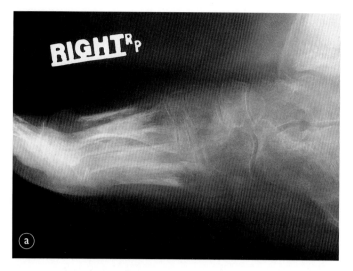

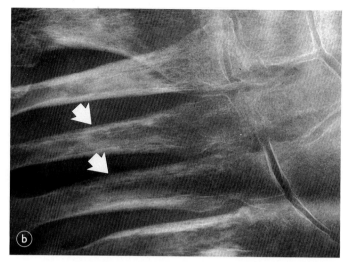

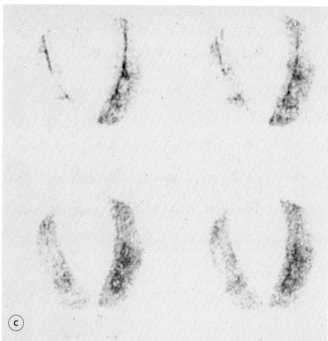

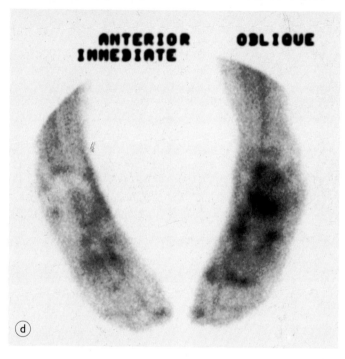

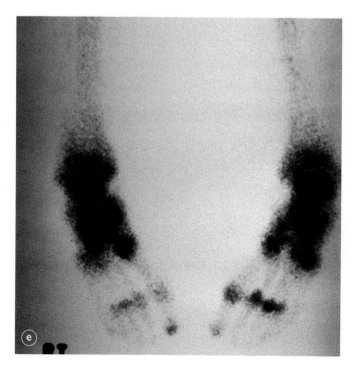

Fig. 8.1. Reflex sympathetic dystrophy of the foot. **a.** Lateral radiograph of the foot. Patchy osteoporosis is greatest in the periarticualar regions, with less severe osteoporosis evident in the metatarsal shafts. **b.** Coned oblique radiograph of the metatarsals (same patient). There are extensive, linear intracortical lucencies (arrows), which mimic a periosteal reaction. The medullary bone has a moth-eaten appearance. **c.** ^{99m}Technetium bone scan, radionuclide angiogram. Select images from angiogram show increased arterial and venous flow to the entire left foot. **d.** ^{99m}Technetium bone scan, blood pool image. Patchy areas of increased activity are seen bilaterally, more prominent on the left. RSD is often bilateral, but one side is usually more severely affected than the other. Interpretation of bone scans depends on comparing one side of the patient with the other; abnormalities on the less affected side should not be overlooked. **e.** ^{99m}Technetium bone scan, 3 hour AP view. Markedly intense radionuclide uptake is present in both feet, greatest in the periarticular regions.

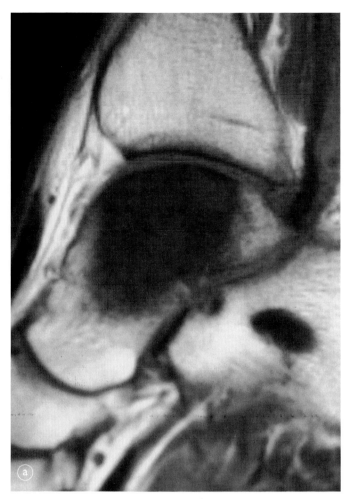 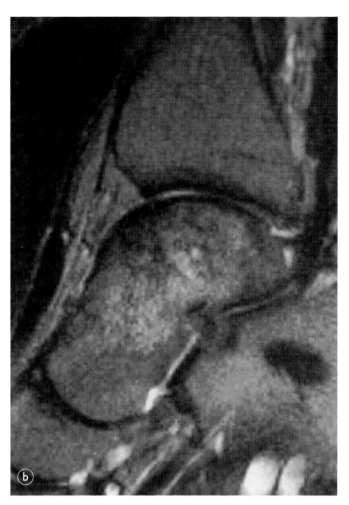

Fig. 8.2. Transient bone marrow edema. Plain radiographs were normal. **a.** Sagittal T1-weighted MRI, SE 500/15. Diffuse low signal intensity is seen throughout much of the talar head and neck. **b.** Sagittal T2-weighted MRI, SE 2000/80. A mottled increase in signal intensity is seen. Avascular necrosis was suspected, and biopsy was performed, which showed no evidence of necrosis. Patient's symptoms resolved without sequelae. (The oval lesion which is low signal intensity on both T1 and T2-weighted images is a bone island in the calcaneus.)

limited distribution, and involvement of the entire foot would be extremely unlikely.

The MRI findings of RSD or transient bone marrow edema are nonspecific. Early avascular necrosis, bone bruise and fracture, and marrow infiltration with tumor should also be considered in the differential diagnosis.

Treatment of RSD

Effective treatment of RSD is aimed at blocking the effects of sympathetic hyperactivity. Physical therapy, steroids and other medications, and sympathetic blocks are used.[1,13] Results are best with early initiation of treatment, while late stages tend to be refractory.

PERIOSTEAL NEW BONE FORMATION

The periosteum forms new bone in response to a wide variety of insults. When a periosteal reaction is seen in the foot or ankle, infection or stress fracture should be considered as the most likely causes. However, there are many other possible etiologies

(Table 8.1, Fig. 8.3). Pseudoperiosteal reaction is a mimic of periosteal reaction and is caused by severe intracortical tunneling in osteoporosis (see Fig. 8.1b).

ACRO-OSTEOLYSIS

Acro-osteolysis refers to resorption of the terminal tufts of the phalanges (Fig. 8.4). Acro-osteolysis is caused by a wide variety of conditions, of which the less uncommon[14] are summarized in Table 8.2

HEEL PAIN SYNDROME (SUBCALCANEAL PAIN)

Heel pain syndrome is a common entity that appears to have several different causes. Table 8.3 lists causes of subcalcaneal heel pain.[15–17]

Heel pain is commonly considered to be due to a nonspecific condition known as plantar fasciitis. Physical examination

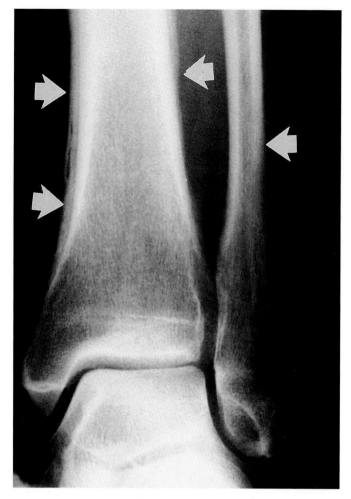

Fig. 8.3. Periosteal reaction due to hypertrophic pulmonary osteoarthropathy in a patient with lung carcinoma. The findings were bilaterally symmetric. A thick periosteal reaction (arrows) is seen along the shafts of the tibia and fibula.

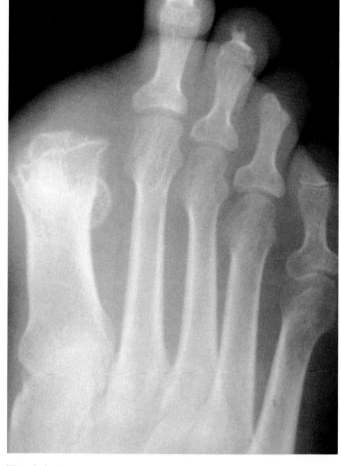

Fig. 8.4. Acro-osteolysis caused by frostbite. AP radiograph. Patient has undergone amputation of the first toe. Severe resorption of the terminal phalanges is seen in the lesser toes.

shows point tenderness over the medial tuberosity of the calcaneus, where the plantar fascia originates. Rupture of the plantar fascia can occur in athletes[18] or following steroid injections for plantar fasciitis.[19]

Nerve entrapment is increasingly recognized as a cause of heel pain. It can occur at the level of the tarsal tunnel (see the discussion on tarsal tunnel syndrome below), along the course of the calcaneal nerve, beneath a heel spur, where the nerve to the abductor digit quinti may become entrapped,[15] or between the abductor hallucis fascia and the fascia of the quadratus plantae muscle. A bursa exists between the origin of the plantar fascia and the heel pad,[16] and subcalcaneal bursitis can develop because of either mechanical factors or inflammatory arthritis.

Imaging of Heel Pain Syndrome

Plain radiographs are usually the only study ordered to evaluate heel pain syndrome (Fig. 8.5). A bony spur at the plantar aspect of the calcaneus may be a sign of plantar fasciitis. However, Tanz[17] found that heel spurs originate at the origin of the flexor digitorum brevis, not the plantar fascia. Graham[16] considers that the spur is a stress reaction at the origin of the

Table 8.1. Causes of periosteal new bone.

Osteomyelitis

Cellulitis or soft-tissue ulcer

Neuropathic joint

Stress or other fracture

Battered child syndrome

Normal tendon insertion

Inflammatory arthritis (especially psoriatic, juvenile rheumatoid arthritis, or Reiter's)

Hypertrophic pulmonary osteoarthropathy (bilaterally symmetric)

Bone tumor

Venous stasis

Familial pachydermoperiostosis (bilaterally symmetric)

Sickle cell dactylitis

Pseudoperiosteal reaction due to osteoporosis

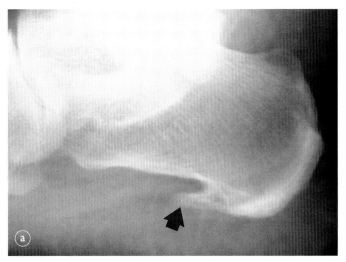
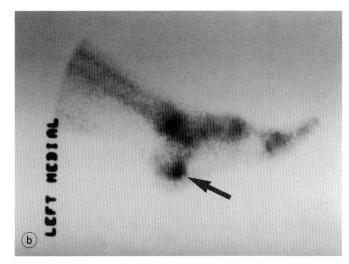

Fig. 8.5. Calcaneal spur. **a.** Lateral radiograph. A well-marginated spur is seen (arrow). **b.** [99m]Technetium bone scan, 3 hour mediolateral view. Uptake is seen at the calcaneal spur, as well as at other sites in the foot (caused by degenerative changes). Flow and blood pool images were normal.

Table 8.2. Causes of acro-osteolysis. (From Resnick and Niwayama.[14])

Vasculitis
Progressive systemic sclerosis (scleroderma)
Thermal (frostbite, burns)
Neuropathic
Hyperparathyroidism
Psoriatic arthritis
Polyvinyl chloride exposure
Congenital (pyknodysostosis, Hajdu–Cheney)

Table 8.3. Causes of heel pain syndrome. (Modified from Bordelon[15] and Graham.[16])

Heel spur formation
Inflammatory arthropathy (erosions, periostitis, rheumatoid nodules)
Plantar fasciitis, plantar fascia rupture
Bursitis and tendinitis
Nerve entrapment (including tarsal tunnel syndrome)
Pronated foot
Painful fat pad
Calcaneal stress fracture
Combinations of these conditions

flexor digitorum brevis; he found that in severe cases, small compression fractures develop at the site of the spur. There is certainly a correlation between heel pain and the presence of a bone spur: only 15% of asymptomatic adults have plantar calcaneal spurs, while 50% of patients with heel pain have spurs.[17] In patients with heel spurs, the spurs are usually bilateral, while only one heel is painful. Heel spurs that project directly inferiorly, as opposed to following the more common horizontal course, have a very high association with heel pain.

Patients with heel pain may have inflammatory arthritis. It is not uncommon to detect radiographic evidence of clinically unsuspected inflammatory arthritis, and all radiographs of the heel should be carefully scrutinized for erosions and periostitis (see Chapter 5, Figs 5.28, 5.29).

[99m]Technetium-MDP bone scans can be used to determine if there is inflammation or perhaps a fracture at a spur[16] (Fig. 8.5). Most asymptomatic spurs will not show increased radionuclide uptake. Patients with a stress fracture of the calcaneus, which may not be evident on plain radiographs, will also have positive bone scans, but in stress fractures the abnormal activity in the posterior portion of the calcaneus is usually more extensive, and is centered within the bone rather than at the site of a spur.

MRI and CT are increasingly used in cases of refractory heel pain. They can identify plantar fasciitis[20] (Fig. 8.6) or inflammatory arthritis (see Chapter 5, Fig. 5.28). More importantly, MRI and CT can identify lesions that are causing tarsal tunnel syndrome, mimicking plantar fasciitis (Fig. 8.7).

Treatment of Heel Pain Syndrome

Most cases of heel pain syndrome due to plantar fasciitis respond to treatment with a soft heel insert and arch support in the patient's shoe, although the pain may take months to resolve. A variety of nonoperative treatments are used to treat this condition, including steroid injections, night splints, and even the use of a short leg cast for about three weeks. Patients with continued pain refractory to nonoperative treatment are considered for surgical decompression of the heel and excision of the spur[21] if present.

TARSAL TUNNEL SYNDROME

The tarsal tunnel is the space between the flexor retinaculum and the underlying bones – the tibia anterosuperiorly, and the

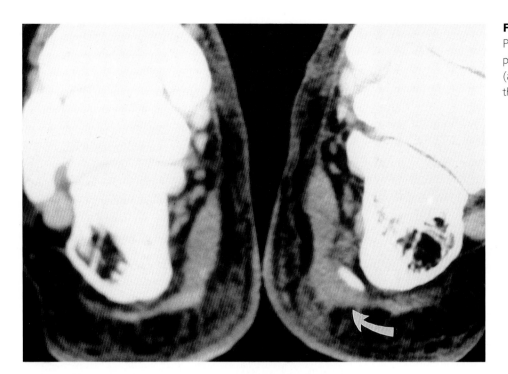

Fig. 8.6. Plantar fasciitis. Coronal CT. Patient has bilateral calcaneal spurs. The plantar fascia on the left is thickened (arrow). Bone scan showed focal uptake at the left calcaneal spur, but not the right.

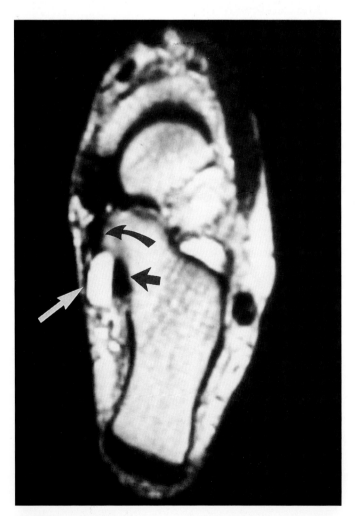

Fig. 8.7. Ganglion cyst causing tarsal tunnel syndrome. T2-weighted MRI. A high signal intensity cyst (white arrow) is located between the flexor digitorum longus (curved black arrow) and flexor hallucis longus (straight black arrow) tendons. MRI was performed to evaluated suspected plantar fasciitis. Plantar fascia were normal.

Table 8.4. Causes of tarsal tunnel syndrome[23,24] (listed from most to least common).

Idiopathic
Traumatic
Bony impingement from talocalcaneal coalition
Ganglion or synovial cyst
Varicosities
Heel varus
Fibrosis
Heel valgus
Diabetes
Obesity
Tight tarsal canal
Hypertrophic or accessory abductor hallucis
Rheumatoid arthritis
Lipoma and other soft tissue tumors
Anomalous artery
Acromegaly
Ankylosing spondylitis
Regional migratory osteoporosis
Flexor digitorum accessorious longus

calcaneus and posterior process of the talus laterally. The posterior tibial tendon, tibial neurovascular bundle, flexor hallucis longus, and flexor digitorum longus are located within the tarsal tunnel, with the posterior tibial artery situated between the flexor digitorum longus and the flexor hallucis longus tendons. Fibrous septae divide the tarsal tunnel into compartments. The flexor retinaculum may begin as far as 10 cm proximal to the medial malleolus, and distally it fans out 10 cm to the anterior portion of the sustentaculum tali. The tunnel is narrowest distally, where the flexor retinaculum blends with the fascia of the abductor hallucis muscle. The posterior tibial nerve divides to form calcaneal branches and the medial and lateral plantar nerves. The point relative to the tarsal tunnel at which branching occurs is variable.[22]

Tarsal tunnel syndrome is caused by compression of the posterior tibial nerve or its branches by the flexor retinaculum.[23–27] Most writers extend the definition to include impingement of the medial and lateral plantar nerves distal to the retinaculum, as they course adjacent to the abductor hallucis muscle. The calcaneal branch of the posterior tibial nerve may arise from the posterior tibial nerve either before or within the tarsal tunnel; isolated impingement of this nerve can occur.

Patients generally present with poorly localized, burning pain and paresthesis on the plantar surface of the foot. Depending on the site of impingement, symptoms may be limited to the heel or to the medial or lateral aspect of the foot. A Tinel's sign, where distal paresthesia is elicited by tapping over the nerve, is often found. The diagnosis is often confirmed with electrodiagnostic studies, but their accuracy has been questioned.[23,26] The most sensitive test, sensory action potentials, have a sensitivity of 90.5%.[28] However, in a retrospective study, Pfeiffer and Cracchiolo[29] could find no correlation between the electrodiagnostic studies in any of their patients, and the results following decompression of the tarsal tunnel.

There are numerous causes of tarsal tunnel syndrome. Cimino[26] tabulated the reported causes of 122 cases from 24 reports in the literature, and I have added to his data 50 cases reported by Takakura.[25] These causes are listed in Table 8.4.

Imaging

MRI is the imaging method of choice to exclude a space-occupying lesion causing tarsal tunnel syndrome[30,31] (Fig. 8.7). The MRI protocol outlined in chapter 7, Table 7.6 for the evaluation of the posterior tibial tendon is recommended. CT can also be used, preferably with both coronal and axial images and intravenous contrast, but it is slightly less sensitive than MRI in the detection of subtle soft tissue masses.

Differential Diagnosis

The symptoms of tarsal tunnel syndrome overlap with those of many other entities, listed in Table 8.5.

Treatment

Patients with biomechanical problems may be treated with orthoses. Nonsteroidal anti-inflammatory drugs are sometimes used. Surgical release of the flexor retinaculum may be needed, with release of the more distal portions of the nerves. Any space-occupying lesion is removed, if present. Pfeiffer and Cracchiolo[29] found that only patients who had a lesion or mass impinging on the nerve seemed to have a uniformly good result from surgical release. Unfortunately, in patients not having such a lesion, there seems to be no foolproof method of establishing the diagnosis and selecting those patients who should definitely benefit from surgical decompression. One of us (AC) now tells

Table 8.5. Differential diagnosis of tarsal tunnel syndrome[24]

lumbosacral radiculopathy
plantar fasciitis
rheumatoid arthritis
peripheral neuritis
diabetic neuropathy
peripheral vascular disease
Morton's neuroma

such patients that the operation is the final test which will determine whether the diagnosis is correct. Therefore, surgical treatment to relieve the pain of tarsal tunnel syndrome should be approached with caution.

ANTERIOR TARSAL TUNNEL SYNDROME

The anterior tarsal tunnel is the space between the inferior extensor retinaculum and the talus and navicular. The deep peroneal nerve and its branches course through the anterior tarsal tunnel deep to the extensor hallucis longus and extensor digitorum longus tendons, and adjacent to the dorsalis pedis artery.

Patients present with paresthesia, aching, and numbness over the dorsum of the foot and the first and second toes. Tinel's sign (distal paresthesia elicited by tapping over the nerve) is positive, and there may be decreased two point discrimination. Causes of anterior tarsal tunnel syndrome include talonavicular osteophytosis, pes cavus, ganglia, fractures, and tightly laced shoes.[32] The condition is rarely seen, even in a large clinical practice.

Imaging

The radiologist should report the presence of plain radiographic findings that can cause tarsal tunnel syndrome (talonavicular osteophytes, fractures, and pes cavus). However, since the anterior tarsal tunnel syndrome is located superficially, and space-occupying lesions should therefore be palpable, advanced imaging is probably not needed.

SINUS TARSI SYNDROME

The sinus tarsi (or tarsal sinus) is the region separating the talus and the calcaneus anterolaterally. It is bordered posteriorly by the posterior facet of the subtalar joint, medially by the middle and anterior subtalar facets, and anteriorly by the talonavicular joint. The posteromedial portion of the sinus, between the posterior and middle subtalar facets, is called the tarsal canal. As detailed in Chapter 1, it contains fat, the artery of the sinus tarsi, the talocalcaneal ligaments (ligament of the tarsal canal and cervical ligament), as well as insertions of the extensor retinaculum.

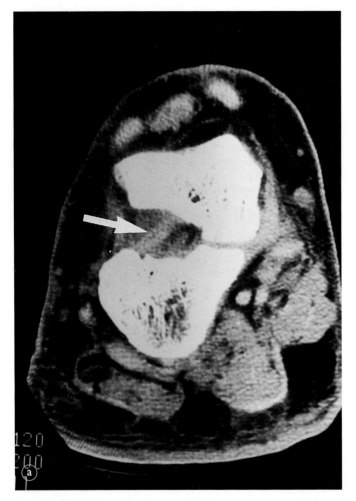
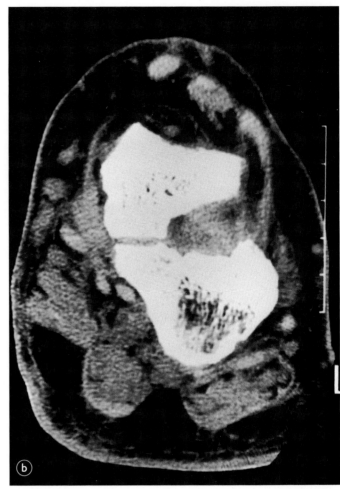

Fig. 8.8. Tarsal sinus syndrome. **a.** Coronal CT through the tarsal sinus on the unaffected side shows a normal cervical ligament (arrow). **b.** Coronal CT of the symptomatic foot shows amorphous soft tissue in the tarsal sinus. Cervical ligament is not visualized. Patient had had chronic lateral hindfoot pain, and 'ankle sprain' in the past.

Sinus tarsi syndrome refers to foot pain localized to the tarsal sinus. The syndrome is most commonly post-traumatic in origin and is caused by inversion injury of the ankle with rupture of the talocalcaneal ligaments.[33–35] It can also occur as a result of a mass in the tarsal sinus.[35,36] It is not an uncommon entity and is increasingly recognized today on advanced imaging techniques.

Patients present with chronic lateral hindfoot pain and localized tenderness. Most patients give a history of ankle sprain, and rupture of the lateral collateral ligaments of the ankle is commonly demonstrated. Rupture of the interosseous talocalcaneal ligaments is difficult to demonstrate on physical examination because it results in minimal detectable instability.[33]

Imaging

In the past, arthrography of the posterior facet of the subtalar joint has been used.[33] The sinus tarsi syndrome was diagnosed arthrographically when there was loss of the usual small joint recesses at the anterior margin of the joint. Studies have not been done to assess the accuracy of this method of diagnosis, but one can infer from MRI findings that its sensitivity is probably low – patients with clinical and MRI evidence of sinus tarsi syndrome do not necessarily show loss of the joint recesses on MRI.

Sinus tarsi syndrome caused by rupture of the interosseous ligaments is evident on CT or MRI[37] when soft tissue or fluid is present within the normally fat-filled tarsal sinus, and the interosseous ligaments are not visible. On CT, 1.5–2 mm thick coronal cuts optimally demonstrate the ligaments, and they should be evident in normal patients (Figs 8.8, 8.9). On MRI imaging, spin echo sequences may not show the ligaments well because of limitation in slice thickness; the accuracy of the study can be improved with 1–2 mm thick three-dimensional full thickness gradient echo images (Fig. 8.10). The MRI protocol outlined in Chapter 7, Table 7.8 for the evaluation of lateral ankle pain can be used. Soft-tissue masses in this area may be more conspicuous on MRI than on CT.

Differential Diagnosis

Other injuries that can cause lateral hindfoot pain should be considered, as outlined in the section on the differential diagnosis

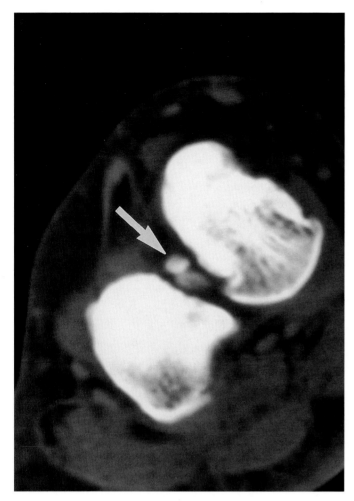

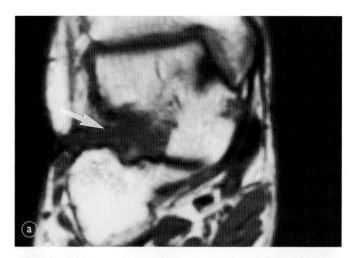

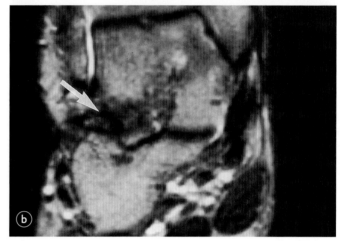

Fig. 8.9. Tarsal sinus syndrome. Coronal CT. Heterotopic ossification (arrow) is seen in the sinus tarsi in this patient with repeated prior traumas and chronic pain. Interosseous ligaments were not visualized.

Fig. 8.10. Tarsal sinus syndrome. Coronal MRI. **a.** T1-weighted sequence, TE 600/18. Amorphous, low-signal material (arrow) is filling the sinus tarsi. **b.** T2-weighted sequence, TE 2200/80. The scar material shows only a mild increase in signal intensity.

of ankle sprain (see Chapter 3, Table 3.4). Arthritis of the ankle or subtalar joint can also mimic sinus tarsi syndrome, as can anterolateral ankle impingement (see Table 7.7).

ANKLE IMPINGEMENT

Ankle impingement can occur because of osteoarthritis (see Chapter 5) or because of impingent by soft tissue structures.

Anterolateral impingement is due to scar tissue formation at the anterolateral aspect of the ankle in patients with chronic ankle sprains. The diagnosis is made arthroscopically.[38] In the several arthroscopically diagnosed cases in which I have performed MRI, MRI was normal.

Posterior impingement of the ankle occurs as the result of a plantar flexion injury, with compression of the flexor hallucis longus (see Chapter 7) or the posterior ankle capsule, or both. This syndrome is associated with the presence of an os trigonum, a fracture of the posterior process of the talus, or a prominent posterior process.[39]

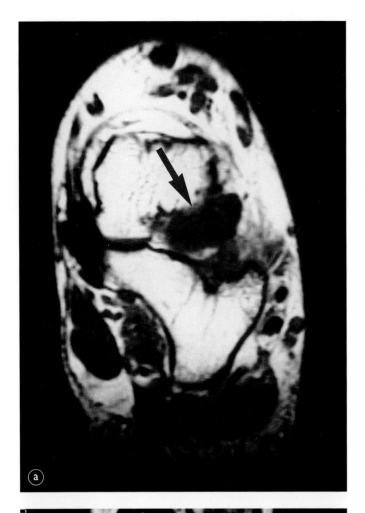

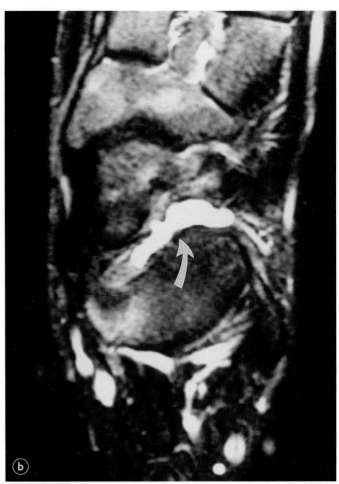

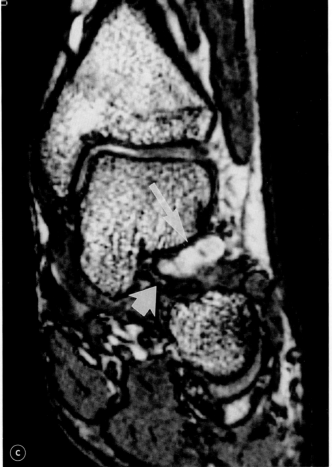

Fig. 8.11. Tarsal sinus syndrome due to a ganglion or synovial cyst extending through the tarsal sinus. Cyst was missed on a prior CT scan, on which only bone windows were photographed. **a.** Coronal T1-weighted MRI, SE 500/16. The cyst (arrow) is low in signal intensity. **b.** Axial T2-weighted MRI, FSE 4000/120. The cyst (arrow), of high signal intensity, extends from the tarsal tunnel anterolaterally. **c.** Coronal, three-dimensional gradient echo image 25/7/60 (1.2 mm slice thickness) shows the cyst (long arrow) adjacent to the cervical ligament of the tarsal sinus (short arrow).

REFERENCES

1. Schwartzman RJ. Reflex sympathetic dystrophy: a review. *Arch Neurol* 1987; **44**: 555–61.

2. Ruggeri SB, Athreya BH, Doughty R, Gregg JR, Das MM. Reflex sympathetic dystrophy in children. *Clin Orthop* 1982; **163**:225–30.

3. Koman LA, Barden A, Smith BP, et al. Reflex sympathetic dystrophy in an adolescent. *Foot Ankle* 1993; **14**:273–7.

4. Genant HK, Kozin F, Bekerman C, McCarty DJ, Sims J. The reflex sympathetic dystrophy syndrome. *Radiology* 1975; **117**:21–32.

5. Kozin F, McCarty CJ , Sims J, Genant HK. Reflex sympathetic dystrophy syndrome: I. Clinical and histological evidence of articular involvement and response to corticosteroid. *Am J Med* 1976; **60**:321–31.

6. Koch E, Hofer HO, Sialer G, Marincek B, von Schulthess GK. Failure of MR imaging to detect reflex sympathetic dystrophy of the extremities. *Am J Roentgenol* 1991; **156**:113–5.

7. Wilson AJ, Murphy WA, Hardy DC, Totty WG. Transient osteoporosis: transient bone marrow edema? *Radiology* 1988; **167**:757–60.

8. Hayes CW, Conway WF, Daniel WW. MR imaging of bone marrow edema pattern: transient osteoporosis, transient bone marrow edema syndrome, or osteonecrosis. *Radiographics* 1993; **13**:1001–11.

9. Reinus WR, Fischer KC, Ritter JH. Painful transient tibial edema. *Radiology* 1994; **192**:195–9.

10. Leguesne M, Kerboull M, Bensasson M, et al. Partial transient osteoporosis. *Skeletal Radiol* 1977; **2**:1–9.

11. Johnson KA. Reflex sympathetic dystrophy syndrome. In: Johnson KA. *Surgery of the Foot and Ankle.* (Raven Press: New York, 1989), 209-19.

12. Genant HK, et al. The reflex sympathetic dystrophy syndrome: A comprehensive analysis using fine-detail radiography, photon absorptiometry and bone and joint scintigraphy. *Radiology* 1975; **117**:21–32.

13. Kozin F, Ryan LM, Carerra GF, Soin JS, Wortmann RL. The Reflex sympathetic dystrophy syndrome (RSDS): III. Scintigraphic studies, further evidence for the therapeutic efficacy of systemic corticosteroids, and proposed diagnostic criteria. *Am J Med* 1981; **70**:23–30.

14. Resnick D, Niwayama G. Osteolysis and chondrolysis. In: Resnick D, Niwayama G. *Diagnosis of Bone and Joint Disorders*, 2nd edn. (WB Saunders: Philadelphia, 1988), 4140–70.

15. Bordelon RL. Subcalcaneal pain: a method of evaluation and plan for treatment. *Clin Orthop* 1983; **177**:49–53.

16. Graham CE. Painful heel syndrome: rationale of diagnosis and treatment. *Foot Ankle* 1983; **3**:261–7.

17. Tanz SS. Heel pain. *Clin Orthop* 1963; **28**:169–75.

18. Leach RE, Jones RP, Silva TF. Rupture of the plantar fascia in athletes. *J Bone Joint Surg [Am]* 1978; **60A**:537–44.

19. Sellman JR. Plantar fascia rupture associated with corticosteroid injection. *Foot Ankle* 1994; **15**:376–81.

20. Berkowitz JF, Kier R, Rudicel S. Plantar fasciitis: MR imaging. *Radiology* 1991; **179**:665–7.

21. Baxter DE, Thigpen CM. Heel pain – operative results. *Foot Ankle* 1984; **5**:16–25.

22. Havel PE, Ebraheim NA, Clark SE, et al. Tibial branching in the tarsal tunnel. *Foot Ankle* 1988; **9**:117–19.

23. Edwards WG, Lincoln CR, Bassett FH III, Goldner JL. The tarsal tunnel syndrome: diagnosis and treatment. *JAMA* 1969; **207**:716–20.

24. Mann RA. Tarsal tunnel syndrome. *Orthop Clin North Am* 1974; **5**:109–15.

25. Takakura Y, Kitada C, Sugimoto K, et al. Tarsal tunnel syndrome: Causes and results of operative treatment. *J Bone Joint Surg [Br]* 1991; **73B**:125–8.

26. Cimino WR. Tarsal tunnel syndrome: review of the literature. *Foot Ankle* 1990; **11**:47–52.

27. Jackson DL, Haglund B. Tarsal tunnel syndrome in athletes: case reports and literature review. *Am J Sports Med* 1991; **19**:61–5.

28. Oh SJ, Savaria PK, Kuba T, Elmore RS. Tarsal tunnel syndrome: electrophysiologic study. *Ann Neurol* 1979; **5**:327–30.

29. Pfeiffer WH, Cracchiolo A. Clinical results after tarsal tunnel decompression. *J Bone Joint Surg [Am]* 1994; **76A**:1222-30.

30. Kerr R, Frey C. MR imaging in tarsal tunnel syndrome. *J Comput Assist Tomogr* 1991; **15**:280–6.

31. Frey C, Kerr R. Magnetic resonance imaging and the evaluation of tarsal tunnel syndrome. *Foot Ankle* 1993; **14**:159–64.

32. Zongzho L, Jiansheng Z, Zhao L. Anterior tarsal tunnel syndrome. *J Bone Joint Surg [Br]* 1991; **73B**:470–3.

33. Meyer JM, Lagier R. Post-traumatic sinus tarsi syndrome: an anatomical and radiological study. *Acta Orthop Scand* 1977; **48**:121–8.

34. Taillar W, Meyer JM, Garcia J, Blanc Y. The sinus tarsi syndrome. *Int Orthop* 1981; **5**:117–30.

35. Kjaersgaard–Anderson P, Anderson K, Soballe K, Pilgaard S. Sinus tarsi syndrome: presentation of seven cases and review of the literature. *J Foot Surg* 1989; **28**:3–6.

36. Light M, Pupp G. Ganglions in the sinus tarsi. *J Foot Surg* 1991; **30**:350–5.

37. Klein MA, Spreitzer AM. MR imaging of the tarsal sinus and canal: Normal anatomy, pathologic findings, and features of the sinus tarsi syndrome. *Radiology* 1993; **186**:233–40.

38. Ferkel RD, Karzel RP, Del Pizzo W, Friedman MJ, Fischer SP. Arthroscopic treatment of anterolateral impingement of the ankle. *Am J Sports Med* 1991; **19**:440–6.

39. Hedrick MR, McBryde AM. Posterior ankle impingement. *Foot Ankle* 1994; **15**:2–8.

9. CONGENITAL FOOT DEFORMITIES

At birth, the feet are usually in a position of equinus, adduction, and inversion, owing to the in utero position of the feet. The infant's foot is highly flexible. As the child begins to walk, the foot becomes pronated, with eversion of the ankle and forefoot abduction (pes planovalgus).[1] The flat appearance of the young child's foot is also partly due to prominent plantar fat. Over the next few years, the normal adult position of the foot tends to become established, owing to decreased joint mobility, greater rigidity caused by increasing ossification of the foot, and greater muscular control.[1]

Evaluation of the axial relationships of the foot in infants and young children is complicated by the incomplete ossification of the foot. Ossification of the talus and calcaneus is usually seen at birth, and the ossification centers of the forefoot are also seen. The cuboid ossification center appears in the first year of life. The navicular and the cuneiforms ossify in early childhood (see Chapter 1, Table 1.1). Prior to its ossification, the position of the navicular must be inferred; it is expected to lie along the same axis as the first metatarsal, but in several congenital deformities it does not have a normal anatomic relationship to the talus.

TERMINOLOGY

By convention, deformities are always described in terms of the malalignment of the distal bone or part of the body relative to the proximal point of reference. Thus, for example, in a varus deformity of the heel, the heel is angled toward the midline, relative to the axis of the tibia (Fig. 9.1).[2]

- abduction – deviation, in the transverse plane, away from the midline of the body;
- adduction – deviation, in the transverse plane, toward the midline of the body;
- calcaneus – increased dorsiflexion of the calcaneus;
- cavus – elevation of the longitudinal arch of the foot;
- equinus – either plantar flexion of the foot (analogous to a horse's hoof), or plantar flexion of the calcaneus;
- planus – flattening of the longitudinal arch of the foot;
- rocker-bottom deformity – reversal of the normal longitudinal arch of the foot;
- valgus – deviation, in the coronal plane, away from the midline of the body;
- varus – deviation, in the coronal plane, towards the midline of the body.

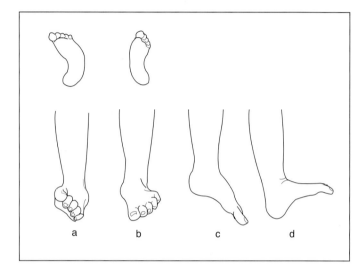

Fig. 9.1. Some congenital deformities of the foot. **a.** Varus deformity. **b.** Valgus deformity. **c.** Equinus deformity. **d.** Calcaneus deformity. (Adapted from Tachdjian.[2])

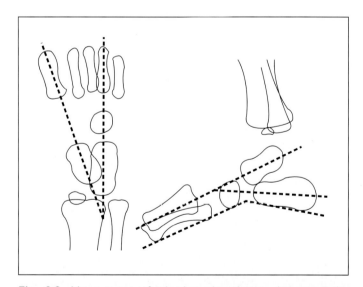

Fig. 9.2. Measurement of talocalcaneal angles. **a.** Anteroposterior diagram. Note the axis of the tibia is in line with the axis of the hindfoot. Lines are drawn along the midline of the talus and calcaneus. **b.** Lateral diagram. The line drawn through the axis of the talus extends through the axis of the first metatarsal if the child is older than five years of age; otherwise, it extends below the axis of the first metatarsal. Note that there is normally slight dorsiflexion of the calcaneus. (Redrawn with permission from Davis and Hatt.[3])

Table 9.1. Normal talocalcaneal angles in childhood. (From Vanderwilde et al.[5])

	mean values in degrees (range)			
	newborn	2 years	4 years	(birth to 9 years)
Anteroposterior	42(27-56)	40(26-50)	34(24-44)	(15-56)
Lateral	39 (23-55)	41 (27-56)	44 (31-57)	(23-56)
Lateral (maximum dorsiflexion)	45 (35-56)	44 (33-54)	33 (32-52)	(25-55)

Table 9.2. Analysis of abnormal angles of the foot.

Radiographic abnormality	local foot deformity	associated with
decreased t-c angle	hindfoot varus	clubfoot neurologic disorders
increased t-c angle	hindfoot valgus	pes planovalgus congenital vertical talus skewfoot calcaneovalgus deformity cerebral palsy other neurologic disorders
plantar flexed calcaneus	equinus	clubfoot congenital vertical talus
dorsiflexed calcaneus	calcaneus	pes calcaneovalgus treated clubfoot pes cavus
plantar flexed foot	equinus of foot	shortened Achilles tendon poliomyelitis other neuromuscular diseases

RADIOGRAPHIC EVALUATION

In children old enough to stand, weight-bearing anteroposterior and lateral radiographs should be obtained. In infants, weight bearing should be simulated by applying pressure uniformly to the plantar surface of the feet. On the anteroposterior radiograph, the tibia should not be oblique relative to the hindfoot. The lateral radiograph should be a true lateral of the ankle.

The axial relationships of the hindfoot are calculated based on the anterior and lateral talocalcaneal angles[3-5] (Fig. 9.2). These

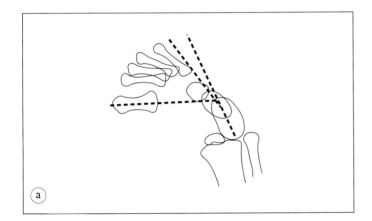

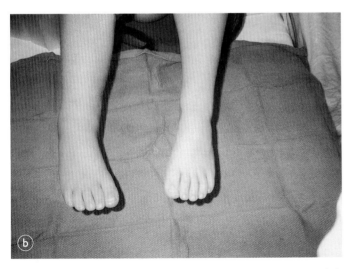

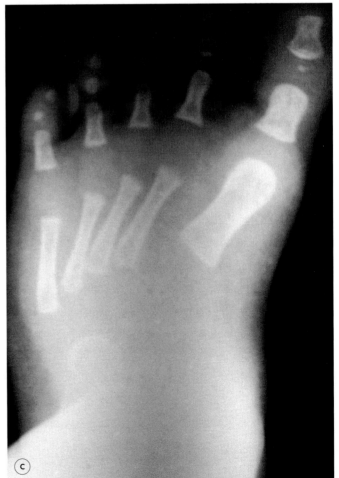

Fig. 9.3. Metatarsus varus. **a.** AP diagram shows that the axes of the metatarsals converge laterally. (Redrawn with permission from Davis and Hatt.[3]) **b.** Photograph of metatarsus varus of the right foot (left side of picture). Compare to the normal left foot. **c.** AP radiograph. Adduction of the forefoot is evident. Talocalcaneal angle is normal.

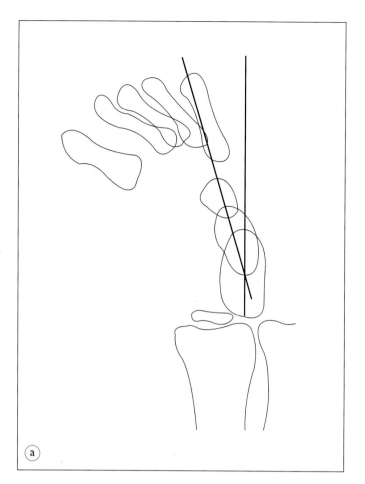

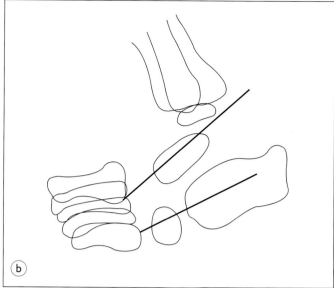

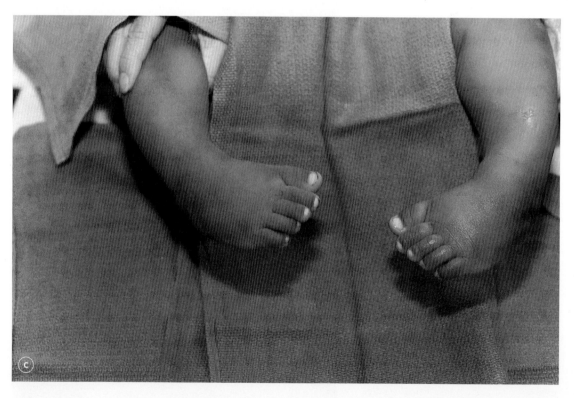

Fig. 9.4. Talipes equinovarus. **a.** AP diagram shows the decreased talocalcaneal angle, and medial deviation of the forefoot. **b.** Lateral diagram shows decreased talocalcaneal angle, and equinus of the calcaneus. (Modified from Davis and Hatt.[3]) **c.** Photograph of bilateral clubfoot deformity. The marked inversion of the foot is evident.

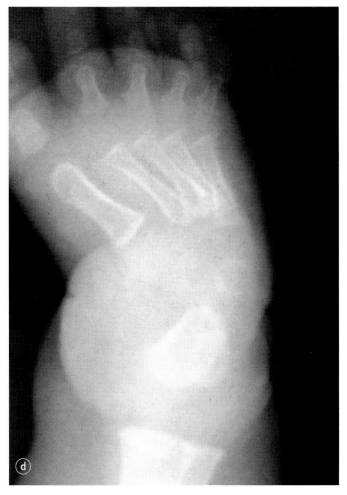

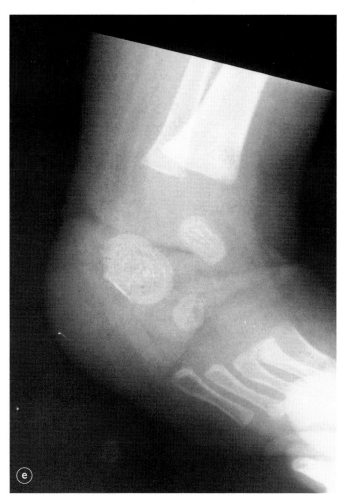

Fig. 9.4 d. AP radiograph. The talus and calcaneus are superimposed. Forefoot inversion is evident both by the medial deviation of the forefoot, and the overlap of the bases of the metatarsals. **e.** Lateral radiograph with forced plantar flexion. There is equinus of the calcaneus, and the talus and calcaneus are approximately parallel. The metatarsals have a ladder-like configuration.

angles vary with a child's age (Table 9.1). Valgus deformity of the hindfoot is present when there is an increase in talocalcaneal angle, and varus deformity is present when there is a decrease in the angle. Stress views may be obtained to determine the extent to which a foot deformity is flexible. Note that the heel is normally in 5–10° of valgus, so valgus alignment of the heel is diagnosed only when the valgus tilt exceeds 10°.[3]

In adults and children older than 5 years of age, a line drawn along the long axis of the talus will normally continue along the axis of the first metatarsal. However, in infants and young children, the talus is more vertically oriented.

Table 9.2 relates radiographic findings to the congenital abnormalities in which they are seen.

TREATMENT OF CONGENITAL DEFORMITIES

When detected early in infancy, many congenital deformities can be treated with progressive casting of the foot. However, if a deformity is not detected early, surgery is often needed.

METATARSUS VARUS (METATARSUS ADDUCTUS)

Isolated metatarsus varus or adductus is a common deformity – it is approximately 10 times as common as clubfoot[6–9] (Fig. 9.3). Metatarsus varus and metatarsus adductus are not interchangeable terms. In metatarsus varus, there is inversion of the foot as well as adduction of the metatarsals. In metatarsus adductus, inversion is absent.

Radiographically, normal bony relationships are seen in the hindfoot, but the metatarsals are adducted, with varying degrees of inversion of the foot. The axes of the metatarsal shafts converge lateral to the calcaneus. Mild deformities may correct on radiographs, owing to the application of plantar pressure.

CLUBFOOT (TALIPES EQUINOVARUS)

Clubfoot occurs in 1–4 per 1000 live births[9] and is slightly more common in males than females. Risk is increased if the child has a first degree relative with clubfoot deformity. Clubfoot is associated with myelomeningocele, arthrogryposis, and tibial

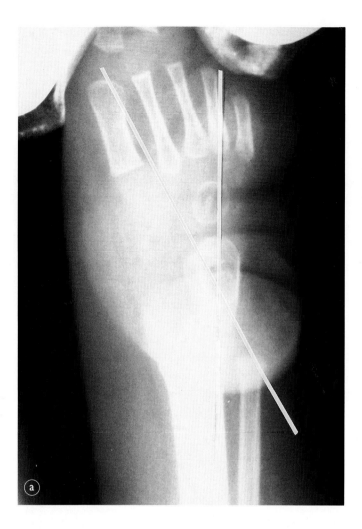

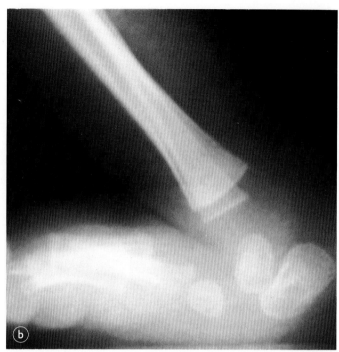

Fig. 9.5. Talipes equinovarus. The forefoot inversion is less severe than in Fig. 9.4. **a.** AP radiograph. **b.** Lateral radiograph.

hemimelia. In clubfoot deformity, the calcaneus is held in an equinus position, the hindfoot is in varus, and there is varus (inversion) of the forefoot (Figs 9.4 and 9.5).

On anteroposterior radiographs, the talus and calcaneus are parallel or superimposed. After the navicular has ossified, it can be seen to be displaced medially. The forefoot is in varus. On the lateral view, the calcaneus is in an equinus position, and the talus and calcaneus are approximately parallel. The metatarsals have a ladder-like configuration, with the weight borne on the fifth metatarsal. Clubfoot deformity can be recognized in utero by ultrasound examination.[10]

CONGENITAL VERTICAL TALUS

Congenital vertical talus is a rare deformity. It is associated with congenital hip dysplasia, congenital scoliosis, spinal dysraphism, trisomies 13–15 and 18, and congenital syndromes. In congenital vertical talus, the talus has a nearly vertical orientation. The talonavicular joint is dislocated dorsally, so that the navicular lies on the neck of the talus. The calcaneus in in equinus and valgus. A rocker-bottom deformity of the foot is seen, with reversal of the normal plantar arch[4,11–13] (Fig. 9.6).

On radiographs, the talocalcaneal angle is increased. There is vertical orientation of the talus, and equinus of the calcaneus. Rocker-bottom deformity is present. There is valgus of both the hindfoot and forefoot.

PES PLANUS

Flat feet can be divided into three categories: static, arthritic, and neuromuscular deformities (Table 9.3). The longitudinal arch of the foot is flattened, and there is a variable degree of hindfoot valgus (Fig. 9.7). Flexible flatfoot is a diagnosis of exclusion. In many children it will resolve spontaneously, although it persists in approximately 10–15% of the population.[1,14]

OTHER CONGENITAL DEFORMITIES

Pes cavus and hallux valgus are discussed in Chapter 10. Skewfoot (Z-foot, serpentine foot, S-shaped foot)[7] is a combination of forefoot adduction and hindfoot valgus. Calcaneovalgus deformity consists of severe dorsiflexion of the foot, with the heel in calcaneus and valgus; abduction and planus of the forefoot are also present.

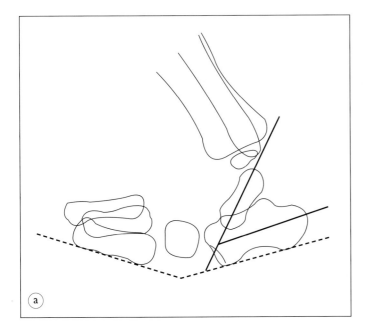

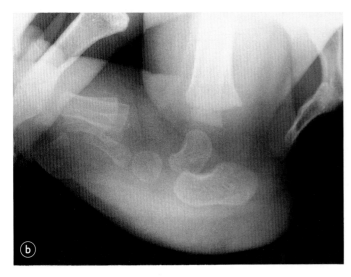

Fig. 9.6. Congenital vertical talus. **a.** Lateral diagram showing increased talocalcaneal angle, and rocker-bottom deformity. (Modified from Davis and Hatt.[3]) **b.** Lateral radiograph. The talus is vertically oriented, and the calcaneus is in equinus. The positions of the first and second metatarsals, and, by inference, the navicular, are dorsal to the head of the talus.

Table 9.3. Causes of flatfoot in children. (From Barry[1] and Eyre-Brook.[13])

Static deformities
  Flexible plantar flexed talus (hypermobile flatfoot)
  Rigid plantar flexed talus (congenital vertical talus)
  Medial deviation of the talonavicular joint
  Z-foot with metatarsus varus
  Calcaneal equinus
  arthritis deformities
  Developmental (tarsal coalition)
  Inflammatory (juvenile rheumatoid arthritis)
  Traumatic ('jumper's foot')
  Degenerative incompetence of the 1st metatarsocuneiform joint
Neuromuscular deformities
  Paralysis
  Posterior tibial tendon rupture, accessory navicular
  Proprioceptive imbalance (mild mental retardation, cerebral palsy, congenital blindness)
  Marfan's, Larsen's syndromes
  Short Achilles tendon

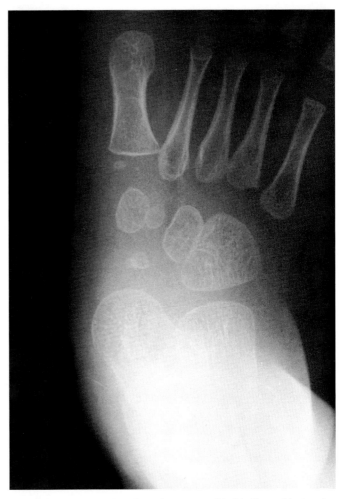

Fig. 9.7. Pes planovalgus in a three year old girl. On weight-bearing radiograph, increase in the talocalcaneal angle is seen. The deformity was bilaterally symmetric.

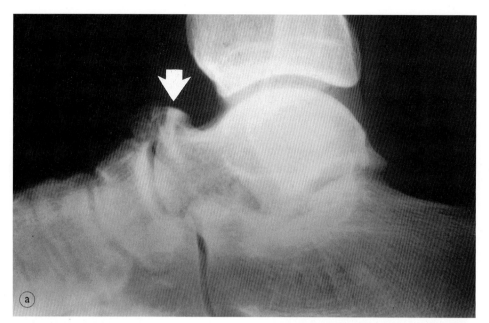

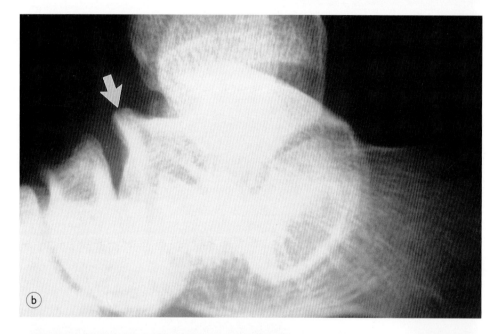

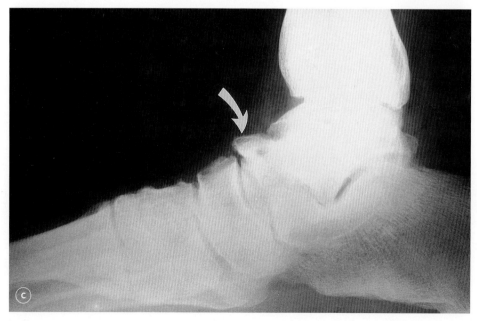

Fig. 9.8. Two examples of talar beaking on lateral radiographs. **a.** Calcaneonavicular coalition. There is a small talar beak (arrow). Note that the coalition itself is not evident on lateral radiograph. **b.** Talocalcaneal coalition. White arrow shows the talar beak. Talar head is hypoplastic. Other signs of talocalcaneal coalition, discussed below, are that the middle subtalar facet is not visible, and the sustentaculum tali is enlarged and misshapen. **c.** Osteophyte of the talovavicular joint in a patient with flexible flatfoot deformity and secondary osteoarthritis, for comparison. Note that the osteophyte (arrow) is located slightly proximal to the joint.

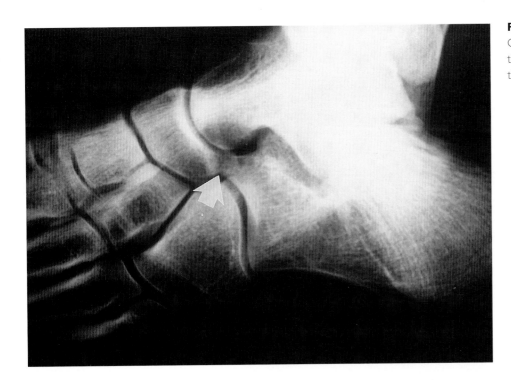

TARSAL COALITION

Tarsal coalition is fusion, either congenital or acquired, of two or more bones of the tarsus. It is thought to affect less than 1% of the population.[15] The fusion may be bony, cartilaginous, or fibrous. Coalitions are often bilateral, and sometimes only one side is symptomatic. The most common type (50%) is reported to be calcaneonavicular, with the second most common being talocalcaneal (35%).[15] However, the advent of CT scanning has increased detection of talocalcaneal coalitions, and they are probably more common than was recognized previously.

Calcaneonavicular coalitions occur between the anterior process of calcaneus and the lateral margin of the navicular. Talocalcaneal coalitions are usually at the middle subtalar facet, but occasionally they involve the posterior and rarely the anterior facet.

Patients present with foot pain. Flatfoot deformity is often but not always present. Valgus of the heel and midtarsal joint are often seen.[16] There may be spasm of the peroneal tendons, which is the source of the old term 'peroneal spastic flatfoot'. Although patients may present in adolescence, many do not develop symptoms until the third and fourth decades of life.[15] Talonavicular coalitions, which are rare, are generally asymptomatic.[17]

Imaging

On lateral radiographs of subtalar or calcaneonavicular coalition, the head of the talus is sometimes hypoplastic, and a talar beak is characteristically seen (Fig. 9.8). A talar beak reflects abnormal hindfoot motion; this is usually due to coalition, but it also occurs occasionally in patients with abnormal alignment and foot mechanics who do not have coalition. It occurs at the most distal dorsal margin of the talus, in contrast to talar osteophytes caused

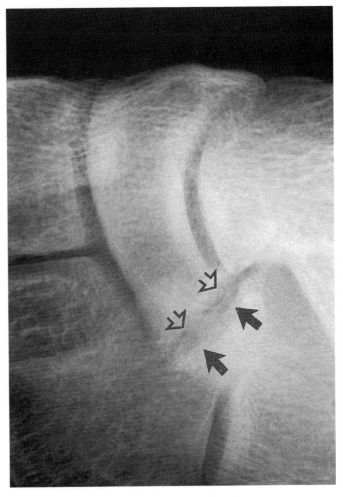

Fig. 9.10. Fibrous or cartilaginous calcaneonavicular coalition. The anterior process of the calcaneus is enlarged, and has a rectangular rather than a triangular anterior termination (closed arrows). It is closely apposed to the lateral margin of the navicular (open arrows).

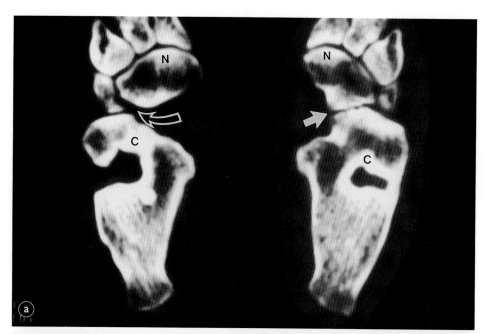

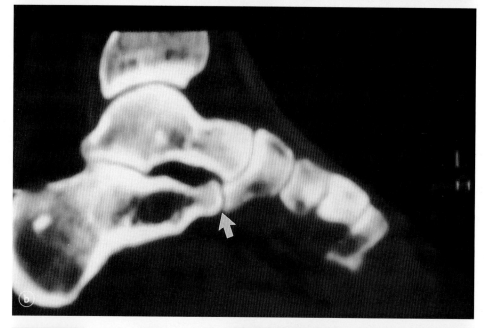

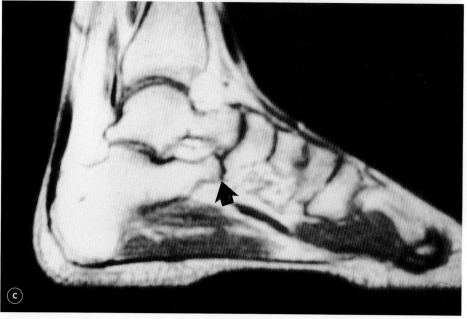

Fig. 9.11. Fibrous calcaneonavicular coalition. **a.** Axial CT. On the normal right side, the anterior calcaneus is slightly separated (open arrow) from the navicular. On the left, the anterior process of the calcaneus is enlarged, and abuts the navicular (closed arrow). The apposing bone margins are serrated. **b.** Sagittally reformatted CT. The abnormal connection between the calcaneus and navicular is well shown (arrow). (Bone islands are present in the talus and calcaneus). **c.** Sagittal T1-weighted MRI, SE 600/28. Appearance is similar to the sagitally-reformatted CT. Arrow points to the coalition.

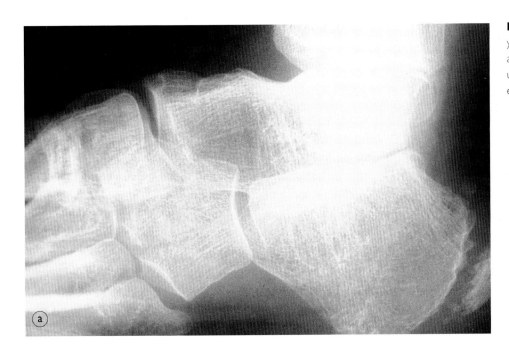

Fig. 9.12. Talonavicular coalition in an 11-year-old boy. Lateral radiograph. Owing to altered stresses, the fused talus and navicular, as well as the calcaneus, are shortened.

by osteoarthritis, which arise just proximal to the articular surface, and the talar ridge (see Chapter 5, Fig. 5.3), which arises at the insertion of the joint capsule of the ankle.[18]

Calcaneonavicular coalitions are usually detectable on oblique plain radiographs. A bony bar between the two bones is the most obvious form (Fig. 9.9). Cartilaginous or fibrous coalitions – imaging cannot reliably distinguish between these two types – are manifest by overgrowth of the anterior process of the calcaneus, and close apposition of the anterior process to the navicular (Fig. 9.10). The apposing bony surfaces tend to have a serrated, sclerotic appearance. CT and MRI can be performed[19] (Fig. 9.11). However, close inspection of the plain radiographs will usually yield the diagnosis.

Talonavicular coalitions (Figs 9.12, 9.13) and most other coalitions are also usually identifiable on routine radiographs.

Talocalcaneal coalitions are more difficult than calcaneonavicular bars to detect on routine radiographs. They usually involve the middle subtalar facet, and examination of the sustentaculum tali on the lateral radiograph can lead one to suspect middle facet coalition. Normally, the sustentaculum is seen as a flat rectangle superimposed on the calcaneus, and on a lateral radiograph obtained with the beam perpendicular to the subtalar joint, the joint space of the middle facet can be visualized. If a middle facet coalition is present, the sustentaculum often appears enlarged and its margins are poorly defined or convex inferiorly; the middle subtalar facet is not visible (Figs 9.8 and 9.14). However, poorly centered radiographs may mimic these findings in normal patients. The Harris or axial view will detect most coalitions involving the middle facet[17] (see Fig. 9.14), but a few subtle coalitions will be missed.

A 'C sign' has been described as evidence of talocalcaneal coalition.[20] It refers to a continuous, C-shaped line formed by the medial outline of the talar dome and the inferior margin of the sustentaculum tali (see Figs 9.8 and 9.14). However, the sign

may be absent in some talocalcaneal coalitions, and can be seen in patients who have a pronated foot but do not have tarsal coalition. [99m]Technetium bone scans can show increased uptake at a nonbony coalition.[21,22]

CT or MRI will readily show subtalar coalition[19,23–25] (Fig. 9.15). It is useful to image both feet, both in order to provide an internal comparison and because coalitions are often bilateral. CT or MRI should be performed in the axial and coronal planes, with 3–5 mm slice thickness. In my experience, the two modalities are of equal accuracy in making this diagnosis, and I usually employ CT because it is less expensive. The MRI diagnosis relies primarily on T1-weighted images, but coronal T2-weighted images are sometimes useful. If high signal is seen on T2-weighted images at the coalition site, this confirms that the coalition is not bony. If CT is done, soft tissue windows are important for evaluating any associated soft-tissue abnormalities. Chapter 8, Fig. 8.11 shows a synovial cyst in the sinus tarsi which occured in a patient with middle facet coalition, but was missed on CT because soft-tissue windows were not obtained.

Rarely, a talocalcaneal coalition affects only the most posterior portion of the middle facet. The findings on CT and MRI are subtle, and can easily be overlooked. It must be remembered that the posterior portion of the sustentaculum tali normally does not articulate with the talus (see Chapter 1, Fig. 1.22d). A coalition is detected in this area by recognizing overgrowth of the talus and close apposition of the talus and calcaneus (Fig. 9.16) in an area where the bones are normally separated by fat. This unusual coalition was included in Harris's landmark description of subtalar coalition,[16] but at that time (which was before the availability of CT) it could not be identified radiographically. A similar condition, a painful accessory articulation at the posterior aspect of the sustentaculum tali, has been called the assimilated os sustentaculi.[26]

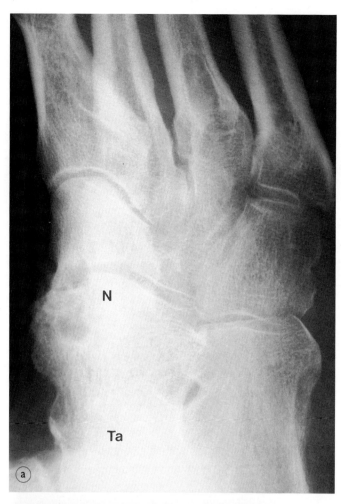

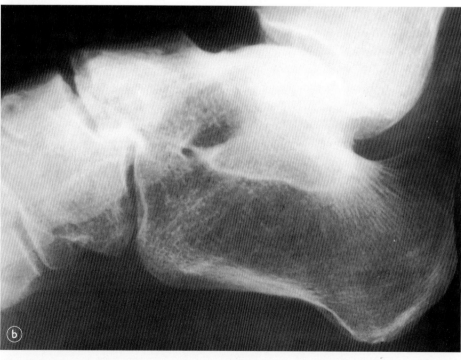

Treatment

If the coalition is discovered before secondary osteoarthritis has developed, it can be excised with good results. However, if osteoarthritis is present, patients are usually treated with surgical fusion.

Fig. 9.13. Complex coalition. **a.** Oblique radiograph. The talus and navicular are fused. Degenerative subchondral cysts at the naviculocuneiform joint are due to increased stress at this articulation. Patient has only four toes. **b.** Lateral radiograph. The posterior and middle subtalar joints are fused, as is the talonavicular joint.

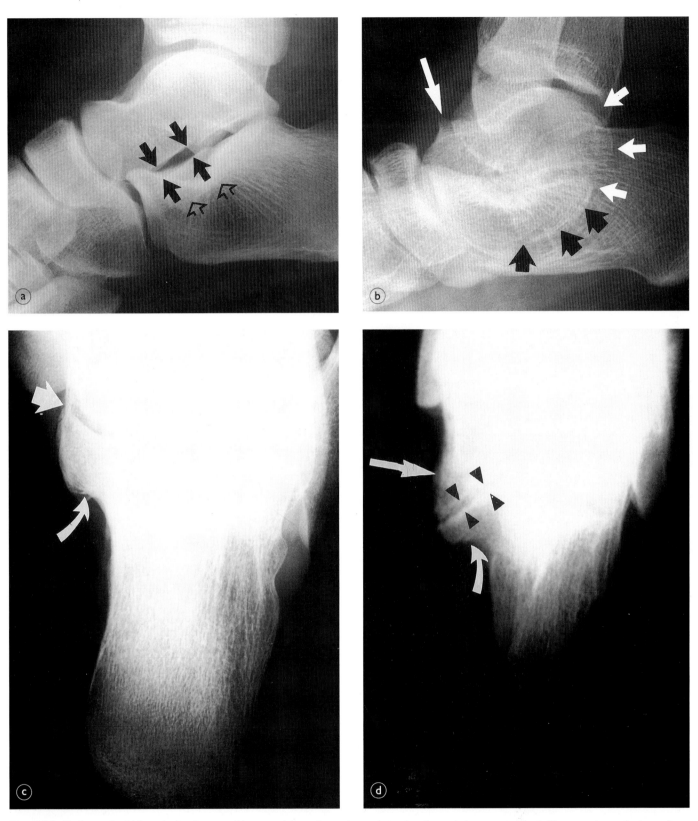

Fig. 9.14. Findings of middle subtalar facet coalition on plain radiographs. **a.** Lateral radiograph in a normal foot. The apposing articular surfaces of the middle facet (closed arrows) are well seen, and slightly overlap the posterior facet. The inferior margin of the sustentaculum tali (open arrows) is visible. The sustentaculum tali has the shape of a flat brick. **b.** Subtalar coalition. A talar beak is evident (long white arrow). The subtalar joint is not visible, and the sustentaculum tali is enlarged and convex inferiorly rather than having a straight margin. A 'C' sign is seen, with an uninterrupted curved line extending from the talar dome to the sustentaculum tali (short black and white arrows). **c.** Harris view in a normal foot. The joint space of the horizontally-oriented middle subtalar facet (straight arrow) is seen, and the articular cortices are smooth and sharply defined. Sustentaculum tali forms a rectangle, with its inferior surface (curved arrow) perpendicular to the medial wall of the calcaneus. **d.** Harris view in a patient with subtalar coalition. There is overgrowth of the medial talus (straight white arrow), and malformation of the sustentaculum tali (curved white arrow). The articulation between the talus and calcaneus is obliquely oriented (black arrowheads) and narrowed. The articular cortices are irregular.

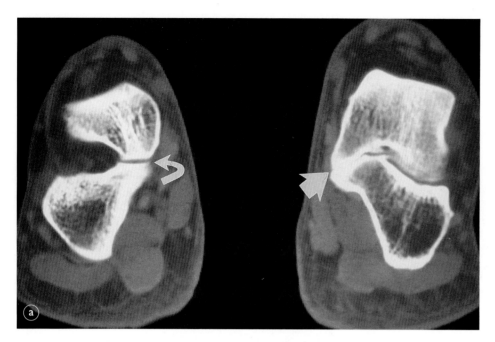

Fig. 9.15. CT and MRI of subtalar coalition (four different cases). **a.** Coronal CT in patient with fibrous coalition of the left middle subtalar facet (straight arrow). There is overgrowth of the medial talus, close apposition of the talus and calcaneus, and enlargement of the sustentaculum tali. Compare the normal right middle facet (curved arrow). **b.** Coronal T1-weighted MRI (SE 600/20) in a patient with bilateral subtalar coalitions. On the right, the coalition is bony and fatty bone marrow can be seen extending across the coalition (curved arrow). On the left, low signal-intensity due to fibrous coalition is present (straight arrow). Overgrowth of both the medial talus and the sustentaculum tali is evident bilaterally. **c.** Oblique axial T1-weighted MRI (SE 550/20) in another patient, who had bilateral bony coalitions. Note that the deformities of the talus and sustentaculum are less evident in the axial plane. **d.** Sagittal T1-weighted MRI (SE 600/20) showing bony middle facet coalition.

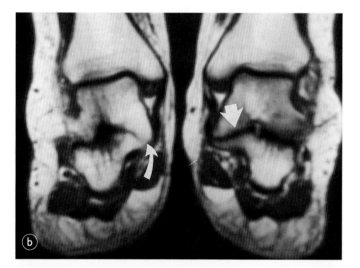

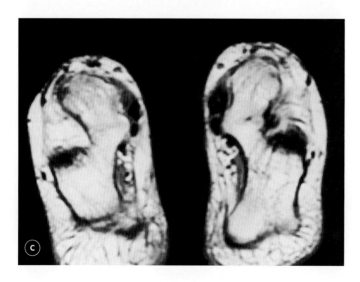

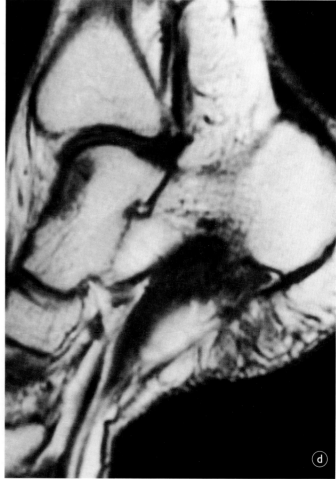

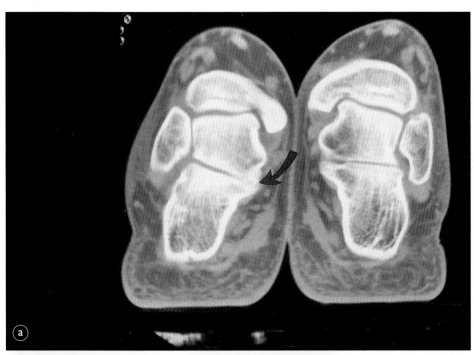

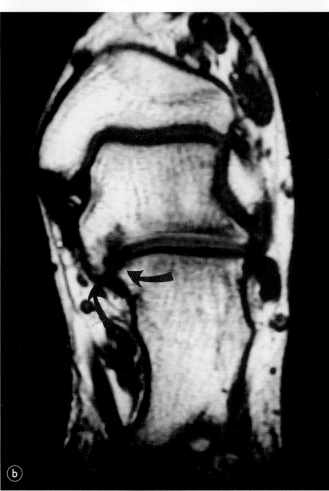

Fig. 9.16. Subtalar coalition limited to the most posterior portion of the sustentaculum tali; both cases surgically proven. **a.** Coronal CT. In the normal left foot, there is slight separation of the talus and sustentaculum. On the right, there is overgrowth of the talus and loss of the normal space between the bones (arrow). **b.** Coronal MRI in another patient. Overgrowth of the medial talus and abnormal articulation with the calcaneus just posterior to the sustentaculum tali are seen (arrow). Bone scan confirmed abnormal activity in this area. Same patient as Fig. 8.11.

REFERENCES

1. Barry RJ, Scranton PE. Flat feet in children. *Clin Orthop* 1983; **181:**68–75.
2. Tachdjian MO. Diagnosis and treatment of congenital deformities of the musculoskeletal system in the newborn and the infant. *Pediatr Clin North Am* 1967; **14:**307–58.
3. Davis LA, Hatt WS. Congenital abnormalities of the feet. *Radiology* 1955; **64:**818–25.
4. Freiberger RH, Hersh A, Harrison MO. Roentgen examination of the deformed foot. *Semin Roentgenol* 1970; **5:**341–53.
5. Vanderwilde R, Staheli LT, Chew DE, Malagon V. Measurements on radiographs of the foot in normal infants and children. *J Bone Joint Surg [Am]* 1988; **70A:**407–12.
6. Ozonoff MB. *Pediatric Orthopedic Radiology*, 2nd edn. (WB Saunders: Philadelphia, 1992), 397–460.
7. Berg EE. A reappraisal of metatarsus adductus and skewfoot. *J Bone Joint Surg [Am]* 1986; **68A:**1185–96.
8. Kite JH. Congenital metatarsus varus. *J Bone Joint Surg [Am]* 1967; **49A:**388–97.
9. Wynne-Davies R. Family studies and the cause of congenital clubfoot: talipes equinovarus, talipes calcaneovalgus and metatarsus varus. *J Bone Joint Surg [Br]* 1964; **46B:**445–63.
10. Benacerraf BR, Frigoletto FD. Prenatal ultrasound diagnosis of clubfoot. *Radiology* 1985; **155:**211–3.
11. Coleman SS, Stelling FH III, Jarrett J. Pathomechanics and treatment of congenital vertical talus. *Clin Orthop* 1970; **70:**62–72.
12. Harrold AJ. Congenital vertical talus in infancy. *J Bone Joint Surg [Br]* 1967; **49B:**634–43.
13. Eyre-Brook AL. Congenital vertical talus. *J Bone Joint Surg [Br]* 1967; **49B:**618–27.
14. Bleck EE, Barzins BA. Conservative management of pes valgus with plantar-flexed talus, flexible. *Clin Orthop* 1977; **122:**85.
15. Stormont DM, Peterson HA. The relative incidence of tarsal coalition. *Clin Orthop* 1983; **181:**28–36.
16. Harris RI. Rigid valgus foot due to talocalcaneal bridge. *J Bone Joint Surg [Am]* 1955; **37A:**169–83.
17. Zeide MS, Wiesel SW, Terry RL. Talonavicular coalition. *Clin Orthop* 1977; **126:**225–7.
18. Resnick D. Talar ridges, osteophytes and beaks: a Radiologic commentary. *Radiology* 1984; **151:**329.
19. Wechsler RJ, Schweitzer ME, Deely DM, Horn BD, Pizzutillo PD. Tarsal coalition: depiction and characterization with CT and MR imaging. *Radiology* 1994; **193:**447–52.
20. Lateur LM, Van Hoe LR, Van Ghillewe KV, et al. Subtalar coalition: diagnosis with the C sign on lateral radiographs of the ankle. *Radiology* 1994; **193:**847–51.
21. Deutsch AL, Resnick D, Campbell G. Computed tomography and bone scintigraphy in the evaluation of tarsal coalition. *Radiology* 1982; **144:**137–40.
22. Goldman AB, Pavlov H, Schneider R. Radionuclide bone scanning in subtalar coalitions: differential consideratons. *Am J Roentgenol* 1982; **138:**427–32.
23. Sarno RC, Carter BL, Bankoff MS, Semine MC. Computed tomography in tarsal coalition. *J Comput Assist Tomogr* 1984; **8:**1155–60.
24. Stoskopf CA, Hernandez RJ, Kelikian A, Tachdjian MO, Dias LS. Evaluation of tarsal coalition by computed tomography. *J Pediatr Orthop* 1984; **4:**365–9.
25. Wechsler RJ, Karasick D, Schweitzer ME. Computed tomography of talocalcaneal coalition: imaging techniques. *Skeletal Radiol* 1992; **21:**353–8.
26. Bloom RA, Libson E, Laz E, Pogrund H. The assimilated os sustentaculi. *Skeletal Radiol* 1986; **15:**455–7.

10. ABNORMALITIES OF ALIGNMENT IN ADULT PATIENTS

MEASURING THE ALIGNMENT OF THE FOOT

The alignment of the foot should be evaluated only on weight-bearing anteroposterior and lateral radiographs. It should be remembered that there is wide variability in the angles measured in normal, asymptomatic feet,[1] and measurements of alignment should not be considered in isolation from the patient's symptoms. Many different angles can be measured to assist in the evaluation of specific mechanical abnormalities of the foot, but these fall outside the purview of the radiologist, and are most appropriately used in a tailored fashion by the orthopedist or podiatrist, in conjunction with the physical examination. The specialist reader is recommended to Klenerman's podiatric text.[2] The radiologist should be familiar with the most important of the normal anatomic angles and their use in diagnosing abnormal alignment. These angles are shown schematically in Fig. 10.1.

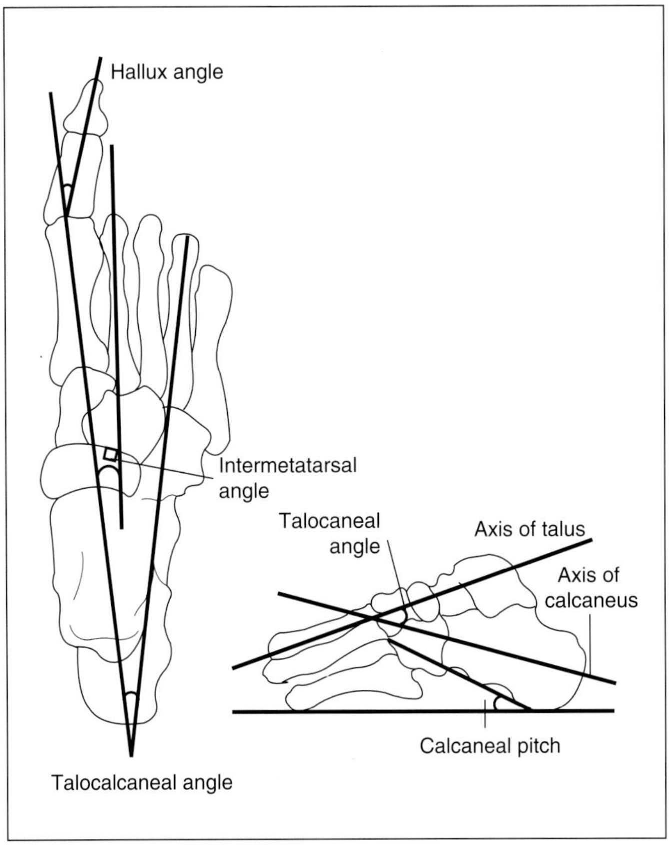

The axes of the foot are assessed by the relationships of the talus, the first metatarsal, and the calcaneus. A lateral view of the foot, which should include the ankle, is most useful in assessing the hindfoot joints, especially the talonavicular and calcaneocuboid joints. This view is also the most helpful in evaluating the relationship between the hindfoot and the midfoot.

A line drawn on the lateral radiograph through the center of the longitudinal axis of the talus should pass through the middle of the longitudinal axis of the first metatarsal. If the axis of the talus extends above the first metatarsal, pes cavus is present, and if below, pes planus. Pes cavus and planus can also be evaluated by the angle of elevation of the calcaneus (calcaneal pitch). This is the angle between a line drawn from the posteroinferior margin of the calcaneus to the anteroinferior margin, and a line drawn along the weight-bearing surface. It should measure 20–30°.[3] The talocalcaneal angle is the angle between the midlongitudinal axes of the talus and calcaneus, and it measures 15–30°.[3]

On the anteroposterior radiograph, the long axis of the talus should bisect the first metatarsal, and the lateral margin of the calcaneus should extend along the fourth metatarsal or between the fourth and fifth metatarsals. The angle between these two axes is called the talocalcaneal angle, and can vary from 15–30° in adult patients.[3] Valgus position of the hindfoot is manifest as an increase in talocalcaneal angle on the anteroposterior and lateral views, while in heel varus, the talocalcaneal angle may be normal or decreased (see Chapter 5, Fig. 5.24).

The angle between the axes of the first metatarsal and first proximal phalanx (hallux angle) should measure less than 10°. A angle greater than 20° indicates significant hallux valgus. The intermetatarsal angle is the angle between the long axes of the first and second metatarsal, and this should measure less than 10°. An increase in the intermetatarsal angle indicates metatarsus primus varus.

PES PLANUS

Pes planus, or flatfoot, is diagnosed when the longitudinal axis of the talus extends below the longitudinal axis of the first metatarsal (Fig. 10.2). The calcaneal pitch is decreased. In its hereditary form, flatfoot is considered a normal variant.[4] Between 7% and 10% percent of the population have a flatfoot deformity

Fig. 10.1. Normal axial relationships of the foot. **a.** AP view. **b.** Lateral view.

Labels in figure: Hallux angle; Intermetatarsal angle; Talocaneal angle; Axis of talus; Axis of calcaneus; Calcaneal pitch; Talocalcaneal angle

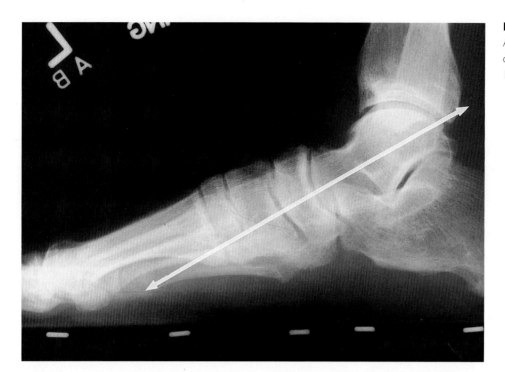

Fig. 10.2. Pes planus. Lateral radiograph. A line drawn through the longitudinal axis of the talus extends below the axis of the 1st metatarsal.

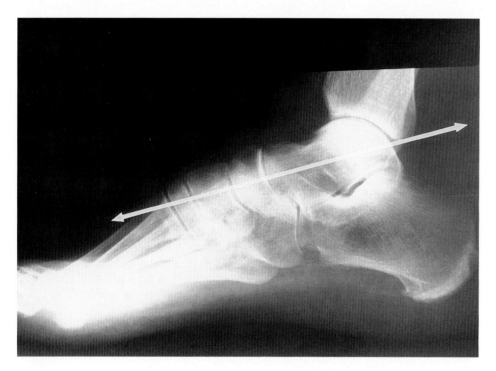

Fig. 10.3. Pes cavus. Lateral radiograph. A line drawn through the longitudinal axis of the talus extends above the axis of the 1st metatarsal.

without other abnormality.[5] Other causes are listed in Table 10.1. Neuromuscular disorders can cause pes planovalgus.[6] Pes planus in children is discussed in Chapter 9.

PES CAVUS

Pes cavus refers to a high longitudinal arch of the foot. The longitudinal axis of the talus extends above the longitudinal axis of the first metatarsal (Fig. 10.3). The heel is in a calcaneus position, with increase in the talocalcaneal angle on the lateral radiograph. It is most often congenital,[7–8] but symptoms are

Table 10.1. Causes of flatfoot deformity.

Normal variant
Tarsal coalition
Posterior tibial tendon rupture
Spring ligament rupture
Rheumatoid arthritis
Neuropathic joint
Neuromuscular disorders
Congenital anomalies (see chapter 9)
Congenital syndromes (Ehler–Danlos, Marfan's)

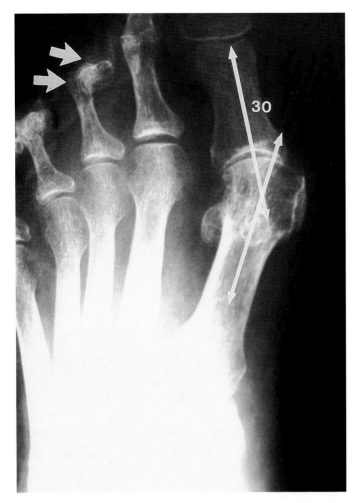

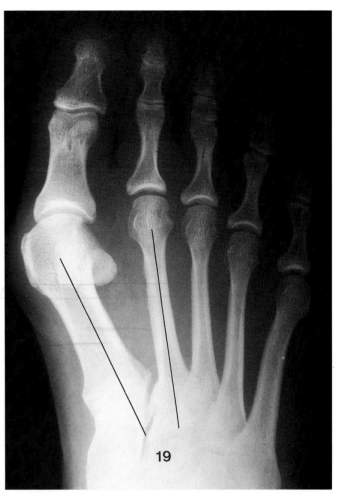

Fig. 10.4. Hallux valgus. AP radiograph. The angle between the axes of the 1st metatarsal and 1st proximal phalanx measures 30°. Note the lateral displacement of the sesamoids of the first metatarsal head. Hammer toe deformities of the lesser toes, with flexion of the proximal interphalangeal joint, often with hyperextension of the distal interphalangeal joint, are seen, and are most evident in the third toe (arrows).

Fig. 10.5. Hallux valgus and metatarsus primus varus. AP radiograph. The angle between the axes of the 1st and 2nd metatarsals measures 19°.

generally absent until adulthood. Causes of pes cavus are listed in Table 10.2.

Patients with pes cavus may complain of fatigue and diffuse discomfort of the foot, or of pain under the metatarsal heads owing to increased pressure. Patients may have altered gait.

HALLUX VALGUS AND METATARSUS PRIMUS VARUS DEFORMITY

The normal angle between the axis of the first metatarsal and that of the first phalanx should measure less than 5–20°. Hallux valgus is diagnosed when the angle exceeds 15° (Fig. 10.4). The term bunion refers to the medial prominence of the head of the first metatarsal. Bursitis often develops in the bursa medial to the first metatarsal head.

Hallux valgus is strongly associated with varus of the first metatarsal (metatarsus primus varus). Metatarsus primus varus is diagnosed radiographically by measuring the angle between the

Table 10.2. Causes of pes cavus (From Samilson and Dillin.[8])

Congenital
Neurologic (spina bifida, Charcot–Marie–Tooth, polio, tethered cord)
Juvenile rheumatoid arthritis
Treated clubfoot
Arthrogryposis

first and second metatarsals (Fig. 10.5). This angle (the intermetatarsal angle) should measure less than 10°.

There is an hereditary predisposition to hallux valgus, but it is most commonly related to women's shoes, with their narrow toe boxes and resultant mechanical pressure on the hallux.[9] Other causes are listed in Table 10.3.

As hallux valgus develops, there is lateral displacement of the sesamoids beneath the first metatarsal head, and the sesamoids no longer lie in their normal grooves beneath the metatarsal

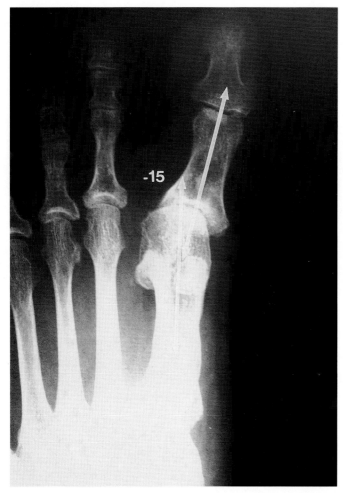

Fig. 10.6. Hallux varus following surgery for hallux valgus. A varus deformity of -15° is present.

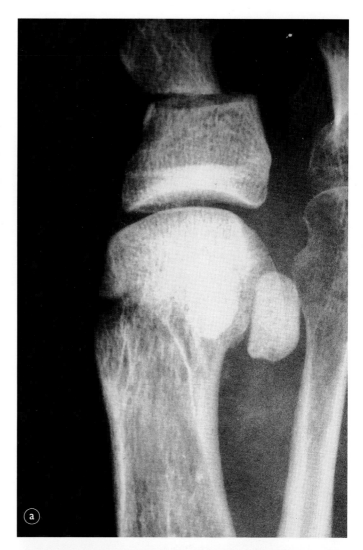

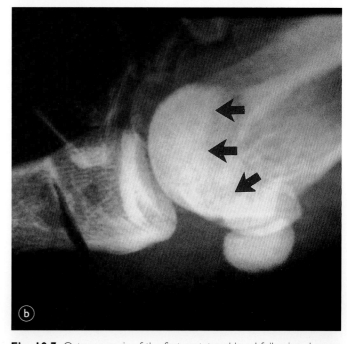

Fig. 10.7. Osteonecrosis of the first metatarsal head following chevron osteotomy. **a.** AP radiograph. The metatarsal head is dense. **b.** Lateral radiograph. The V-shaped (chevron) configuration of the healed osteotomy is evident (arrows). There is an osteotomy of the proximal phalanx.

head (Figs 10.4, 10.5). The severity of this displacement can be evaluated on sesamoid views of the toes. Lateral subluxation of the metatarsophalangeal joint develops, and this can be expressed as a percentage of the joint surface. Hallux valgus causes pressure on the lesser toes, especially the second, and leads to flexion deformities of the lesser toes, with hyperextension of the metatarsophalangeal joints, and to subluxation or dislocation of the second metatarsophalangeal joint.[10]

There is a wide variety of operations to repair hallux valgus and metatarsus primus varus. Simple excision of the medial prominence of the metatarsal head (bunionectomy) tends to cause early recurrence of the deformity, and is usually done in

Table 10.3. Causes of hallux valgus.

Hereditary predisposition

Mechanical factors

Metatarsus primus varus

Rheumatoid arthritis

Marfan's syndrome

Traumatic: rupture of medial ligaments of first metatarsophalangeal joint conjuncton with other surgery. The McBride procedure adds resection of the fibular sesamoid, and suturing of the conjoined adductor hallucis tendon to the metatarsal head. The Mitchell osteotomy is an osteotomy of the metatarsal neck; a modification of this is the Chevron osteotomy, which has the shape of an inverted V (Fig. 10.7). Proximal osteotomies can also be performed and are used when metatarsus primus varus is present. In the Lapidus procedure, the metatarsus primus varus deformity is corrected and the first tarsometatarsal joint is fused. Osteotomies of the first proximal phalanx may be performed.

Complications of hallux valgus surgery can occur. Overcorrection of hallux valgus can lead to hallux varus (see Fig. 10.6). Osteonecrosis of the first metatarsal head may develop as the result of a distal osteotomy[11] (see Fig. 10.7).

HALLUX VARUS

Hallux varus usully occurs as a result of inflammatory arthropathy or surgery for hallux valgus. An idiopathic, flexible varus deformity has been described in adults;[12] this is correctable with modifications in the patient's shoes.

FLEXION DEFORMITIES OF THE TOES

Flexion deformities of the interphalangeal joints are a common abnormality. They are often related to shoes with narrow toe boxes, and can also occur secondary to rheumatoid arthritis. The hammer toe deformity is flexion of the proximal interphalangeal joint, often with hyperextension of the distal interphalangeal joint. The hammer toe is often congenital. When it is an aquired deformity, it is often secondary to hallux valgus deformity (see Fig. 10.4). The mallet toe is flexion of the distal interphalangeal joint. The claw toe is fixed or flexible flexion of the proximal and distal interphalangeal joints, and dorsal subluxation of the metatarsophalangeal joint. The cock-up toe shows hyperextension and subluxation of the metatarsophalangeal joint (see Chapter 5, Figs 5.13, 5.21).

REFERENCES

1. Steel MW, Johnson KA, DeWitz MA, Ilstrup DM. Radiographic measurements of the normal adult foot. *Foot Ankle* 1980; **1:**151–8.

2. Klenerman L (ed). *The Foot and its Disorders*, 3rd edn. (Blackwell Scientific: Oxford, 1991).

3. Weissman BNW, Sledge CB. *Orthopedic Radiology*. (WB Saunders: Philadelphia, 1986), 625–70.

4. Ritchie GW, Keim HA. Major foot deformities: Their classification and x-ray analysis. *J Can Assoc Radiol* 1968; **19:**155–66.

5. Harris RI, Beath T. Etiology of peroneal spastic flat foot. *J Bone Joint Surg [Br]* 1948; **30B:**624–34.

6. Barry RJ, Scranton PE Jr. Flat feet in children. *Clin Orthop* 1983; **181:**68–75.

7. Weseley MS, Barenfeld PA, Shea JM, et al. The congenital cavus foot: a follow-up report. *Bull Hosp J Dis* 1982; **47:**217–29.

8. Samilson RL, Dillin W. Cavus, Cavovarus and calcaneocavus: an update. *Clin Orthop* 1983; **177:**125–32.

9. Edgar MA, Klenerman L. Hallux valgus and hallux rigidus. In: Klenerman L (ed). *The Foot and its Disorders*, 3rd edn. (Blackwell Scientific: Oxford, 1991), 57–86.

10. Coughlin MJ. Second metatarsophalangeal joint instability in the athlete. *Foot Ankle* 1993; **14:**309–19.

11. Meier PJ, Kenzora JE. The risks and benefits of distal first metatarsal osteotomies. *Foot Ankle* 1985; **6:**7–17.

12. Granberry WM, Hickey CH. Idiopathic adult hallux varus. *Foot Ankle* 1994; **15:**197–205.

11. TUMORS AND TUMOR-LIKE CONDITIONS

A detailed discussion of bone and soft-tissue tumors is beyond the scope of this book. There are several excellent texts, including those by Hudson,[1] Dahlin and Unni,[2] and Mirra,[3] which detail the radiologic criteria for the differential diagnosis of tumors. This chapter discusses how to analyse the features of bone and soft-tissue tumors, describes briefly the most common tumors seen in the foot and ankle, and discusses the diagnosis of conditions that mimic tumors.

RADIOGRAPHIC EVALUATION OF BONE TUMORS

Bone tumors can be divided into those that are definitely radiographically benign, those that are intermediate, and those that are radiographically malignant.

Benign bone tumors are usually well-demarcated ('geographic') lesions. A distinct margin is seen between the tumor

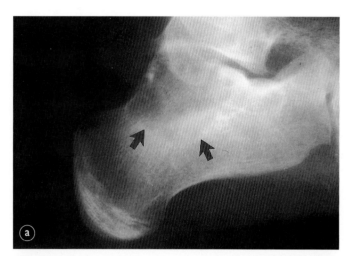

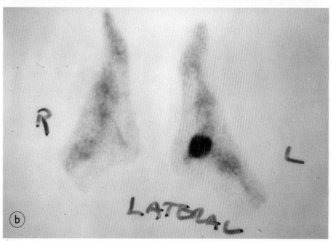

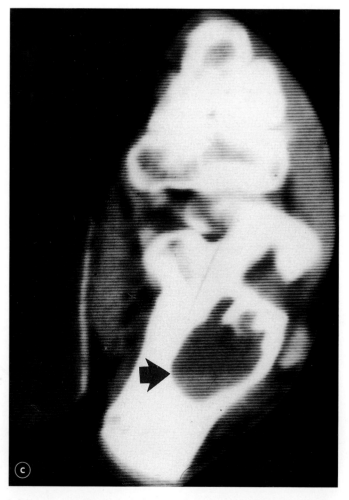

Fig. 11.1. Chondroblastoma of the calcaneus. **a.** Lateral radiograph. The lytic lesion is well-marginated (arrows). It has a characteristic location for chondroblastoma, adjacent to the subtalar joint. **b.** Lateral ^{99m}technetium-MDP bone scan shows markedly increased uptake in this benign tumor. **c.** Axial CT, soft tissue window. A fluid-fluid level is seen (arrow). These can be found in aneurysmal bone cysts as well as chondroblastomas.

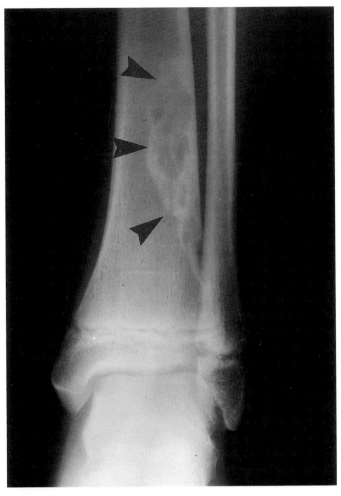

Fig. 11.2. Nonossifying fibroma of the distal tibia. The lesion has a multilobular appearance, and is elongated relative to its width. Margin is sclerotic.

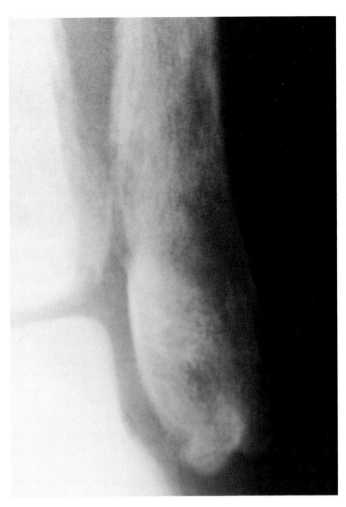

Fig. 11.3. Primitive neuroectodermal tumor of the fibula. The boundaries of the permeative tumor are poorly defined, but loss of bone density is obvious.

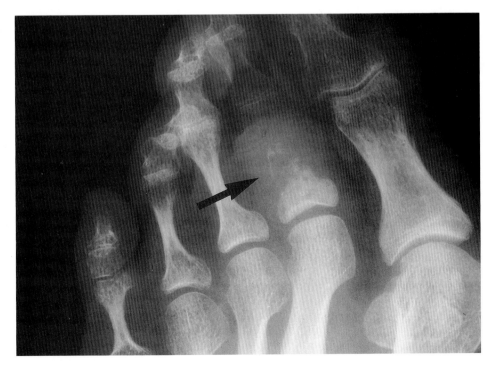

Fig. 11.4. Lymphoma involving the second proximal phalanx (arrow). The majority of the bone is destroyed, with a rim of subcortical bone seen distally, and a permeative process evident in the base of the phalanx.

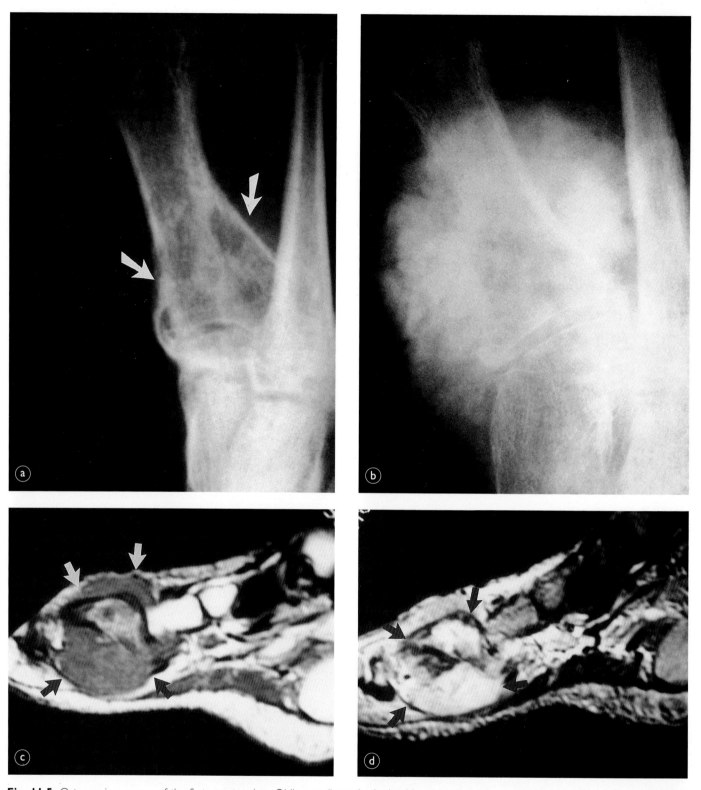

Fig. 11.5. Osteogenic sarcoma of the first metatarsal. **a.** Oblique radiograph obtained because the patient complained of foot pain. An ill-defined lucency is seen in the proximal metatarsal, and periosteal new bone (arrows) is faintly visible. Findings were missed. **b.** AP radiograph 2 months later. The tumor has grown into the soft tissue surrounding the metatarsal, and has developed dense, amorphous ossification. Findings are diagnostic of osteogenic sarcoma. **c.** Sagittal T1-weighted MRI (SE 550/20) along the axis of the first ray. The large soft-tissue mass (arrows) has a deceptively innocent appearance of encapsulation. **d.** Sagittal T2-weighted (SE 2000/80) image slightly medial to (c). Mass (arrows) is hyperintense to fat.

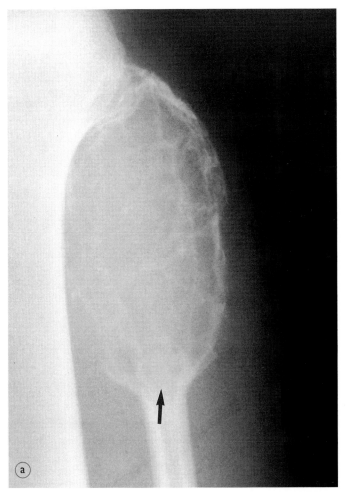
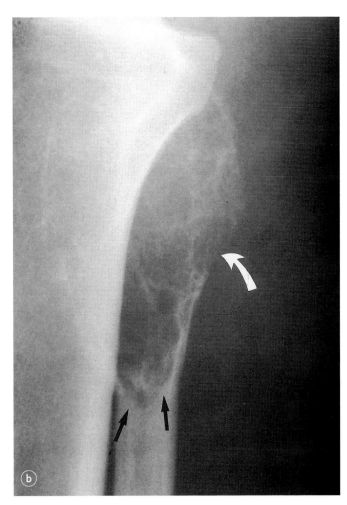

Fig. 11.6. Giant cell tumor of the proximal fibula. **a.** AP radiograph. **b.** Lateral radiograph. There is a sharp zone of transition between the tumor and the host bone (black arrows). The bone appears expanded because of reactive periosteal new bone formation which occured as the tumor slowly grew. Giant cell tumors are more aggressive than most other benign tumors, and cortical breakthrough may be seen (white arrow).

and the host bone, and the transition zone between the tumor and the host bone is narrow (Fig. 11.1). If the lesion is very slow-growing, a reactive rim of sclerosis often develops around the tumor (Fig. 11.2). If a benign tumor grows larger than the original size of the affected bone, the host bone develops a shell of appositional periosteal new bone around it, resulting in an expanded appearance of the bone (see Figs 11.1c and 11.6). Chondrosarcoma is the only malignant tumor that will expand the shaft of a long bone.

Malignant bone tumors may be either primary or metastatic. Metastases are rare below the knee, except for those from carcinomas of the lung, breast, or kidney. Malignant tumors typically have a permeative or moth-eaten appearance, owing to infiltration by the rapidly-growing tumor between trabeculae of host bone (Figs 11.3–11.5). The zone of transition with the host bone is therefore wide. The tumor often breaks through the cortex of the bone (see Fig. 11.4). Periosteal reaction tends to be either multilaminar or spiculated (see Fig. 11.5). Osteomyelitis mimics a malignant tumor, owing to its permeative appearance and cortical breakthrough. Aneurysmal bone cyst and giant cell tumor are two nonmalignant bone

tumors which can sometimes show cortical breakthrough as well.

Intermediate tumors, which are locally aggressive but do not metastasize, include desmoplastic fibroma, osteoblastoma, aneurysmal bone cyst, and chondroblastoma. Giant cell tumors are best included in this category, although rarely they may metastasize. Radiographically they have an appearance intermediate between the benign and the malignant tumors (Fig. 11.6). They are geographic lesions, but they usually do not have a sclerotic margin. The tumor may break through the cortex, raising the suspicion of a malignancy.

The cell type of a bone tumor can sometimes be determined by analysis of the tumor matrix. Enchondromas usually develop internal calcifications in the pattern of punctate dots and small rings (Figs 11.7 and 11.8), although radiographically visible calcifications may be absent in enchondromas of the digits (Fig. 11.8b). In chondrosarcomas (rare in the foot), the calcifications tend to have a 'windblown' appearance because of destruction of an underlying enchondroma by the malignant tumor. Osteoblastomas and osteosarcomas form amorphous foci of bone (Fig. 11.5).

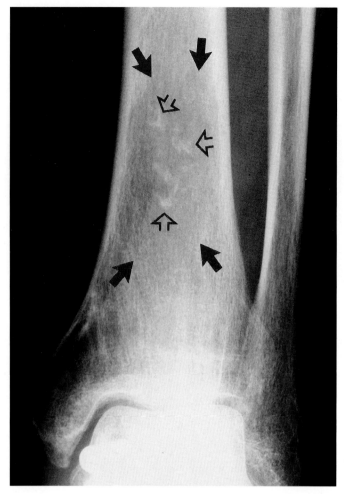

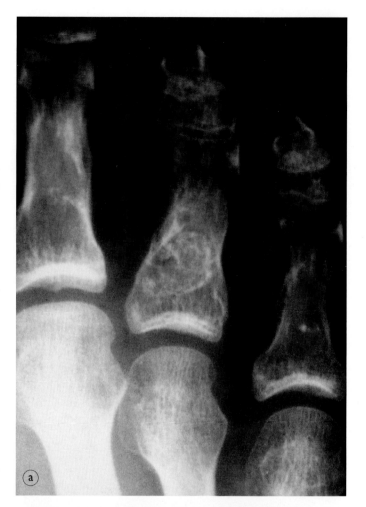

Fig. 11.7. Enchondroma of the distal tibia. AP radiograph. Margins are well-defined, but nonsclerotic (solid arrows). Punctate foci of calcified cartilage are evident centrally (open arrows).

Advanced Imaging of Bone Tumors

If a tumor is clearly benign by plain radiographic criteria, and the patient is asymptomatic, advanced imaging is not needed. Advanced imaging with bone scan, CT, or MRI is performed for the further evaluation of tumors if their benignity is uncertain, or in order to ascertain the extent of a malignant tumor.

Bone scans

99mTechnetium-MDP bone scans are of very limited utility in determining whether a tumor is benign or malignant. Most benign tumors, including nonossifying fibroma, enchondroma, and even some bone islands, will show increased uptake on single phase bone scan (see Fig. 11.1). Osteoid osteoma and osteoblastoma will show markedly increased blood flow as well as increased delayed activity. Most malignant tumors will show increased blood flow, but blood flow may be normal in some low-grade tumors, such as grade I chondrosarcomas.

CT

CT is the imaging method of choice when plain radiographs are equivocal in assessing a bone tumor (see Fig. 11.1). Tumor

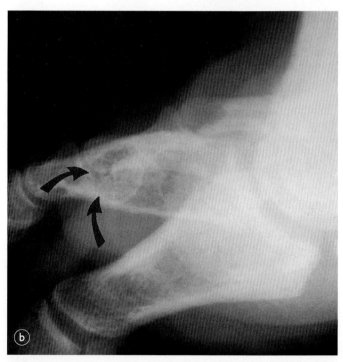

Fig. 11.8. Phalangeal enchondromas. **a.** Enchondroma of the fourth proximal phalanx. AP radiograph. There are central calcifications, as well as a calcified rim. **b.** Enchondroma of the second proximal phalanx in another patient. Lateral radiograph. The proximal phalanx of the second toe is expanded by a geographic process with a well-defined border (arrows). Radiographically apparent calcifications are absent in this case.

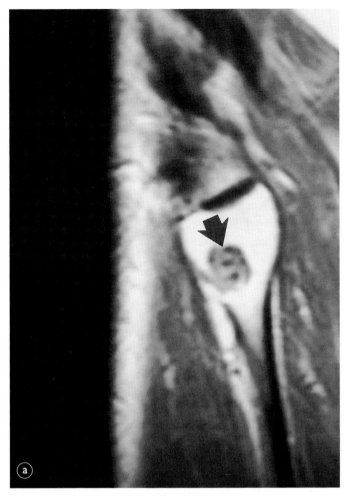
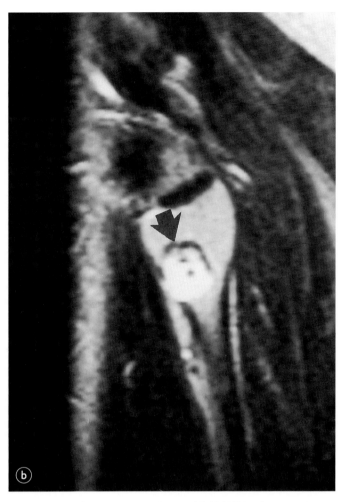

Fig. 11.9. Enchondroma of the proximal fibula, showing a typical MRI appearance. **a.** Sagittal balanced image, SE 2200/20. Arrow points to the enchondroma, which is of intermediate signal intensity, and contains two punctate foci of low-signal intensity calcifications. **b.** Sagittal T2-weighted image, SE 2200/80. The cartilaginous portion of the enchondroma is of high signal intensity, while the calcific foci remain low in signal intensity. Note that the superior margin of the tumor has a thick, low-signal intensity border, while the inferiorly the border is of high signal intensity. This phenonemon is due to chemical shift artifact.

matrix is more easily seen on CT than on plain radiographs. Subtle areas of cortical breakthrough and destruction of bone trabeculae can be identified. The marrow extent of the tumor can be seen if soft-tissue windows are obtained.

MRI

MRI is also used to evaluate bone tumors (Fig. 11.5). Unlike CT, it does not reliably show tumor matrix, but the characteristic calcifications of an enchondroma are often visible (see Fig 11.9). MRI will show the marrow extent of tumors, areas of cortical breakthrough and any associated soft tissue mass.

Radiographic Characteristics of the Most Common Bone Tumors of the Foot and Ankle

Nonossifying fibroma (fibrous cortical defect, fibrous metaphyseal defect)

A nonossifying fibroma is not truely a bone tumor but a proliferative stress response within the bone occuring at sites of tendon attachment.[4] It is most commonly seen in adolescent patients, although it can be identified later in life. It should not be diagnosed in other areas where there are no tendinous attachments, such as the talus. In the ankle, it is most common at the lateral aspect of the tibia.[5]

The lesion is oval in shape, and subcortical in location (see Fig. 11.2). It has a lobular contour, and can become quite elongated. There is a sclerotic margin. Despite its name, the nonossifying fibroma eventually heals with bone formation. A healed nonossifying fibroma can appear dense.

Enchondroma

An enchondroma is a benign cartilage proliferation that can be seen in a patient of any age. Multiple enchondromas occur in Ollier's disease and are associated with abnormal bone growth. Approximately 8% of solitary enchondromas occur in the foot and ankle.[6] Occasionally, but rarely in the foot and ankle, the enchondroma can dedifferentiate to chondrosarcoma. Chondro-sarcomatous transformation should be suspected if the patient has pain at the site of the enchondroma. Pain in an enchondroma can also be caused by pathologic fracture, or the enchondroma may be an incidental finding in a patient who has pain for a different reason.

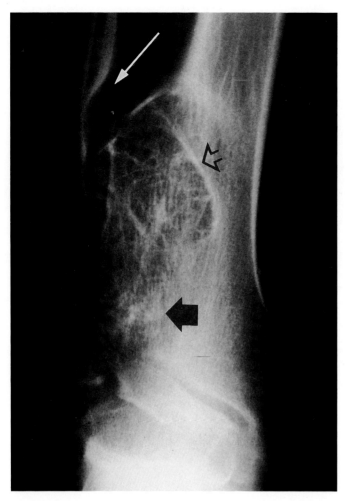

Fig. 11.10. Osteochondroma of the distal tibia. In this case, the tumor has a broad-based origin from the tibia, and is termed a sessile osteochondroma. There are normal trabeculae in this expansile lesion, and a small island of cartilage is also seen (black arrow). The lateral cortex of the tibia flares over the osteochondroma. The apparent sclerotic margin superomedially (open arrow) is created by the margin of the osteochondroma posterior to the tibia. This large osteochondroma has caused erosion of the medial aspect of the fibula (white arrow). There is undergrowth of the lateral tibial metaphysis and epiphysis, resulting in slanting of the distal tibial articular surface.

Radiographically, enchondromas are well-defined, geographic lesions in which rings and dots of calcification can often be seen, although calcifications are less common in enchondromas of the digits (Figs 11.7–11.8). An enchondroma can expand the shaft of a small bone such as a finger or toe; however, if bone expansion is seen in a large tubular bone, chondrosarcoma should be suspected. If a patient has pain, but there is no plain radiographic evidence of malignant degeneration, a CT should be performed to look for subtle areas of marrow infiltration or cortical breakthrough. MRI shows a lesion whose signal characteristics are primarily those of cartilage, usually with foci of calcification visible (Fig 11.9).

Osteochondroma (osteocartilaginous exostosis)

The osteochondroma is the most common benign bone tumor. Approximately 5% of osteochondromas are seen in the foot and ankle. An osteochondroma arises when a subperiosteal portion of the cartilaginous growth plate fails to involute and continues to grow along the shaft of a bone. It forms a mass of mature, normal bone that projects from the surface of the host bone and is capped by cartilage. Because of its pattern of growth, on radiographs it will be seen always to point away from the joint (Figs 11.10, 11.11). It merges with the underlying medullary bone. Small islands of cartilage may be left behind as the osteochondroma grows, so that both enchondroma and osteochondroma are present. The exostosis may present in a subungual location. If the osteochondroma develops in the epiphysis, it is termed Trevor's disease. A syndrome called multiple osteochondromatosis (see Fig. 11.11) results in growth disturbances in addition to osteochondromas.

Osteochondromas are commonly asymptomatic, but patients may present with a palpable mass or pain. Pain can be due to fracture of the exostosis, pressure on adjacent structures, bursitis in the bursa that usually forms adjacent to the cartilage cap, or chondrosarcomatous degeneration. Chondrosarcomatous degeneration is very rare in solitary lesions in the appendages. If it is suspected, MRI can be performed to evaluate the thickness of the cartilage cap; chondrosarcoma should be suspected if the cap measures more than 2 cm.

Simple (unicameral) cyst

In the foot, simple or unicameral bone cysts characteristically occur in the central portion of the calcaneus[8] (Fig. 11.12). Simple cysts must be differentiated from pseudocysts which occur in this location because of local rarefaction of trabeculae in the region (see Chapter 1, Fig. 1.15). The intra-osseous lipoma is an uncommon lesion which may occur in this location and may calcify centrally.[9]

Bone island (enostosis)

A bone island is an ectopically placed round or oval island of cortical bone located within spongy bone. It can occur in any bone. It is an asymptomatic lesion, and is rarely seen in children. Most bone islands are between 2 mm and 2 cm in size.[10] Radiographically, it is a sclerotic lesion with a 'brush border' or trabeculae merging with the surrounding bone trabeculae (Fig. 11.13). Multiple bone islands may be seen in the painless condition known as osteopoikilosis.

Giant cell tumor

A giant cell tumor is a tumor of intermediate aggressiveness originating in the epiphysis in adult patients. Approximately 4% of giant cell tumors occur in the distal tibial epiphysis, and they are rarely seen in the metatarsals and hindfoot.[11]

Radiographically, a giant cell tumor is a geographic lesion without a rim of sclerosis. It originates in an eccentric location in the epiphysis and usually grows into the metaphysis. The bone may be expanded, and cortical breakthrough is not uncommon (Fig. 11.6).

Epidermoid inclusion cyst

Epidermoid inclusion cysts are seen in the terminal tuft of a digit, where they cause a well-defined bone erosion (Fig. 11.14). An intraosseous ganglion or glomus tumor can have the same appearance.

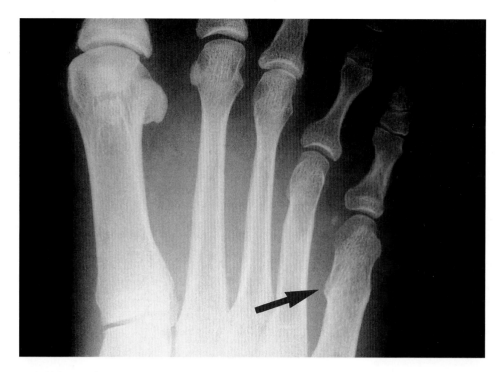

Fig. 11.11. Osteochondroma of the fifth metatarsal in a patient with multiple osteochondromatosis. The fourth and fifth metatarsals are shortened, a common finding in this syndrome. A small osteochondroma (arrow) deforms the contour of the 5th metatarsal shaft.

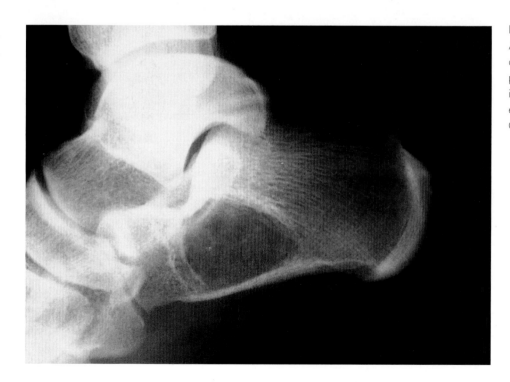

Fig. 11.12. Simple cyst of the calcaneus. A well-marginated lucency is located centrally within the calcaneus. Patient presented with pain; a fracture line is seen immediately anterior to the cyst. A different case of calcaneal cyst is shown in Chapter 1, Fig. 1.15.

DIFFERENTIAL DIAGNOSIS OF BONE TUMORS

Other benign conditions can mimic either benign or malignant tumors. The most common of these is osteomyelitis, which can appear malignant because of its permeative appearance, cortical breakthrough, and periosteal reaction. A Brodie's abscess is a more focal, well-defined infection, and the patient may not have symptoms of osteomyelitis.

Stress fracture is probably the entity most commonly confused with bone tumor. The fracture line may not be apparent on plain radiographs, there may be local osteoporosis simulating a lytic lesion, and a prominent periosteal reaction can raise the suspicion of bone tumor. Osteoid osteomas are rare in the foot, but the radiographic suspicion of an osteoid osteoma may be raised because the dense reactive bone surrounding a stress fracture can have a similar appearance to an osteoid osteoma. However, osteoid osteomas have a round nidus centrally, which is usually radiolucent, while a stress fracture show a linear lucency surrounded by sclerosis (see Fig. 3.20). A careful history should be obtained relating to whether the onset of pain was sudden (fracture) or insidious (tumor), and whether the patient had

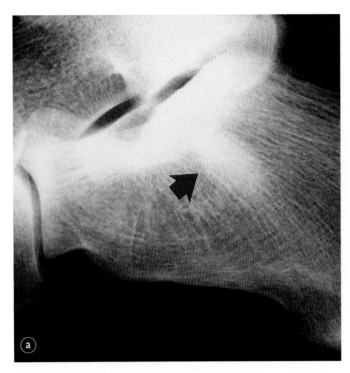

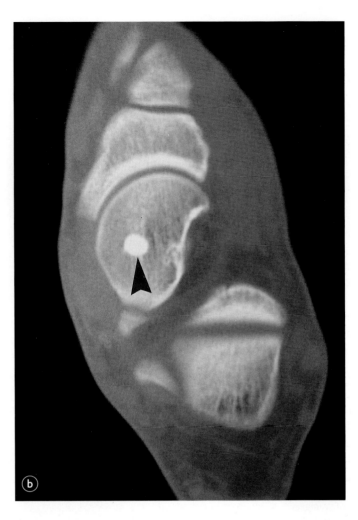

Fig. 11.13. Bone islands. **a.** Lateral radiograph. The sclerotic lesion (arrow) in the central calcaneus merges with adjacent trabeculae. **b.** Axial CT in a different patient shows a bone island (arrowhead) of the talus.

Fig. 11.14. Epidermoid inclusion cyst. AP radiograph shows a well-defined lytic lesion (arrow) in the distal phalanx of the third toe.

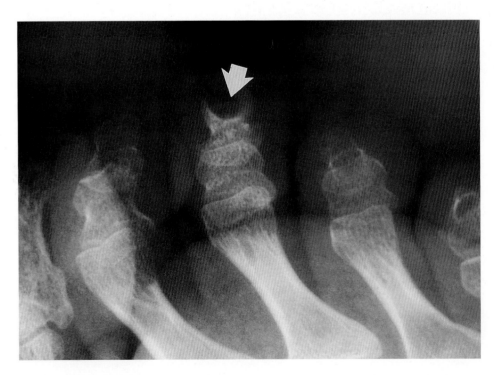

recently engaged in increased activity. In addition, tumor-related pain is often worse at rest, while pain due to a stress fracture increases when the patient is active. Often by the time that a patient is referred to the radiologist for evaluation of a suspected bone tumor, repeat plain radiographs will show a healing, nonpathologic fracture. If that is not the case, or if the patient is unwilling to wait 1–2 weeks to follow the abnormality radiographically, the fracture line can be identified by multidirectional tomography, CT, or MRI.

Occasionally, disuse osteoporosis may be mistaken for tumor. A distinction can be made radiographically because disuse osteoporosis involves multiple bones throughout the affected foot, whereas tumor is almost always limited to one bone, or rarely two adjacent bones.

Neuropathic joints can mimic tumor, especially when prominent new bone formation is present (see Chapter 5). However, unlike most tumors, neuropathic joint disease involves at least two contiguous bones and is centered on the joint.

Periosteal reaction in isolation does not indicate that a tumor is present. It occurs not only with tumors, but also with many other conditions, listed in chapter 8, Table 8.1.

SOFT-TISSUE TUMORS

Imaging is of much more limited use in the diagnosis of soft-tissue tumors than in the evaluation of bone tumors. Plain radiographs are typically unhelpful, although destruction of adjacent bone implies a more aggressive tumor.

The characteristics of benign and malignant soft-tissue masses show significant overlap on both CT and MRI (Fig. 11.15). In general, imaging is limited to defining the extent of tumor.[12–14] It should be noted that the extent of tumor may be slightly overestimated on MRI because of high-signal intensity edema on T2-weighted images surrounding the tumor.

There are several soft-tissue tumors where a specific imaging diagnosis can be made:[12–17]

- synovial and ganglion cysts;
- hemangioma;
- lipoma, fibrolipoma, hamartoma;
- Morton's neuroma; and
- plantar fibromatosis and desmoid tumor.

Synovial and Ganglion Cysts

Synovial cysts and ganglion cysts are fairly common in the foot and ankle. On MRI, they show homogeneous, low-signal intensity on T1-weighted images, and homogeneous high-signal intensity on T2-weighted images (Figs 11.16 and 11.17). The mass is sharply marginated. On CT, cysts are of low attenuation (generally 0–20 HU).

Hemangioma

The hemangioma has a heterogenous appearance on MRI (Figs 11.18 and 11.19). Areas of high-signal intensity may be seen on T1-weighted images because of stagnant blood. Areas of signal void may be seen on both T1 and T2-weighted sequences if

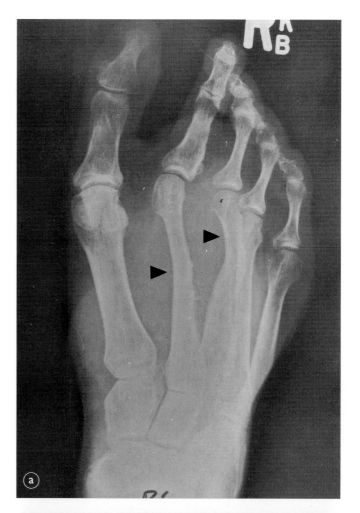

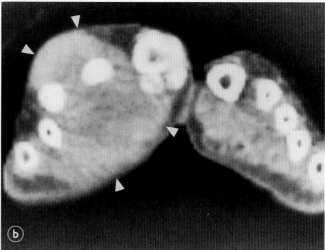

Fig. 11.15. Desmoid tumor of the foot. **a.** AP radiograph of amputation specimen shows remodeling (arrowheads) of the shafts of the second and third metatarsals due to the relatively slow-growing soft tissue mass. **b.** Coronal CT shows the large size and infiltrative nature of the mass (arrowheads); the plantar musculature was almost entirely infiltrated by tumor.

there is significant blood flow. Hemangiomas are usually poorly defined relative to the adjacent musculature, and a significant degree of surrounding edema is seen. It is uncommon in most hemangiomas to visualize phleboliths or draining veins,[11] but

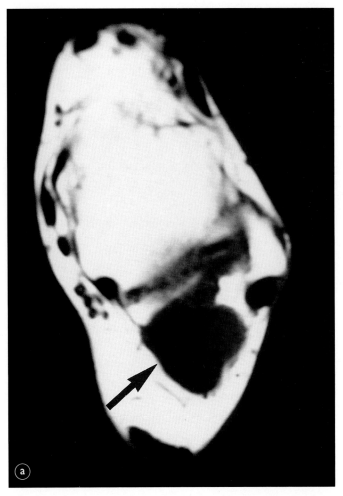
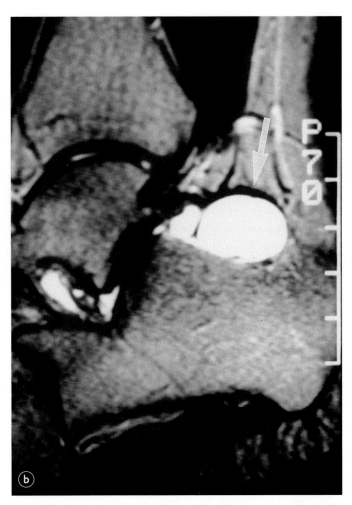

Fig. 11.16. Synovial cyst of the subtalar joint. **a.** Axial T1-weighted (SE 550/18) MRI. A lobular mass (arrow) of low signal intensity is seen posterior to the talus. **b.** Sagittal T2-weighted (SE 2200/80) MRI. The mass is seen to be associated with the posterior subtalar joint. The apparent thickening of its margin superiorly (arrow) is due to chemical shift artifact.

they are sometimes seen in arteriovenous malformations (Fig. 11.19).

Lipoma, Fibrolipoma, Hamartoma

The lipoma is a benign neoplasm of mature fat cells. It has a purely fatty appearance on both CT and MRI. If areas of soft-tissue are seen within a suspected lipoma, the lesion could represent either a benign fibrolipoma (Fig. 11.20), a hamartoma, or a liposarcoma.[14,17] Infants and children may present with a hamartoma involving the bones and soft-tissues of a digit; this condition is known as macrodystrophia lipomatosa (Fig. 11.21).

Morton's neuroma

Morton's neuroma is a common condition involving a plantar digital nerve.[18] It is probably produced by pressure of the overlying transverse metatarsal ligament on the nerve. It is not a true neuroma, as the enlargement of the nerve is produced by a perineural fibrosis. The mass is usually seen between the third and fourth or the second and third metatarsal heads. Patients present with tenderness between the toes, and plantar pain which may radiate into the toe and is relieved by rest, or wearing wider, low-heeled shoes.[18,19] The diagnosis is usually made clinically, and injection of a local anaesthetic is a good test. MRI should be reserved for cases which are very difficult clinically. The neuroma is often difficult to see. It is of low signal intensity on T1-weighted image, and isointense or hypointense to fat on T2-weighted image. It enhances slightly with gadolinium.[20]

In order to optimize visualization of these small lesions, Erickson et al[20] describe using both an oblique coronal scan plane perpendicular to the metatarsophalangeal joints, and an oblique axial plane obtained from the oblique coronal plane and angled to include the first and fifth metatarsals in the same image.

Differential diagnosis of Morton's neuroma includes stress fracture, degenerative and inflammatory arthritis, injury of the plantar plate, and Freiberg's infraction.[21-23]

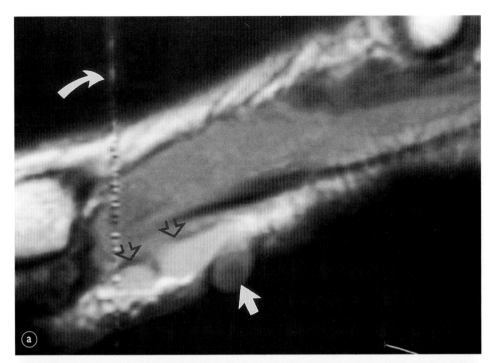

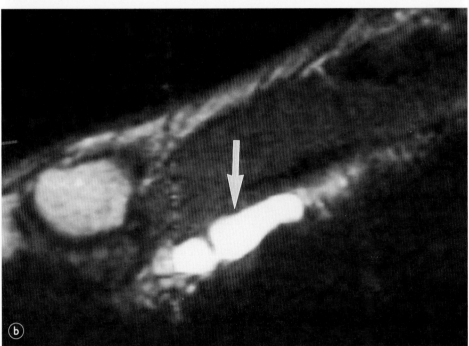

Fig. 11.17. Ganglion cyst of the first toe. MRI was performed to evaluate a palpable mass. **a.** Sagittal balanced image, SE 2000/20. The bilocular cyst (open arrows) is of homogeneous, intermediate signal intensity. A line of arterial pulsation artifact is seen (curved white arrow). The palpable mass was marked with a vitamin E capsule (white arrow). Note that the capsule is not visible on the T2-weighted image. **b.** Sagittal T2-weighted image, SE 2000/80. The mass is high in signal intensity, homogeneous and smoothly marginated.

Plantar Fibromatosis and Desmoid Tumor

Fibromatosis, or desmoid tumor, is an aggressive, nonmetastasizing tumor of fibroblastic origin. It recurs if incompletely excised, and severe cases may eventually require amputation (Figs 11.15, 11.22). It often occurs in the plantar fascia, and in this location it is known as plantar fibromatosis.[24] The diagnosis is usually made clinically, and the mass usually does not require surgical excision.[25] However, if the mass is enlarging or painful, or if multiple masses are present then further investigation is warranted. It is best evaluated by MRI.[26–27] On MRI, plantar fibromatosis is seen to be closely associated with the plantar aponeurosis, and it has infiltrative margins. On T1-weighted images, it is isointense or slightly hyperintense to adjacent muscle; on T2-weighted images, the majority of lesions are also isointense or only slightly hyperintense. In a small number of cases, the lesion is hyperintense on T2-weighted images, but the signal intensity remains less than that of fluid.[27] MRI is essential in evaluating a plantar mass should it recur following surgical excision (Fig. 11.22). Recurrent or multiple lesions may be fixed to the dermis, requiring skin excision and application of a skin graft, and this can be seen on MRI. In addition, any deeper penetration of the fibroma, along the septae which extend to the metatarsals, can be identified.

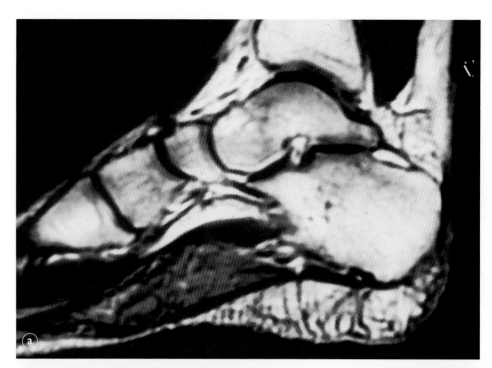

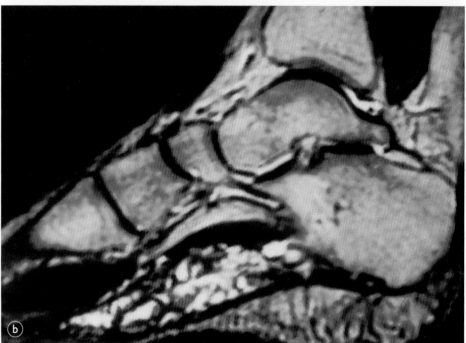

TUMOR-LIKE CONDITIONS OF BONE AND SOFT TISSUE

Bone Infarcts

Bone infarcts are a painful, but generally self-limited, necrosis of the shaft of a bone. The causes of bone infarcts are identical to those of avascular necrosis (see Chapter 5). Complications of infarction are uncommon, although there may be superinfection since the dead bone is an inert nidus for bacteria, and rarely sarcomatous transformation can occur.[28]

Early bone infarcts show a permeative appearance on radiographs.[29] A unilaminar periosteal reaction is often seen. 'Splitting' of the cortex may develop. Later in their course, granulation tissue forms around the periphery of the infarct.[28,30] This calcifies and is evident radiographically as a serpentine line (Fig. 11.23). Irregular areas of calcification may develop within the infarct.

Bone infarcts have a distinctive appearance on MRI (Fig. 11.24). The central portion of the infarct has variable areas of fat and fibrosis. The necrotic fat is indistinguishable in signal from normal fatty marrow, showing high signal intensity on T1-

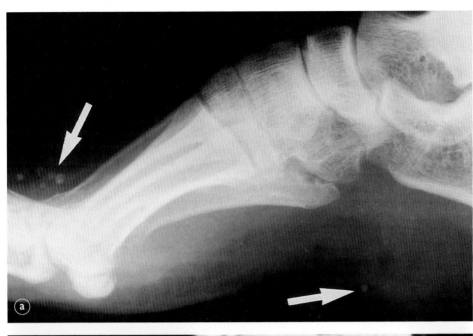

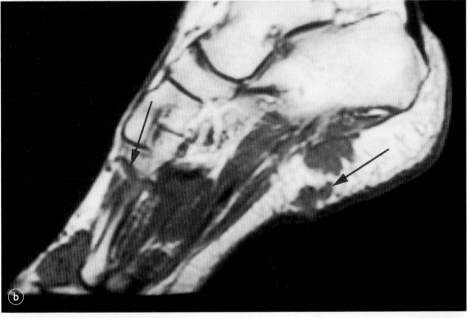

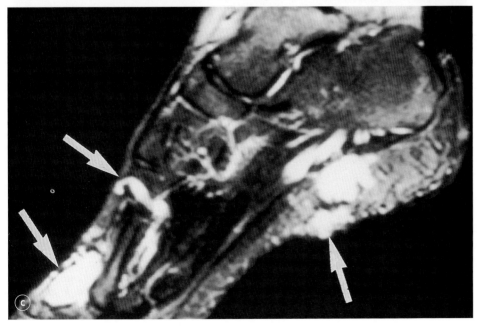

Fig. 11.19. Arteriovenous malformation. **a.** Lateral radiograph. Several phleboliths are seen (arrows). **b.** Sagittal T1-weighted image, SE 550/20. Dilated veins are somewhat difficult to discern on this sequence (arrows). **c.** Sagittal T2-weighted image, FSE 4000/102. Dilated veins (arrows point to several of those visible) are high signal intensity due to slow flow.

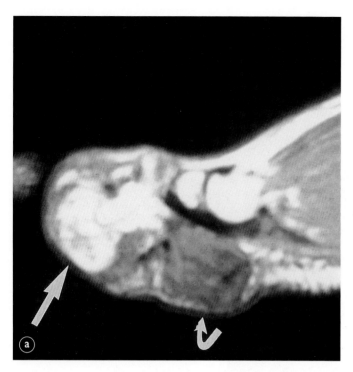
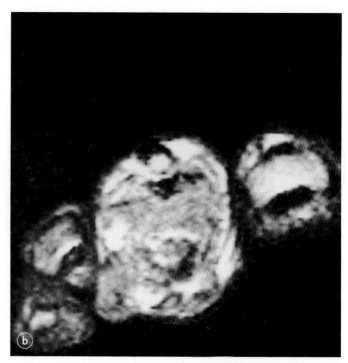

Fig. 11.20. Fibrolipoma of the toe. Lesion had been stable for many years; MRI was performed prior to excision to enable patient to wear conventional shoes. **a.** Sagittal T1-weighted MRI SE 600/15. About one-half of the mass shows the signal intensity of fat (straight arrow), while half has intermediate signal intensity caused by fibrous tissue (curved arrow). Fibrous tissue may also be low in signal intensity. **b.** Coronal T2-weighted MRI SE 2200/90. Although the signal intensity of the fatty component decreases on this sequence, the intensity of some of the fibrous tissue increase.

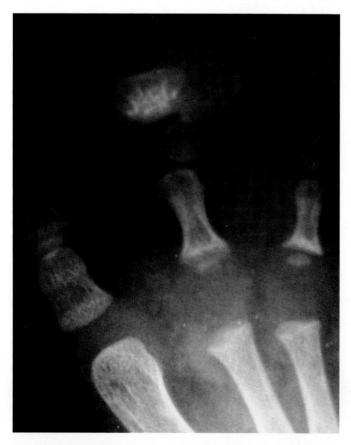

Fig. 11.21. Macrodystrophia lipomatosa. There is marked overgrowth of the bones and soft tissues of the second toe. The same appearance may occur in neurofibromatosis.

weighted images, which decreases on T2-weighted images. Fibrotic areas are of intermediate signal intensity, variably increasing on T2-weighted images.[29] Sometimes an infarction is cystic and fluid characteristics are seen, with uniform low signal intensity on T1-weighted images which increases markedly on T2-weighted images. A well-defined rim of low-signal intensity is seen surrounding a mature bone infarct.

The radiologist is often asked, especially if the patient has sickle cell disease, whether superinfection of an infarct is present. Unless cortical breakthrough is seen, there are no reliable imaging signs which can be employed to detect osteomyelitis superimposed on a bone infarct.

Paget's Disease

Paget's disease occurs in as many as 3% of people of European descent,[31] usually after the age of 40. It can affect any bone. It is a condition probably of viral origin[32] in which vastly accelerated osteoblastic activity occurs, resulting in bone lysis, and is followed by disorganized bony repair and increased bone turnover. Paget's disease almost always starts at one end of a bone and progresses to the other end. Paget's disease may be asymptomatic, and is often discovered on bone scans performed for other reasons (e.g. a search for metastases). However, it can be extremely painful, especially if multiple bones are involved. Pagetic bone is weak, and may fracture or develop a bowing deformity due to microfractures.

The initial radiographic finding in Paget's disease is a lytic lesion of bone that originates in the epiphysis and extends along the shaft of the bone. A 'flame edge' of lytic bone is seen at the

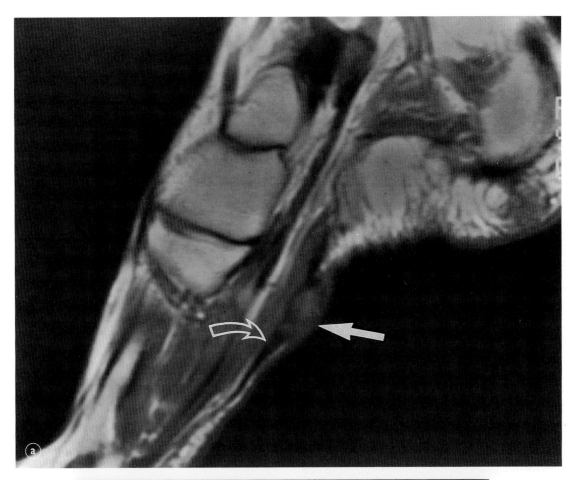

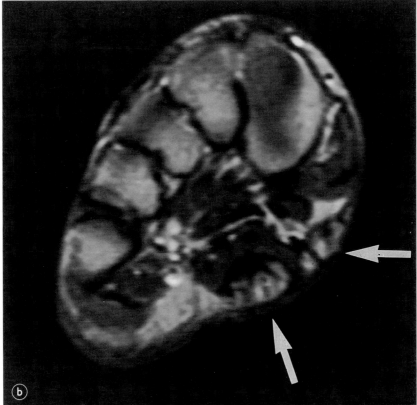

Fig. 11.22. 48-year-old woman with recurrent plantar fibromatosis. **a.** Sagittal balanced MRI, SE 2000/20. The mass can be seen to arise from the plantar fascia (open arrow). Invasion of the dermis can be seen (closed arrow). **b.** Coronal T2-weighted MRI, SE 2000/80. The mass (arrows) shows only a slight, heterogeneous increase in signal intensity on T2-weighted images.

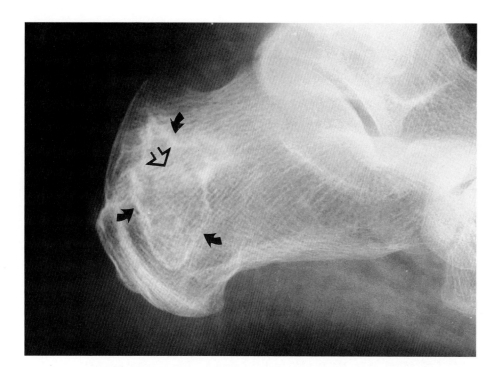

Fig. 11.23. Infarct of the calcaneus in a patient with systemic lupus erythematosis. Lateral radiograph. The infarct is outlined by a serpentine calcified border (arrows). An area of calcification is seen centrally (open arrow).

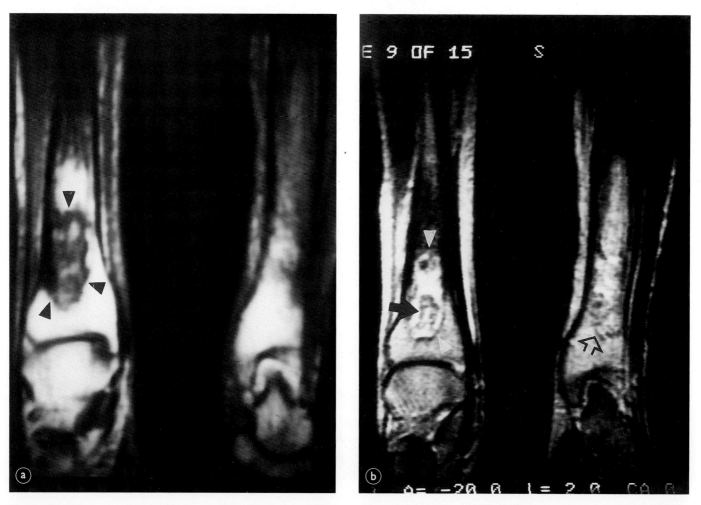

Fig. 11.24. Infarcts of the distal tibias in a patient with sickle cell disease. **a.** Coronal T1-weighted MRI SE 600/28. A serpentine line (arrowheads) delimits an infarct of heterogeneous signal intensity. **b.** Coronal MRI SE 2000/80. High signal areas relative to the fatty marrow probably represent granulation tissue. Fat signal (black arrow) is lower in signal intensity. Arrowheads show margins of infarct. A less well-defined infarct is evident in the contralateral tibia (open arrow).

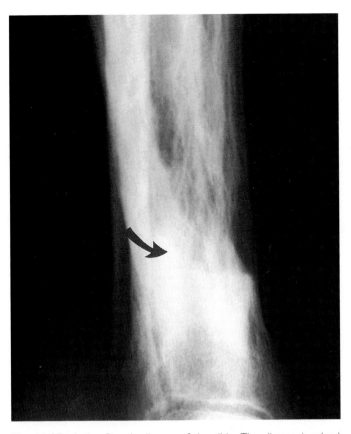

Fig. 11.25. Active Paget's disease of the tibia. The disease involved almost the entire tibia, sparing the distal end. A lytic area is seen at the advancing edge (arrow). More proximally, the trabeculae are thickened and irregular, and the entire bone is enlarged.

advancing margin (Fig. 11.25). In the reparative phase, thickened, disorganized trabeculae are seen, and the bone is often enlarged (Figs 11.25, 11.26). The Pagetic bone shows markedly increased activity on bone scan, unless the disease is long-standing and 'burned-out'. Rarely, sarcomatous degeneration can develop and a superimposed destructive process is seen on radiographs.

Melorheostosis

Melorheostosis is a disease of unknown cause that results in irregular thickening of cortical bone, usually involving one limb[33] (Fig. 11.27). It appears to follow a sclerotomal distribution.[34] It may be asymptomatic or it may cause severe pain.

Myositis Ossificans

Ossification can develop in the soft tissue in response to injury, and can mimic tumor. Early in its development, myositis ossificans shows only a hazy, amorphous mass of bone (Fig. 11.28). If the patient has a history of trauma, the lesion should be watched for several weeks; sequential radiographs will show development of a rim of mature ossification around the mass. Not all patients will remember a traumatic episode, however. If the mass is excised, it is important for the pathologist to identify that ossification begins at the periphery and proceeds centrally, in order to differentiate myositis ossificans from a soft-tissue osteosarcoma, which has more mature ossification centrally than at its periphery.[35]

Pigmented Villonodular Synovitis

Pigmented villonodular synovitis is a proliferative condition of synovium, and is discussed in Chapter 5.

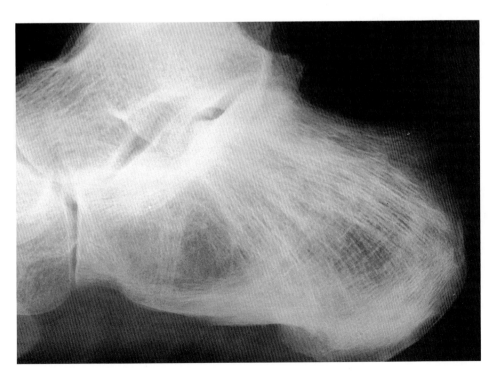

Fig. 11.26. Paget's disease of the calcaneus. The calcaneus is enlarged, and trabeculae are thickened. The normal relative lucency or 'pseudocyst' in the anterior calcaneus (see also Chapter 1, Fig. 1.15) is accentuated by the increased density of the bone in the remainder of the calcaneus.

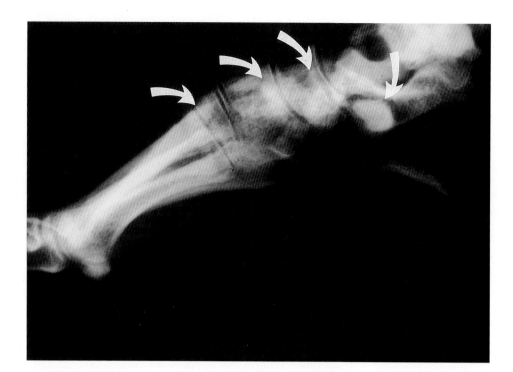

Fig. 11.27. Melorheostosis of the foot. Lateral radiograph. Sclerotic cortical bone is seen in several adjacent bones (arrows).

Xanthoma

Xanthomas may occur in the Achilles tendon in patients with hypercholesterolemia (see Chapter 7, Fig. 7.2). They are commonly bilateral. The abnormality is confined to the substance of the tendon.

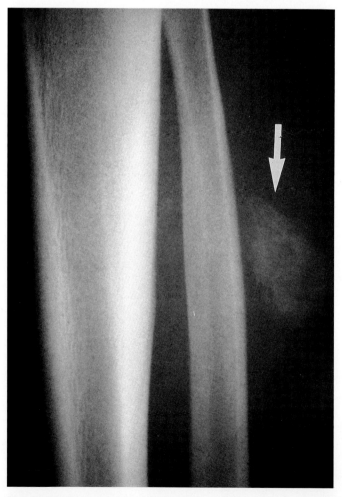

Fig. 11.28. Early myositis ossificans of the calf. Lateral radiograph. A hazy cloud of bone is seen in the soft tissue. The mass was excised and shown histologically to be myositis ossificans.

REFERENCES

1. Hudson TM. *Radiologic–Pathologic correlation of Musculoskeletal Lesions.* (Williams and Wilkins: Baltimore, 1987).

2. Dahlin DC, Unni KK. *Bone Tumors: General Aspects and Data on 8,542 Cases*, 4th edn. (Charles C Thomas: Springfield, Illinois, 1986).

3. Mirra JM, Picci P, Gold RH. *Bone Tumors: Clinical, Radiologic, and Pathologic Correlations*, 2nd edn. (Lea and Feibiger: Philadelphia, 1989).

4. Videman T. An experimental study of the effects of growth on the relationship of tendons and ligaments to bone at the site of diaphyseal insertion. *Acta Ortop Scand Suppl* 1970; **131:** 7–22.

5. Ritschl P, Karnel F, Hajek P. Fibrous metaphyseal defects – determination of their origin and natural history using a radiomorphological study. *Skeletal Radiol* 1988; **17:**8–15.

6. Dahlin DC, Unni KK. *Bone Tumors: General Aspects and Data on 8,542 Cases*, 4th edn. (Charles C Thomas: Springfield, Illinois, 1986), 35.

7. Dahlin DC, Unni KK. *Bone Tumors: General Aspects and Data on 8,542 Cases*, 4th edn. (Charles C Thomas: Springfield, Illinois, 1986), 20.

8. Smith RW, Smith CF. Solitary unicameral bone cyst of the calcaneus: a review of twenty cases. *J Bone Joint Surg [Am]* 1974; **56A:**49–56.

9. Milgram JW. Intraosseous lipomas: Radiologic and pathologic manifestations. *Radiology* 1988; **167:**155–60.

10. Mirra JM, Gold RH, Picci P. Osseous tumors of intramedullary origin. In: Mirra JM, Picci P, Gold RH. *Bone Tumors: Clinical, Radiologic, and Pathologic Correlations*, 2nd edn. (Lea and Feibiger: Philadelphia, 1989), 182.

11. Mirra JM. Giant Cell Tumors. In: Mirra JM, Picci P, Gold RH. *Bone Tumors: Clinical, Radiologic, and Pathologic Correlations*, 2nd edn. (Lea and Feibiger: Philadelphia, 1989), 942–1020.

12. Kransdorf MJ, Jelinek JS, Moser RP, et al. Soft-tissue masses: diagnosis using MR imaging. *Am J Roentgenol* 1989; **153:**541–7.

13. Wetzel LH, Levine E. Soft-tissue tumors of the foot: value of MR imaging for specific diagnosis. *Am J Roentgenol* 1990; **155:**1025–30.

14. Crim JR, Seeger LL, Yao L, et al. Diagnosis of soft-tissue masses with MR imaging: can benign masses be differentiated from malignant ones? *Radiology* 1992; **185:**581–6.

15. Berquist TH, Ehman RL, King BF, Hodgman CG, Ilstrup DM. Value of MR imaging in differentiating benign from malignant soft-tissue masses: study of 95 lesions. *Am J Roentgenol* 1990; **155:**1251–5.

16. Kaplan PA, Williams SM. Mucocutaneous and peripheral soft-tissue hemangiomas: MR imaging. *Radiology* 1987; **163:**163–6.

17. Kransdorf MJ, Moser RP, Meis JM, Meyer CA. Fat-containing soft-tissue masses of the extremities. *Radiographics* 1991; **11:**81–106.

18. Alexander IJ, Johnson KA, Parr JW. Morton's neuroma: a review of recent concepts. *Orthopedics* 1987; **10:**103–6.

19. Mann RA, Reynolds JC. Interdigital neuroma – a Critical clinical analysis. *Foot Ankle* 1983; **3:**238–43.

20. Erickson SJ, Canale PB, Carrerra GF, Johnson JE, et al. Interdigital (Morton) neuroma: High–resolution MR imaging with a solenoid coil. *Radiology* 1991; **181:**833–6.

21. Yao L, Do HM, Cracchiolo A, Farahani K. Plantar plate of the foot : Findings on conventional arthrography and MR imaging. *Am J Roentgenol* 1994; **163:**641–4.

22. Gould JS. Metatarsalgia. *Orthop Clin North Am* 1989; **20:**553–62.

23. Thompson FM, Hamilton WG. Problems of the second metatarsophalangeal joint. *Orthopedics* 1987; **10:**83–9.

24. Lee TH, Wapner KL, Hecht PJ. Current concepts review: plantar fibromatosis. *J Bone Joint Surg [Br]* 1993; **75B:**1080–4.

25. Cracchiolo A. Plantar fibromatosis. In Helal B, Myerson M, Rowley D, Cracchiolo A. *Surgery of Disorders of the Foot and Ankle*, 2nd edn. (Martin Dunitz: London, 1995).

26. Keigley BA, Haggar AM, Ganba A, et al. Primary tumors of the foot: MR imaging. *Radiology* 1989; **171:**755–9.

27. Morrison WB, Schweitzer ME, Wapner KL, Lackman RD. Plantar fibromatosis: A Benign aggressive neoplasm with a characteristic appearance on MR images. *Radiology* 1994; **193:**841–5.

28. Mirra JM. Fibrohistiocytic tumors of intramedullary origin. In: Mirra JM, Picci P, Gold RH. *Bone Tumors: Clinical, Radiologic, and Pathologic Correlations*, 2nd edn. (Lea and Feibiger: Philadelphia, 1989), 691–799.

29. Munk PL, Helms CA, Holt RG. Immature bone infarcts: findings on plain radiographs and MR scans. *Am J Roentgenol* 1989; **152:**547–9.

30. Edeiken J, Hodes PJ, Libschitz HI, Weller MH. Bone ischemia. *Radiol Clin North Am* 1967; **5:**515–29.

31. Mirra JM. Paget's disease. In: Mirra JM, Picci P, Gold RH. *Bone Tumors: Clinical, Radiologic, and Pathologic Correlations*, 2nd edn. (Lea and Feibiger: Philadelphia, 1989).

32. Mirra JM. Pathogenesis of Paget's disease based on viral etiology. *Clin Orthop* 1987; **217:**162–70.

33. Werner MS, Scheimer RA. Melorheostosis: a review of the literature and case report. *J Am Podiatry Assoc* 1987; **77:**96–8.

34. Murray RO, McCredic J. Melorheostosis and the sclerotomes: A Radiological correlation. *Skeletal Radiol* 1979; **4:**57–71.

35. Mirra JM. Osseous soft tissue tumors. In: Mirra JM, Picci P, Gold RH. *Bone Tumors: Clinical, Radiologic, and Pathologic Correlations*, 2nd edn. (Lea and Feibiger: Philadelphia, 1989), 1550–86.

12. SYSTEMIC DISORDERS AFFECTING THE FOOT

OSTEOPOROSIS

Osteoporosis refers to bone that is qualitatively normal, but quantitatively deficient. It can occur as a generalized condition or be limited to one area. Generalized osteoporosis occurs normally with aging ('senile osteoporosis'), and is accelerated in women because of decreased estrogen production following menopause. It can also be due to medications such as steroids and heparin, to malnutrition and generalized debilitation, to hyperparathyroidism and other endocrine abnormalities, or to congenital diseases such as osteogenisis imperfecta.[1] Local osteoporosis has a wide range of causes (Table 12.1). Osteoporosis increases the risk of fractures.[2-3] Stress fractures due to normal stress on osteoporotic bone are known as insufficiency fractures (see Chapter 3).

Imaging Evaluation

Plain radiographs are not sensitive to the detection of osteoporosis, as loss of 30–50% of bone mineral density is required before the decrease in density is evident. Two types of osteoporosis can be distinguished radiographically – acute and chronic.

Table 12.1. Causes of focal osteoporosis.

Disuse (e.g. after trauma, or due to paralysis)
Osteomyelitis
Reflex sympathetic dystrophy
Tumor

In acute osteoporosis (Fig. 12.1), the bone has a patchy, 'moth-eaten' appearance. Intracortical tunneling can be seen. Both subperiosteal and endosteal resorption of bone are often evident. Acute osteoporosis most commonly occurs because of disuse (e.g. as a result of immobilization for fracture treatment). The Hawkins sign, a subcortical lucency in the talar dome (see Chapter 4, Fig. 4.10) is a sign of disuse osteoporosis. Acute osteoporosis may also reflect infiltration of bone marrow with infection or tumor. A radiographic appearance of acute osteoporosis is seen in the syndromes of transient osteoporosis and reflex sympathetic dystrophy (see Chapter 8).

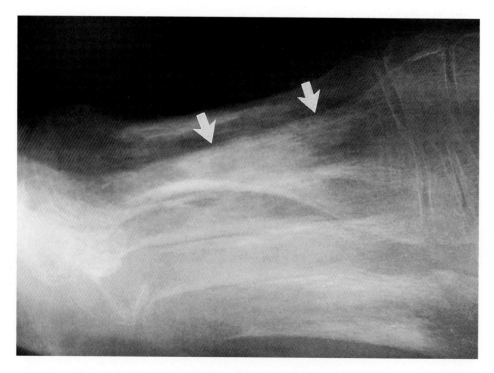

Fig. 12.1. Acute osteoporosis due to disuse. Lateral radiograph of the metatarsals. The bone marrow has a moth-eaten appearance. Intracortical tunneling (arrows) can be seen. Osteoporosis is most severe in the periarticular regions.

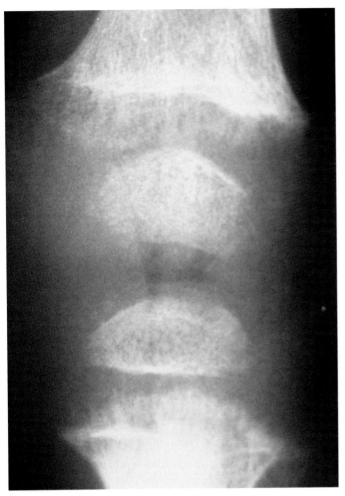

Fig. 12.2. Rickets in a two-year-old girl. AP radiograph of the knee. Radiographic changes are usually most prominent at the knee. There is fraying of the metaphysis , and the cortical margins of the epiphysis are indistinct.

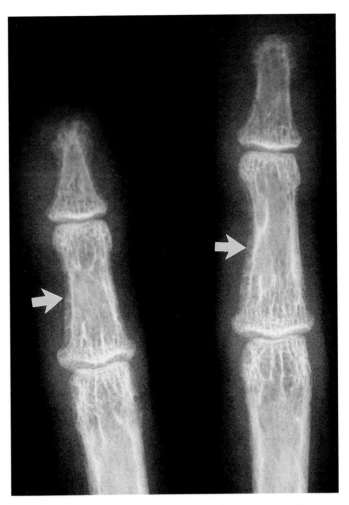

Fig. 12.3. Primary hyperparathyroidism involving the hand. AP radiograph. There is severe subperiosteal bone resorption, most prominent on the radial side of the middle phalanx (arrows). There is also resorption of the terminal tufts.

In chronic osteoporosis (see Chapter 4, Figs 4.32–4.33), the bone cortex is thinned. Secondary (nonweight-bearing) trabeculae are resorbed, resulting in increased prominence of primary trabeculae, and an overall decrease in bone density.

Since plain radiographs are an insensitive measure of osteoporosis, several methods have been developed to quantitate bone mineral density. These include single-photon and dual-photon absorptiometry, dual-energy X-ray absorptiometry, and quantitative computed tomography.[4–5]

RICKETS AND OSTEOMALACIA

Rickets and osteomalacia result from deficient vitamin D in the diet (rare today), or more commonly deficient absorption or metabolism of vitamin D. Deficient vitamin D activity causes bone formation to be qualitatively and quantitatively deficient.[6] In the growing child, this deficiency is manifest as rickets, and results in severe abnormalities centered around the growth plate (Fig. 12.2). In osteomalacia, blurring of bone trabeculae is seen, and there is loss of distinction between the bony

medulla and cortex. Looser's lines are pseudofractures that develop in osteomalacia. They are perpendicular to the cortex of the bone, along its concave aspect, and are often bilaterally symmetric. They rarely occur in the tibia or metatarsals.

HYPERPARATHYROIDISM AND RENAL OSTEODYSTROPHY

Primary hyperparathyroidism occurs as a result of hyperplasia, adenoma, or rarely carcinoma of the parathyroid gland. There is net loss of bone mineral density, and serum calcium levels are elevated. Approximately 10–25% of patients develop bone complaints.[7–8]

Secondary hyperparathyroidism refers to increased activity of the parathyroid gland caused by chronic hypocalcemia, most commonly from chronic renal failure and hyperphosphatemia. It is part of a complex of bone abnormalities referred to as renal osteodystrophy: secondary hyperparathryoidism, osteomalacia, and bone sclerosis.[7]

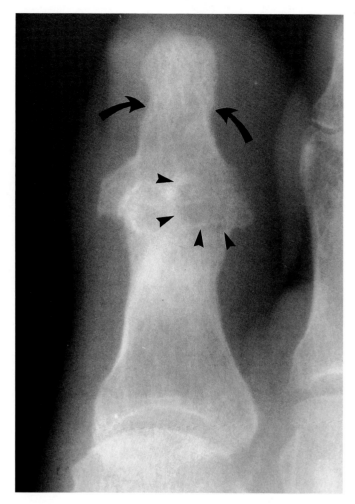

Fig. 12.4. Renal osteodystrophy affecting the interphalangeal joint of the first toe. AP radiograph. The interphalangeal joint is subluxed, and a large erosion is present (arrowheads). Subperiosteal bone resorption is seen in the distal phalanx (curved arrows).

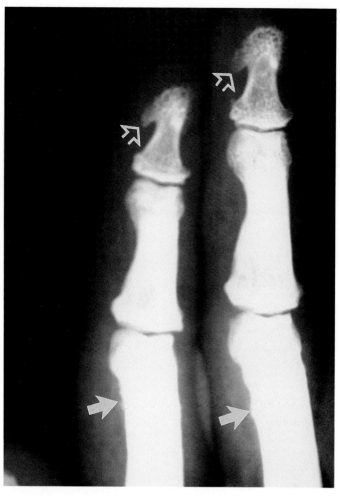

Fig. 12.5. Acromegaly of the hand. There is overgrowth of the terminal tufts (open arrows). Periosteal new bone (closed arrows) is seen along the shafts of the phalanges. Joint spaces are slightly widened.

Radiographic Findings

Most patients with primary hyperparathyroidism are diagnosed today before the development of radiographic signs of hyperparathyroidism.[8] Most cases seen radiographically are due to secondary hyperparathyroidism in patients with chronic renal failure. Resorption of subperiosteal cortical bone and subligamentous bone, as well as generalized osteoporosis, are seen in both primary and secondary hyperparathyroidism (Fig. 12.3). There may be erosion of the ungual tuft (acro-osteolysis). Erosive changes develop at joints both in the spine and digits (Fig. 12.4). Soft-tissue calcification can occur.

ACROMEGALY

Acromegaly is caused by hypersecretion of growth hormone in adult patients. Growth hormone hypersecretion in the mature skeleton stimulates periosteal and endosteal bone formation, thickening and ossification of cartilage, thickening of soft tissues, and organomegaly. The onset of symptoms is insidious. Patients

may present with headaches, visual loss, back pain, or pain in large joints such as the shoulders, hips and knees. Raynaud's phenomenon may be present.

Radiographs of the hands and feet show widened joint spaces (often with secondary osteoarthritis), overgrowth of the terminal tufts, enlargement of the sesamoids, and soft-tissue thickening (Fig. 12.5). Bony proliferation at tendon insertions is seen. The metatarsal shafts may be widened because of periosteal new bone formation. Thickening of the subcalcaneal heel pad has been used as a sign of acromegaly,[9,10] but it should be remembered that heel thickness is greater in men than women and increases with increasing body weight. A heel pad thicker than 23 mm in a man, or 21.5 mm in a woman suggests acromegaly.

ACCELERATED OR DELAYED SKELETAL MATURATION

Bone growth, and epiphyseal development and fusion may be altered by both systemic and local conditions, as outlined in Tables 12.2–12.4. Note that causes of a single shortened bone

Table 12.2. Causes of delayed skeletal maturation.

Addison's disease
Chronic illness
Chronic renal failure
Congenital syndromes
Hypogonadism
Hypopituitarism
Hypothyroidism
Malnutrition

Table 12.3. Causes of accelerated skeletal maturation.

Generalized accelerated maturation
　Hypergonadism
　Hyperthyroidism
　McCune–Albright syndrome
　Neuromuscular disorders
　Pituitary and adrenal tumors
　Albright's hereditary osteodystrophy (pseudohypoparathyroidism)
　Sexual precocity
Accelerated maturation limited to one or several growth centers
　Infectious arthritis
　Juvenile rheumatoid arthritis
　Trauma
　Hyperemic tumor

Table 12.4 Causes of local bone overgrowth or shortening.

Local bone overgrowth
　Klippel–Trenauney–Weber syndrome
　Macrodystrophia lipomatosa
　Mafucci's syndrome
　Neurofibromatosis
Shortened bone
　Juvenile rheumatoid arthritis
　Infection
　Trauma to the physeal plate
　Osteochondromatosis
　Enchondromatosis
　Albright's hereditary osteodystrophy
　Other congenital syndromes

(Table 12.4) overlap with causes of accelerated bone maturation (Table 12.3), since the latter condition often leads to bone shortening.

The most common causes of abnormal bone maturation are endocrine abnormalities. Trauma may lead to premature fusion involving only a portion of an epiphysis, resulting in asymmetric bone growth. There are numerous congenital syndromes that affect bone growth. These can be investigated radiographically by the use of Taybi and Lachman's text.[7]

REFERENCES

1. Resnick D, Niwayama G. Osteoporosis. In: Resnick D, Niwayama G. *Diagnosis of Bone and Joint Disorders*, 2nd edn. (WB Saunders: Philadelphia, 1988), 2023–85.
2. Cummings SR, Kelsey JL, Nevitt MC, O'Dowd KJ. Epidemiology of osteoporosis and osteoporotic fractures. *Epidemiol Rev* 1985; **7:**178-208.
3. Hui SL, Slemenda CW, Johnston CC Jr. Age and bone mass as predictors of fracture in a prospective study. *J Clin Invest* 1988; **81:**1804-9.
4. Melton LJ, Eddy DM, Johnston CC Jr. Screening for osteoporosis. *Ann Int Med* 1990; **112:**516-28.
5. Johnson CC, Slemenda CW, Melton LJ. Clinical use of bone densitometry. *New Engl J Med* 1991; **324:**1105-9.
6. Pitt MJ, Rickets and Osteomalacia. In: Resnick D, Niwayama G. *Diagnosis of Bone and Joint Disorders*, 2087–2126.
7. Resnick D, Niwayama G. Parathyroid disorders and renal osteodystrophy. In: Resnick D, Niwayama G. *Diagnosis of Bone and Joint Disorders*, 2219–85.
8. Silverberg SJ, Shane E, de la Cruz L, et al. Skeletal disease in primary hyperparathyroidism. *J Bone Min Res* 1989; **4:**283–91.
9. Gonticas SK, Ikkos DG, Stergiou LH. Evaluation of the heel pad as an aid to diagnosis of acromegaly. *Radiology* 1964; **82:**418–24.
10. Kho KM, Wright AD, Doyle FH. Heel pad thickness in acromegaly. *Br J Radiol* 1970; **43:**119–22.
11. Taybi, Lachman. *Radiology of Syndromes, Metabolic Disorders, and Skeletal Dysplasias*, 3rd edn. (Year Book Medical Publishers: Chicago, 1990).

INDEX

Note: Numbers in bold denote pages containing illustrations